The Making of Modern Hospitals in Central Europe between the Enlightenment and the Second World War

Clio Medica

STUDIES IN THE HISTORY OF MEDICINE AND HEALTH

VOLUME 109

The titles published in this series are listed at *brill.com/clio*

The Making of Modern Hospitals in Central Europe between the Enlightenment and the Second World War

Edited by

Zdeněk Nebřenský
Daniela Tinková

BRILL

ISSN 0045-7183
ISBN 978-90-04-75505-5
ISBN 978-90-04-75506-2 (PDF)
DOI https://doi.org/10.1163/9789004755062

Library of Congress Control Number: 2026934827

Brill and Koninklijke Brill BV are part of De Gruyter Brill.
www.degruyterbrill.com

Questions about General Product Safety Regulation: productsafety@degruyterbrill.com

Cover illustration: The plan of the Zagreb hospital in the nineteenth century, s.d. No legend available. In HDA-904, plan no. 112, © Ivana Horbec.

Contents

Preface

This volume originated in the spring of 2023, when preparations began for the organization of the conference "Hospitals and the Institutionalization of Healthcare in Central and Eastern Europe in the Long 19th Century." The conference took place in June of the same year thanks to the generous support of the German Historical Institute in Warsaw, which cooperated closely with the Faculty of Arts and Philosophy at Charles University in Prague. The impetus for the conference was the concept of the hospital as a specific space that is constantly changing. With the "spatial turn" in the social and cultural sciences, space gained importance as a historical factor. Usually, space in the geographical sense meant a universal and infinite area or concrete surface of the earth on which things were located. Historical approaches to space oscillated between geopolitics, social space, and mental maps. However, some (art) historians pointed out that space and place could also be a physical arrangement of things which created the material framework in which people lived and worked. This approach therefore encompassed not only the demarcation of the state territory, a regional unit, or an administrative district, but also the layout of neighborhoods, locations in the streets, sites of individual houses and buildings such as hospitals.

The consistent historicization and empirical examination of the "birth of the clinic" in the age of reason and the manifold interrelationships between science, technology and society seemed to be a novelty for Central and Eastern European hospital history, which experienced its heyday in Western historiography almost fifty years ago. In reading the conference abstracts, preparing the program and presenting the individual papers, it became clear that the concept of the hospital as a transforming "liminal" place cannot be separated from other issues. The most important were the extent to which state, regional and municipal authorities intervened in the construction and layout of hospitals and how they influenced the form and operation of hospitals. As the authors of this volume argue, the institutionalization of healthcare on its way to medical modernity was accompanied not only by epistemic communities and progressive healing practices, but also by members of religious orders and poorly paid ordinary staff. Without this personnel's help and voluntary work the operation of many hospitals in Central Europe could not have run smoothly until the end of the nineteenth century.

Readers can learn more about related problems in the individual chapters. The authors would like to take this opportunity to thank the institutions and colleagues without whom the publication of this volume would not have been possible. Half of the texts were written thanks to the support of research foundations, without which historical work in Central Europe would be difficult to imagine today; acknowledgments and references to the relevant research projects can be found in the respective chapters. In addition to grants that enable historians to access primary sources in archives and libraries and sometimes critically reflect on their topics at conferences with interested scholars, there are universities and academies where historical knowledge is cultivated. The Medical University of Vienna, where one of the editors spent five months clarifying individual details of hospital history with Professor Herwig Czech and his team, played an indispensable role in the development of this volume. The editors would like to thank Brill Publishing for including the volume in the Clio Medica series and especially Bogdan C. Iacob and Melissa Allieri for their exemplary assistance in the preparation for its production. Two anonymous reviewers provided important feedback and helped to significantly improve the structure and terminology of the final version. For multilingual place names, the editors have tried to list all variants in the first mention and then the current one.

Figures, Maps and Tables

Figures

Maps

Tables

Notes on Contributors

Piotr Franaszek
(Ph.D.) is a professor at the Institute of History of the Jagiellonian University in Kraków. His main areas of research are the social and economic history of Poland and the modern world. He has published extensively on the history of the oil industry and the history of public health in the 19th and 20th centuries.

Eva Hajdinová
(Ph.D.) is a lecturer in early modern history at the Faculty of Arts of Charles University in Prague. She is co-editor of several volumes and has published numerous articles on the cultural, social, and religious history of pre-modern Europe. She is the author of a monograph comparing the religious life of clandestine Protestants in Bohemia and the Huguenots in Languedoc in the 18th century.

Ivana Horbec
(Ph.D.) works as a senior researcher at the Croatian Institute of History. She has edited numerous volumes and published several books on the political, medical and legal history of the early modern Habsburg Monarchy. Her monographs on the history of public healthcare and state building in enlightened absolutism have been honored with the National Science Award and the Croatian historians' Prize.

Martynas Jakulis
(Ph.D.) is an associate professor of History at Vilnius University, where he teaches and researches the social and economic history of East Central Europe. He has published a monograph on the history of hospitals in early modern Vilnius as well as numerous articles on the history of health care and poor relief in the Grand Duchy of Lithuania.

Janka Kovács
(Ph.D.) is a research fellow at the ELTE Research Centre for the Humanities, Institute of History (Budapest). She studied English and History at the Eötvös Loránd University in Budapest. Her research focuses on the history of the psy-sciences in Hungary in the 18th and 19th centuries. Her recent monograph focuses on the early history of the disciplinarization of the psy-sciences and the medicalization of psychological knowledge in Hungary.

Ingrid Kušniráková

(Ph.D.) is a senior researcher at the Institute of History of the Slovak Academy of Sciences v. v. i. She focuses on the social and ecclesiastical history of early modern Hungary, with an overlap into the mid-19th century. Among other works, she is the author of the monographs Piae fundationes. *Pious Foundations and Their Importance for the Development of Early Modern Hungarian Society* (2009) and *Behind the Orphanages Gates. The Care for Children in the First Hungarian Orphanages (1750–1815)* (2019).

Zdeněk Nebřenský

(Ph.D.) is a historian at the Regional Museum – Prague East. He worked at the German Historical Institute in Warsaw and was also an assistant professor at the Medical University of Vienna. He has published monographs, thematic issues, and many articles on the history of Central Europe in a globalized world.

Ludwig Pelzl

(Ph.D.) holds a doctorate from the European University Institute in Florence. He is a postdoctoral researcher and currently Marie Skłodowska-Curie fellow at Harvard University. He is preparing his first monograph and has published widely on early modern social history of Europe with a focus on the history of old and calendar ages.

Pavlína Pončíková

(M.A.) is the curator of the History of Biological Sciences and Genetics Collection at the Moravian Museum. She studied history and museology at Masaryk University in Brno and has published several articles on the life and times of Gregor Mendel and Mendel's research. She is co-author of the *Iconographia Mendeliana* (2022).

Barbora Rambousková

(M.A.) is a doctoral candidate at the Institute of History at the University of Pardubice and at the Universidad Autónoma de Madrid as part of a joint degree program. She is interested in the social history of medicine in the 19th and first half of the 20th century. Her dissertation focuses on the changing relationships between doctors and patients, the development of the social status of doctors, and the professionalization of the medical market.

Daniela Tinková
(Ph.D.) is an associate professor of History at the Faculty of Arts, Charles University in Prague. She is the author of several monographs focusing mainly on the European and Bohemian Enlightenment, the French Revolution, and the history of science and medicine. Her most recent works include the comprehensive history of Enlightenment in the Bohemian lands.

Introduction

Zdeněk Nebřenský

Although modern hospitals and healthcare facilities have been critically studied for nearly seventy years, the history of hospitals in Central Europe has been investigated only sporadically. Historians have generally focused on the history of the General Hospital in Vienna, recognizing that J. P. Frank had a major influence on the operation of several university clinics in the region.[1] Many other hospitals, particularly in land capitals and provincial towns, not to mention convent hospitals, are absent from English-language books on history of modern hospitals. Moreover, Central Europe was often associated with approaching cholera and plague epidemics that sent shivers down the spine.[2] Even nuanced histories of medicine assumed that Central European hospitals were not so different from Western hospitals as to require specifical analysis. This conclusion may be correct, but it was drawn in a very arbitrary way. It is based neither on a sound knowledge of the academic literature nor on solid historical research.

This volume attempts, at least in part, to fill an existing gap in the history of modern medicine by examining Central European hospitals between the Enlightenment and the outbreak of the Second World War. The early modern charitable guest houses have long received much attention from historians. The history of biopolitics in the age of extremes and post-imperial changes in health care outside the home, before the welfare states took over hospital care, has also been richly studied.[3] Less researched, however, is the period in which caregiving infirmaries and hospitals for patients with accurately diagnosed illnesses overlapped. The transition from one type to the other may not have been obvious or without conflict, as in some cases there was institutional and spatial continuity between both. The variability of individual hospitals can

1 Guthrie, *A History of Medicine*, 260. Risse, *Mending Bodies, Saving Souls*, 257–288. Lesky, Das Wiener Allgemeine Krankenhaus, 23–37.

2 Bynum, *Science and the Practice*, 59, 77, 221. Lindemann, *Medicine and Society*, 204.

3 Weindling, *Health, Race and German Politics*. Lambert, Eugenics and Lysenkoism, 115–132. Mircheva, Fighting Social Pathology, 16–43. Gawin, Early Twentieth-Century Eugenics, 1–15. Mogilner, Racial Psychiatry, 99–133. Stauter-Halsted, Bio-Politics between Nation and Empire, 134–160. Clark, Doyle, Imperial and post-imperial healthcare, 617–834.

 | HTTPS://DOI.ORG/10.1163/9789004755062-002

hardly be reduced to a common denominator manifested in a single historical moment and geographical location.[4]

If one follows the previous conclusions of historical research, the volume does not share the "big bang theory" of the sudden rise of the modern hospital. Of course, there were several leading health institutions that transformed themselves from early modern almshouses into clinics of Leiden type.[5] Given the scope and level of healthcare in both types of institutions and the people they admitted, many modern facilities could be established independently of older predecessors. Hospitals were built under specific socio-cultural conditions, which could differ from one another.[6] Provincial hospitals with trained chief physicians could be a model for hospitals in the capital. This volume therefore traces the (micro)history of the individual imperial, municipal and church hospitals as well as the institutions for the mentally ill in from a longer perspective. It explores the decades of competition and coexistence between different types of institutional provision, only some of which were ultimately successful.

The volume raises the question of how Central European rulers, court officials, provincial authorities, urban elites and physicians dismantled caregiving facilities and promoted the establishment of new healthcare institutions. It asks how the idea of building a hospital in a city came about, who promoted it and who opposed it, and what the reasons for this were. How difficult was it to raise the funds to build and run the hospital? The volume is interested in the factors that contributed to the development of the hospitals, the organization and the application of medical knowledge within their walls. It broadens the view of provincial hospitals as a multi-centered network of activities that were intertwined in various ways with the imperial medical agenda and epistemic communities. It looks into the chronology and dynamics of the emergence of medical modernity. It examines how the nexus between politics, medicine and charity functioned in Central Europe. In this respect, the volume seeks to provide a basis for comparison with broader regional and continental transformations.[7]

The driving force behind institutional provision was the tension between medical knowledge and political economy. The book argues that despite

4 Faure, The Social History of Health, 437–451. Labisch, Spree, Die Kommunalisierung des Krankenhauswesens, *Kommunalisierung*, 9, 11–12.

5 Risse, *Mending Bodies, Saving Souls*, 4. Vogel, *The Transformation of the American Hospital*, 40–41.

6 Reinarz, *Health Care in Birmingham*, 11–12.

7 Topp, *Freedom and the cage*, 4. Cetinoglu, A History of the Barbados General Hospital, 96–97. See also *From Western Medicine to Global Medicine*, ed. Harrison, 2.

familiarity with Western medical knowledge in Central Europe, political reluctance, a lack of economic resources and personnel shortage slowed its appropriate application. Enlightenment rulers aimed to break the structure of traditional communities and dominate them. As these were long-term struggles to enforce centralization measures in the administration and financing of health care, state authorities could not initially provide an adequate substitute for communal welfare and folk healing practices. Especially urban and church institutions retained their indispensability until the second half of the nineteenth century. Without their support, modern medical knowledge and health care would not have advanced so far.

Due to the economic shortages that undermined their development, provincial and convent hospitals remained smaller facilities that were easier to administer and could therefore adapt more quickly to the changing demands of modern healthcare. Their individual approach to patients and their trained staff sometimes resulted in astonishingly high cure rates. After the constitutional reforms of the Habsburg Monarchy in the late 1860s, which further strengthened the autonomy of provinces and enabled the emancipation of national culture and scholarship, young doctors embarked on an educational journey to Western Europe and quickly made careers in provincial hospitals. They were able to experiment with and introduce new medical knowledge and practices, albeit to a lesser extent than they themselves would have liked.

This volume prefers the term Central Europe. Concepts such as Western and Eastern Europe were defined geopolitically. They refer to the legacy of the Cold War and are therefore ahistorical for the period examined in this volume.[8] East Central Europe is understood geographically as the region between the Baltic and the Adriatic, and it is debatable whether it includes Würzburg, where one of the important Enlightenment hospitals was located.[9] Central Europe stands for the German-speaking world, German-identifying people as well as non-German speakers who lived in the historical regions of the German Empire, the Habsburg Monarchy and Switzerland.[10] In addition to this last, somewhat general definition, the individual chapters of the volume aim to show that Central Europe encompasses more than just the German and Habsburg (hereditary) lands themselves. Drawing on previous debates, the volume points out that Central Europe was first and foremost a space interwoven with rich social ties and intellectual connections stretching from Zagreb, Buda

---

8 Ther, Beyond the Nation, 64–66.

9 *East Central Europe* – journal of social sciences and humanities with a focus on the region between the Baltic and the Adriatic.

10 See also Bryant, Habsburg History, 56–65.

and Pest via Vienna and Prague to Brno, Kraków and Vilnius.[11] Intra-regional and transnational mobility of people, ideas and policies went far beyond Dresden and Würzburg. They reached leading medical institutions across the Rhine border, as the chapters of the volume demonstrate.

Historical studies of healthcare institutions that existed in land capitals and provincial towns are still a formidable challenge, as the examples of individual hospitals in this volume show. In the last years of the seventeenth century and the first half of the eighteenth century, the *Bürgerspital zum Heiligen Geist* in the southern German city of Würzburg was the scene of a decades-long conflict between the municipality and the city ruler, the prince-bishop, over the purpose and effects of corrodies (*Spitalpfründen*), a specific form of institutional provision. The initiative to establish a general hospital in Vilnius, which fell under the rule of the Russian Empire after the third partition of the Polish-Lithuanian Commonwealth in 1795, was supported by the imperial administration, but local actors – representatives of religious orders, urban elites, and medical practitioners – played a decisive role in the process. A special place among the provincial hospitals in Galicia was occupied by St. Lazarus Hospital in Cracow/Kraków, whose origins date back to the Enlightenment, when its ambiguous status led to disputes between ecclesiastical, academic, and municipal authorities.

In the Kingdom of Hungary, which was part of the Habsburg Monarchy, the St. Roch's Hospital in Pest was the first healthcare institution to be founded and operated independently of the older convent caregiving facilities in the 1770s. Due to a lack of financial resources, the support of the Viennese court was crucial for the construction of the hospital. The establishment of the new hospitals in the Croatian lands in the late eighteenth century was no less of a challenge, as the health facilities there had to contend with the military and civilian requirements of the imperial border regions. In 1792, provincial representatives, excited by the vision of modern health care, pushed for the establishment of a general hospital in Zagreb, but lack of funds delayed construction for decades. The early history of the institutionalization and professionalization of psychiatry in Buda was marked by unrealized plans. These, however unsuccessful they may have been, are worth examining in more detail, as they show how official and professional attitudes towards the mentally ill changed in the second third of the nineteenth century.

Despite competition from the General Hospital in Prague, the health care in the province and the city could not do without the convent hospitals of the

11 Csáky, Middle Europe/Central Europe, 9–16.

Hospitaller Brothers of St. John of God and the Sisters of Mercy of St. Elisabeth until the middle of the nineteenth century. At a time when public healthcare facilities were overcrowded and struggling with financial difficulties, there was always a free place in the carefully managed convent hospitals. The *Irrenanstalt* in Prague became the best-run institution of its kind in the entire monarchy and served as a model for similar institutions. It was transformed from an institution based mainly on disciplinary measures and methods of subjugating patients into an institute that strove to improve the mental state of hospitalized persons. The wealth of advanced medical knowledge and practices acquired by the doctors may not have been sufficient for the long-term operation of a modern psychiatric facility, as the history of the Provincial Institute for the Mentally Disordered People in Brno showed. Many politicians could not get away from the idea that psychiatric premises were not only institutions of confinement but also medical sites. In the long run, political friction over the construction and operation of hospitals was not that unusual.

1 Institutionalization

There is no consensus among historians on the extent to which the Enlightenment hospitals adopted the principles of modern healthcare institutions. Many historians see these hospitals as health institutions in quotation marks ("institutions") and prefer to distinguish between early modern hospitals, smallpox quarantine facilities, alms-, pest- and poorhouses, leprosaria, asylums, and plague infirmaries.[12] These facilities were more concerned with isolating and caring for the sick than treating them. Patients entered their gates because they were often forced to do so and not always voluntarily. Their medical component may not have been immediately apparent because social control prevailed, although the rigid separation of hospitals into social and medical purposes seems somewhat artificial.[13] Similarly, the individual chapters in this volume argue that the German, Habsburg, and Polish-Lithuanian charitable and health institutions were intended to replace almshouses for all categories of socially dependent people. They combined a restrictive and a curative focus,

12 Kinzelbach, Leprosaria. In *Tracing Hospitals Boundaries*, eds. Stevens Crawshaw, Benyovsky Latin, Vongsathorn, 46–66. See also *The Hospital in History*, ed. Granshaw, Porter, 150.

13 Bernard, The Limits of Absolutism, 194. Risse, Before the Clinic Was "Born", 75–96. *Health Care and Poor Relief*, ed. Grell, Cunningham, Roeck, 11. Cetinoglu, A History of the Barbados General Hospital, 100. *Altın, Psychiatry, Space, and Time*, 67–89.

practicing a kind of preventive medicine and thus treating society as a whole (for additional insight on this topic also see chapter by Horbec).

The moral mission originally associated with the church hospitals as caregiving facilities for disabled, the elderly, the homeless and the mentally ill continued. However, the individual chapters in the volume refine the approach by which the authorities sought to maintain public order through hospitals. The authorities understood public health institutions as a biopolitical tool to influence the behavior of the poor, but at the same time they promoted the idea of a specialized medical place for people with precisely diagnosed illnesses. It cannot be overlooked that even disciplinary institutions such as the sanitary cordons, enforced by the armed forces and controlled by court officials included an elaborate network of guardhouses staffed by hygienists, physicians and surgeons. Protocols were developed in quarantine stations to isolate the infected for treatment and to involve medical staff in dealing with health issues. These measures were potentially long-lasting and later became health observances that affected almost every member of society (for additional insight on this topic also see chapters by Kušniráková, Tinková, Kovács, Jakulis, Franaszek).[14]

There were at least two competing medical concepts that distinguished between health care with and without walls. According to the first concept, home care was primarily intended for the poor. Hospitals were designed to be a place of rehabilitation and healing. This was supposed to reduce the growing number of potential inpatients by limiting them to the most severe cases. As a result, the sick remained at home in the care of their families. It was believed that they were better off at home, being cared for by loving relatives and visited by district doctors. Kinship lent an extraordinary importance to their emotional relationships, and illness at home offered the individual an escape from the daily routine. Practitioners, in turn, struggled to abstract patients from their surroundings and to follow the physiological progression of their illnesses undisturbed by social factors. They saw personal relationships as burden, because they upset the balance in the family thus impaired and delayed the patient's recovery. Overworked persons could not help when the sickness struck. New forms of housing offered less space and privacy (for additional insight on this topic also see chapters by Tinková, Kovács).[15]

Impatient with the pace, the Central European sovereigns tried to accelerate the changes in health care. Instead of constructing a new building, some formed

14 Lovejoy, *The Hospital and Society*, 536. Risse, *Mending Bodies, Saving Souls*, 268.

15 Bernard, The Limits of Absolutism, 193–194. Vogel, *The Transformation of the American Hospital*, 43–49. Risse, *Mending Bodies, Saving Souls*, 266–267.

almshouses were simply converted into hospitals, ordering the use of existing objects. The Hôtel Dieu in Paris was imitated, even though it was already in a very dilapidated state at the time. This was done against the advice of court physicians and scholars, who pointed out that the monastery buildings with inner courtyards were unsuitable for medical care. Rectangular or square buildings did not meet hygiene requirements, as corners and enclosed spaces contributed to air stagnation. The larger buildings would not provide adequate ventilation (for additional insight on this topic also see chapters by Hajdinová, Kovács, Jakulis, Franaszek).[16] The poor and elderly, who had previously been housed in charitable facilities, were simply moved to new premises. The cost saving achieved by placing patients into confined spaces led to a higher mortality rate (for additional insight on this topic also see chapters by Hajdinová, Tinková, Jakulis).

2 Medical Knowledge

The requirements for public hygiene based on the neo-Hippocratic miasma theory influenced the structural and organizational form of the hospitals and led to a change in their character, the social composition of patients and ultimately their external and internal form. In Central Europe, the idea of preserving the population and human kindness removed the old stigmas attached to unwed mothers, people with disabilities and persons with venereal diseases. The premises for the treatment of syphilis played a special role in the development of hospitals. Syphilis was the first known chronic disease whose symptoms disappeared after a simple two-month treatment. The institutions for syphilitics were designed as medical facilities for the diagnosis and treatment of diseases (for additional insight on this topic also see chapter by Kušniráková).[17] This was not a novelty of any kind in Vilnius, as the general hospital simply continued the work of the earlier caregiving institutions, although the patients were not treated by the merciful brothers, but by the medical staff of the general hospital (for additional insight on this topic also see chapter by Jakulis).

---

16 Thompson, Goldin, *Hospital*, 105, 108. Risse, *Mending Bodies, Saving Souls*, 266. Henderson, *The Impact of Hospitals*, 16.

17 Lovejoy, The Hospital and Society, 539–540. Jütte, Vom Hospital zum Krankenhaus, "*Einem jeden Kranken*", 31–50. *Health Care and Poor Relief*, 11. Stauter-Halsted, Moral Panic and the Prostitute in Partitioned Poland, 557–581. Czech, Venereal Disease, Prostitution, and the Control of Sexuality in World War II Vienna, 64–78.

In Göttingen, Vienna and other university cities in Central Europe, official commissions studying the problems of public health and hygiene recommended far-reaching education reforms with changes to medical school curricula. They shared the opinion that the most important prerequisite for successful health care is a sufficient number of qualified and trained doctors. The hours of clinical teaching in the final year of study were increased and practical training took place in hospitals. Individuals who were previously destined for the priesthood had changed careers and started studying medicine instead. The nursing staff originally recruited from religious orders was gradually replaced by lay attendants, who were more or less evenly distributed between the sexes. Corps of professionals, medical practitioners and midwives were trained at the bedside. Nurses were to be paid a higher wage than to ordinary servants to prevent bribery, which was known to occur in infirmaries (for additional insight on this topic also see chapter by Horbec).[18]

From the late eighteenth century, Habsburg physicians followed French models and introduced a classification of diseases, even though, it was not necessarily suitable for use in all hospitals: traditional descriptions could not be mechanically transferred to contemporary categories. Removed from their families and treated in way that neglected their needs, patients almost became specimens. Based on the recommendations of local trustees (priests, practitioners, reeves), they could be classified according to their ailments and assigned to the appropriate hospital ward. The identification as curable and incurable patients was of central importance. To maintain 'morality', each gender was assigned to a separate part of the building. Distribution within the hospital was determined by income, which was reflected in the standard of material care. The more affluent were offered comfortable lodgings and privacy. The general hospital and the ward for the mentally ill shared a common chapel (for additional insight on this topic also see chapters by Hajdinová, Tinková, Kovács, Jakulis).[19]

Moral therapy produced a compromise solution, the so-called 'bourgeois home' instead of a castle, monastery or workhouse, which separated patients not only by gender, but also by rank and intellectual ability, circumstance and status. In addition, the staff – especially the nursing and medical personnel

18 Bernard, The Limits of Absolutism, 194–195. Thompson, Goldin, *Hospital,* 107–109, 113–115. Vogel, *The Transformation of the American Hospital,* 41–43. Risse, *Mending Bodies, Saving Souls,* 261–263. Henderson, *The Impact of Hospitals*, 16–18. Schlumbohm, "The Pregnant Women are here for the Sake of the Teaching Institution", 59–78.

19 Thompson, Goldin, *Hospital,* 113. Bernard, The Limits of Absolutism, 200. Vogel, *The Transformation of the American Hospital,* 43–48. Risse, *Mending Bodies, Saving Souls,* 266–267. Henderson, *The Impact of Hospitals*, 18.

who were responsible for supervising the inmates – were housed in central apartments. The organization of gardens, rooms and common areas was to be harmonized. Great emphasis was placed on community activities, which were considered fundamental to the successful recovery of the mentally disabled. Games, workshops and leisure activities were aimed at men, while women were expected to perform domestic tasks in the kitchen and laundry. Educated and religious patients could engage in spiritual activities and had a library and musical instruments at their disposal. Works that served the running of the mental asylum and supplemented its equipment was paid for and patients could take these earnings with them on discharge (for additional insight on this topic also see chapters by Hajdinová, Tinková, Kovács, Jakulis).

The French Revolution and the Napoleonic Wars transformed medicine no less than the economy and society. They removed hospitals from the aegis of the church and left them in the hands of secular, scientifically oriented authorities. The folk wisdom and naturopathy anchored outside the hospitals was called into question. Doctors who trained at universities and performed surgical procedure contributed to the spread of new medical knowledge. Many of them furthered clinical instructions for medics and city dwellers, who were more closely monitored and medically examined than before. The medical practices that developed in a particular political context, gradually expanded, especially as physicians sought to adopt the ideals of progressive clinical institutions.[20]

A clear distinction emerged between the 'care' provided of incurable people and 'treatment', which introduced new methods such as drugs for patients who were deemed curable. Nevertheless, humoral theory and dietetic practices prevailed in some hospitals for decades, so that the level of medical care and nursing stagnated rather than improved. The suppressed revolution of 1848 paralyzed the work of many important associations and forums of the medical community. If there was any significant change in treatment, it did not occur until the late 1850s. By this time, however, a younger generation of doctors was making study trips to Western Europe and was eager to learn about the medical knowledge and practices there (for additional insight on this topic also see chapters by Hajdinová, Tinková, Kovács).

Hospitals were opened to physicians with superior education and academic aspirations, who had familiarized themselves with the latest medical developments on their travels abroad. As far as mental health care was concerned, inspiration came mainly from France: the first mental health doctors spent time in Paris, where they met a humane approach to the custody and care of

20 Ackerknecht, *Medicine at the Paris Hospital*, 75.

people with mental disorders. The Habsburg and Polish-Lithuanian "insane asylums" were influenced by the reforms in Saxony, where the first university department of psychiatry was founded. The doctors undertook a journey that could be used in the planning process of a new, purpose-built asylum. They visited both older, more prestigious, state-run institutions and smaller, newer private institutions, which became one of the cradles of the new psychiatric care and scholarship (for additional insight on this topic also see chapters by Tinková, Kovács).[21]

Clinical medicine based on anatomy and pathology was a further step in the development of modern hospitals. Equipped with the most advanced theoretical knowledge, doctors set out with considerable criticism of the adaptability of numerous health technologies. Medical discoveries such as antisepsis and asepsis represented a qualitative intervention in the development of hospitals, which were transformed from an instrument of general state–imposed protection against disease into a place where one could receive individualized and predictable medical assistance in the event of illness. The wards were to be vacated by patients from time to time to allow for proper cleaning and ventilation of the premises and to paint or whitewash the walls to rid the rooms of any residue of contagion. To avoid the risk of cross-infection, each inmate was to be allocated their own bed, although this was rarely possible in crowded urban areas inhabited by new arrivals (for additional insight on this topic also see chapters by Hajdinová, Kovács, Jakulis, Franaszek).[22]

From the mid-nineteenth century onwards, the training of female doctors and midwifes, their employment in hospitals, their relationship with patients and their treatment were harmonized. The public was divided on the issue of maternity wards and foundlings, where male doctors examined women in detail and their bodies were used to train medical students. The ambiguous attitude of the authorities led to progress in the medical education of women and women were admitted to medical colleges. The first-degree programs were established to teach female doctors for example at the University of Zürich, where Bohemian students Bohuslava Kecková and Anna Bayerová graduated in the early 1880s. Some healthcare institutions like the maternity hospital in Chernivtsi/Czernowitz set up midwifery schools that gave lectures in various

21 Lafferton, *Hungarian Psychiatry*.

22 Risse, Before the Clinic Was "Born", 75–96. Colin Jones, The Construction of the Hospital Patient, *Institutions of Confinement*, 55–56. Porter, *Health, Civilization, and the State*, 3. Lindemann, *Medicine and Society*, 120–123. Sechel, Networks of Medical Knowledge, 207–214. Krász, The Circulation of Medical Knowledge, 268–295. Hüntelmann, The shifting politics in public health, 636–662. Kisacky, *Rise of the Modern Hospital*, 79 ff.

vernacular languages and trained nurses for local facilities, so that patients no longer had to wait for the services of overworked ward matrons. Young, diligent trainees could be hired as private nurses as the number of doctors practicing in their surgeries and patients' homes increased.[23]

3 Political Economy

In earlier times, almshouses and hospitals were built without any prior thought as to their location, and in most cases, they were simply built near existing churches. Only by chance some of them were built near the city walls or gates, which had little to do with the incentive to strengthen the fortifications or isolate the poor and sick from the rest of the population. Some buildings of older palaces or houses were conveniently integrated into the structure of the general hospitals. The central urban location was essential for practical, prestigious and symbolic reasons, but the hospitals could also be deliberately moved from densely populated area to the outskirts of the city as exemplified by most health institutions examined in this volume.[24] The aim was to physically relocate patients suffering from communicable diseases that were considered dangerous to society. This location made it possible to create large gardens and construct multi-story buildings grouped around a corridor with enclosed rooms on the first floor around a central courtyard. The interiors of the hospital were equipped with a sophisticated system of sanitation, heating and air circulation (for additional insight on this topic also see chapters by Hajdinová, Tinková, Jakulis).

As healthcare facilities selectively admitted sick people with acute illnesses, hospitalism became an important issue in any debate about architecture and internal management. Similar to Western European clinics, also in Central European hospitals, mortality was inversely related to the size of the hospital. Building smaller institutions and straightforward facilities without side wings were considered more appropriate. A larger capacity required separate buildings arranged in rows, the so-called corridor and pavilion type of hospital, which only became reality a century later. An amphitheater was built to prevent surgical procedures from being performed in the wards in front of the terrified patients. In response to the needs of populated cities with their growing burden of trauma, a separate emergency room was also established.

23 Lovejoy, The Hospital and Society, 549. Johanson, Autocratic Politics, 426–443. Hilber, Obstetric expertise, 668–669.

24 Kisacky, Restructuring Isolation, 6. Moran, Topp, Introduction, *Madness*, 7.

In addition, hospitals were often supplemented by separate facilities for the mentally ill, women, and orphans. Particular attention was paid to maternity and foundling homes (for additional insight on this topic also see chapters by Hajdinová, Kovács, Jakulis, Franaszek).[25]

Such an arrangement spread throughout Central Europe, however, provincial and hospital officials carefully watched the costs of such treatment. The bipartite structure of hospital management contradicted the belief that administrators should be subordinate to medical control to ensure the curative role of the hospital. Conflicts repeatedly arose between the administrators and the doctors who wanted to transform the hospital into a medical facility with outreach functions, drug distribution and smallpox vaccinations. But medical progress had not eliminated the fearsome ravages of smallpox. Especially during the Napoleonic Wars, most of the Central European hospitals had to give up their status as a source of any medical care because they were unable to cope with smallpox epidemics, forcing the administration to revert to the older format of temporary plague stations. The overcrowded hospitals quickly lost their order and turned into a confusing dumping ground for infected people who were unclear whether they had already died or were still alive (for additional insight on this topic also see chapters by Kušniráková, Hajdinová).[26]

Two fundamental characteristics of hospitals were originally lifelong care and short-term treatment. Medical circles increasingly argued that permanently socially dependent persons and curable patients in hospitals were at odds with each other. They demanded that hospitals should abandon their traditional role of helping the poor and focus entirely on health care. At the same time, hospitals could not ignore the poor, as their relative numbers were increasing as society changed (for additional insight on this topic also see chapter by Nebřenský).[27] The discussion about health care quickly shifted from the conceptual level to how it should be administered and financed. Patients were divided into four classes in the hope that the first and second classes would contribute to the cost of treating the third and fourth classes. These plans proved unrealistic, because the expected potential payers never materialized. Barely less than a tenth of the inmates paid a

25 Thompson, Goldin, *Hospital*, 107–109, 113–115. Risse, *Mending Bodies, Saving Souls*, 261–264, 266. Henderson, *The Impact of Hospitals*, 18.

26 Lovejoy, The Hospital and Society, 553. Cotoi, Cholera, Health for All, Nation-Building, 161–187. Blackthorne-O'Barr, Journals of the Plague Year, 203–230.

27 Frieden, Russian Physicians, passim.

daily contribution (for additional insight on this topic also see chapters by Tinková, Kovács).[28]

The emergence of the hospital as a healthcare facility was determined by the public: Hospitals could not be built unless citizenry accepted them. The mobilization of national movements may have led to a general consensus that the hospital ("insane asylum") should be built at society's expense. It was also possible that national fundraising campaigns would not be sufficient, and the monarch contributed to the construction of the hospital from his private coffers (for additional insight on this topic also see chapters by Kovács, Franaszek). Although welfare and health care did not cease to be sources of legitimacy for the emperor (and the monarchy), the imperial authorities ceded some of their powers to the individual provinces in the early 1860s. However, the takeover of the hospitals and asylums by the provincial authorities was a gift from the Danais, as they had to shoulder not only the administration but also their financing. This slowed down the development of the hospitals. While the emperor had been able to support the introduction of new medical and curative practices until then, the provincial authorities were primarily concerned with the costs of running hospitals (for additional insight on this topic also see chapters by Tinková, Nebřenský).

In the early twentieth century, advances in medicine and surgery made Central European hospitals a center for therapy and diagnosis for patients of all classes. Hospitals freed themselves of their charitable mission and overcame the fears of the public. They were no longer the guardians of the poor but became medical and curative institutions serving citizens with health insurance. Many of the private and corporate sick funds were later incorporated into the public health insurance funds after statutory health insurance was introduced. The aim was to prevent the free disposal and misappropriation of funds, which prompted some industrialists to hand over the hospitals to the municipalities. The humanitarian ideal was often overridden by the harsh realities of property values and financial concerns. These were the reasons for the changes in hospital provision, caused by the drive saving money (for additional insight on this topic also see chapters by Franaszek, Rambousková).[29]

---

28 Thompson, Goldin, *Hospital*, 113. Risse, *Mending Bodies, Saving Souls*, 263–265. Henderson, *The Impact of Hospitals*, 19. Lane, *A Social History of Medicine*, 84–85. Lovejoy, The Hospital and Society, 547, 553–554. Dross, *Krankenhaus und lokale Politik*, 57.

29 Lovejoy, The Hospital and Society, 536, 549, 554. Labisch, Stadt und Krankenhaus. In *"Einem jeden Kranken"*, 253–296.

The First World War had a severe impact on public health insurance, causing most funds to go bankrupt. As part of the post-war reconstruction and nation-building, the Central European governments increased their intervention to maintain health care standards. A broad wave of national solidarity, along with foreign aid and support from expatriate communities, contributed to the development of medical knowledge and practices that had emerged in former provincial hospitals. These became the health care institutions of the new capitals and were intended to serve as showcases of national medicine. Medical universities admitted more students, some of whom had completed internships abroad. In Kraków, Prague and Zagreb, new buildings were constructed for newly established specialized departments, employing growing numbers of doctors and nurses. Hospital operations have become more professional, from registering patients at the reception desk to their initial examination, determining the diagnosis, and assigning them to a room in the appropriate ward. Economic crises, especially the Great Depression of the early 1930s, halted the reconstruction of hospitals built during imperial times and disrupted plans for new ones. The rise of authoritarianism also affected hospitals. A younger generation of doctors, dependent on patron-client relationships, became politically radicalized and attacked their older, dissenting and Jewish colleagues to dismiss them from the positions. The doors to the hospital, conceived as a bureaucratic institution integrated into the war machine where there is no place or time for mercy, were opened.

CHAPTER 1

On the Eve of Modernization: Enlightenment Reforms of Institutional Provision in Germany at the Example of the Bürgerspital in Würzburg

Ludwig Pelzl

The last years of the eighteenth and the first of nineteenth century are a watershed for Central European institutional provision and its hospital structures. Enlightened absolutism, the back and forth between revolutionary and counter-revolutionary reforms, and the modernizing impulses of the early nineteenth century profoundly transformed the political governance and hospital administration, if not (generally) its affluence. These changes have been extensively documented in the historiography and are evident in many of the other contributions to this volume.[1] The present article shifts this chronology slightly, turning to the last years of the seventeenth century and the first half of the eighteenth century, a period firmly rooted in the political practice of the *ancien régime*. It studies a debate on reform of institutional provision in said time frame at the *Bürgerspital zum Heiligen Geist* in the southern German city of Würzburg. Mired in a decades-long conflict between the municipality and the city's lord, the prince-bishop of Würzburg, the purpose and implications of corrodies, a specific form of institutional provision, were extensively discussed as part of a local power struggle.[2] In light of the great transformations of hospital governance starting in the later eighteenth century, this clash at the eve of modernization helps measure to what extent Enlightenment ideas about the rationalization of hospital care had already made inroads and informed proposals for change. Simultaneously, it seeks to highlight how the desire for reforms was imbued by the traditionalist logic of early modern society still defining its playing field. This will help set subsequent reforms into perspective.

1 Ulbricht, 'The Debate about Foundling Hospitals': 211–56; Risse, *Mending Bodies*, chap. 5; Frohman, *Poor Relief and Welfare*, chaps 2–3; Brown, 'Medicine, Reform and the "End" of Charity': 1353–88.

2 The respective rulers of the prince-bishopric of Würzburg involved in the conflict were Johann Gottfried II. von Guttenberg (reg. 1684–1698), Johann Philipp Franz von Schönborn (reg. 1719–1724), Karl Philipp von Greiffenclau zu Vollrads (reg. 1749–1754).

 | HTTPS://DOI.ORG/10.1163/9789004755062-003

For this purpose, the article has selected a little studied type of hospital care, so called corrodies, which were used for old age retirement in early modern Germany. They exhibited a series of characteristics which made them stand out from other, more well-known forms of early modern institutional provision, such as almsgiving. Unusual in their design, they resembled rather life annuities than Christian charity but were frequently offered by hospitals all over early modern Europe and especially eighteenth-century Germany. Precisely this form and these addressees were imbued with the logic of early modern institutional provision. They sparked, however, repeated criticism at the same time, opening a window into how contemporaries conceived of the aim and purpose of hospital care. The article starts by describing how the hospital scheme of corrodies functioned in the first section and how it makes certain features of pre-1800s institutional provision more tangible in the second. The studied specific institution, the Bürgerspital zum Heiligen Geist in Würzburg, and very common source types in the study of early modern German hospitals in general and corrodies in specific will be presented in the third. The final section analyzes the reforms in Würzburg during the first half of the eighteenth century.

1 Corrodies as Tools of Early Modern Institutional Provision

The term "corrody" is not self-evident and thus warrants a definition. It refers to a relationship between an individual and a charitable institution in which the former is admitted being housed and fed by the latter. Often the relationship is transactional, regularly also contractual, as the individual basically purchases the right of board and bread from the institution. Virtually always the arrangement is struck for the remainder of the individual's life. In the early modern era, in Germany and elsewhere, these arrangements were frequently used for institutional provision: An individual, recognizing that his or her working days were numbered, found the opportunity to invest their savings into such a corrody. In return, the buyer, or 'corrodian' henceforth, obtained material security of being fed, housed and clad for the rest of his days. The risk of outliving one's savings and spending the last phase of one's life in ignominious poverty was thus averted.

The term corrody has been used by English scholarship to describe such arrangements in the context of late medieval monasticism. Its etymological origin lies in a Medieval French word meaning provisions, such as for travels.[3]

3 Stuckert, *Corrodies in the English Monasteries*, 7–9.

The usage of this English term in continental scholarship has allowed for an increasingly international and comparative literature, capable of aligning phenomena in different European contexts with each other. 'Corrody'/'Corrodian' will thus be preferred to the local terminology.[4] Other European languages in fact know other terms for such arrangements, such as *proveniers* in Dutch, *donnés* in French, or *commessi* or *dedicati* in Italian.[5] Early modern Germans (and Würzburgers) would have referred to such arrangements as a "Pfründe", and to the individual as a "Pfründner". Literally translated to English as 'prebend' or 'prebendary', they denoted a large typology of legal relationships associated with the payments of rents.[6] In fact, corrodies have been likened to life annuities which existed in an array of different forms and contexts in early modern Europe.[7] Normally, however, life annuities were paid out in cash and not necessarily linked to institutional care.[8] If German contemporaries wanted to specifically refer to a hospital corrody, they called it a "Spitalpfründe". This was also because the hospitals played a much bigger role in admitting corrodies than monasteries in the early modern period. Corrodies thus integrated into urban institutional provision.

Besides the case of the Bürgerspital of Würzburg, the evidence for the presence of corrodies in early modern Germany is overwhelming. A strong historiographical interest in institutional histories has provided us with many accounts of single hospitals. These works primarily studied the administrative structure of the hospitals as well as the charitable policies carried out by them over time. The main chronological focus has been on the late Middle Ages and the sixteenth century, but there are significant studies focused on the eighteenth century, too. Social historians have tried to understand the social background of those who retired to a hospital. Economic historians have attempted to understand hospital finances, among others calculating the profitability of corrodies and their place in the institutional budget.[9] Local historians have analyzed through corrodians how a hospital's policies

4 See for example Pelzl, Zuijderduijn, 'Saving the Best for Last?', 326–49.

5 Miramon, *Les 'Donnés' Au Moyen Âge*. Redon, 'Autour de l'hôpital Santa Maria Della Scala', 17–34. Zuijderduijn, "Good Fresh Air and Expert Medical Service", 195–213.

6 Becker, 'Pfründe', in *Handwörterbuch*, 1743–45; Becker, 'Laienpfründe', *Handwörterbuch*, 1353–55.

7 Bell, Sutcliffe, 'Valuing Medieval Annuities', 142–57. For the history of life annuities see Poitras, 'The Early History of Financial Economics', chap. 6.

8 For a discussion of the advantages of corrodies compared to cash annuities see Pelzl, Zuijderduijn, 'Or Do You Prefer Cash?', 237–55.

9 Pelzl, 'Altersvorsorge', 207–34. Heimpel, *Die Entwicklung*. Militzer, *Das Markgröninger Heilig-Geist-Spital*. Sonderegger, 'Wirtschaften mit sozialem Auftrag', 191–216.

affected local communities.[10] Evidence for this exists all over Germany, with a focus on the South which was more prosperous and urbanized in the Renaissance.[11] There are excellent accounts of these, for the example in southern German cities of Regensburg, Bamberg, Forchheim, Rottweil, Tübingen or Memmingen.[12] The Würzburg corrody scheme operated in a way comparable to other schemes in southern Germany. What makes it stand out is the fact that between the late seventeenth century and the early eighteenth century, it became the bone of contention in a power struggle which impelled several actors to make explicit arguments about its purpose and raison d'être, which is rare for other hospitals.

The institutional historiography has often accurately described that the corrodies targeted mainly elderly individuals. Even if hospitals admitting corrodians might resemble modern retirement homes *ante litteram*, the very idea of retirement, as a separate phase at the end of life characterized by withdrawal from social duties and labor, was unknown.[13] For material reasons, it was not an option for most. Individuals approaching old age could take several measures to ensure their material wellbeing in the last years of their lives. The common challenge was that much of the urban population lived off of their income from labor. Only the highest echelons of society could rely on returns on investments to make a living. The vast majority of occupations consisted in physical labor, and again, only few, such as priests, lawyers or scribes, were not fully dependent on their physical force. Insufficient medical care and the poor labor conditions to which men were exposed since adolescence could accelerate the deterioration of health, diminishing the individual's ability to earn a living the older they became. The question at which calendar age one was considered old in the early modern period eludes a general answer: Symbolically, the age of 60 was sometimes chosen, as for example demonstrated by the "steps of life" or "life stairs" visual genre which subdivided the life course in steps of ten years.[14] For all that is known from the corrodians themselves, physical decline could set in considerably earlier than this.

10 Holzwart-Schäfer, 'Pfründner und Bedürftige im Esslinger Katharinenspital', 7–35.

11 Ohngemach, 'Spitäler in Oberdeutschland', 255–91.

12 Neumaier, *Pfründner. Die Klientel des Regensburger St. Katharinenspitals*. Reddig, *Bürgerspital und Bischofsstadt*. Besold-Backmund, *Stiftungen und Stiftungswirklichkeit*. Ohngemach, *Stadt und Spital. Das Rottweiler Hl.-Geist-Spital*. Aderbauer, *Vom Pfründnerheim zur Arbeits- und Armenanstalt*. Lambacher, *Das Spital der Reichsstadt Memmingen*.

13 Whilst the concept of retirement, understood as a workfree period in old age, was unknown, the problem of old age provision was very evident. This paper uses the term 'retirement' anachronistically to denote its functional equivalence to modern retirement.

14 Ehmer, 'The Life Stairs: Aging, Generational Relations, and Small Commodity Production in Central Europe'. In *Ageing and Generational Relations over the Life Course*, ed. Hareven, 55.

The most well-known mechanism of care provision has been family support. According to this logic, parents were taken care of by their sons and daughters, moving in with them and/or being fed by them. The parent generation could offer the prompt transfer of the inheritance as an incentive, as well as whatever minor works, they were still able to contribute, such as help with child-rearing. Particularly in rural settings, the transmission of the farm could be sanctioned by a contract which could then include such provisions.[15] While this was undeniably true for some, it is more than dubious to what extent this can be considered a general fallback option for the majority of the old. After all, the vagaries of fortune stood in the way of this: Some were childless or, in times of rampant child mortality, had lost their children long before old age. Some, in fact, had never married.[16] Children could move away or simply lack the means to sustain their parents, especially when they themselves had numerous children, let alone personal grudges or conflicts. Some retirement contracts hint at the family feuds that could emerge when the role of oldest male coincided no longer with that of the main breadwinner.[17] Likewise, supplication letters, which will be discussed later in more detail, anecdotally hint at the complicated family situations. The 68-year-old couple of Claus and Maria Dettelbacher bemoaned that the no children anymore to take care of them.[18]

Very few occupational groups, such as priests, state bureaucrats, or military veterans, could also find specific retirement institutions at their disposal, provided by their employer.[19] Personal servants who had for many years loyally served a lord could hope for generosity out of personal gratitude. If any savings were available to the elderly, other options could pop up; the aging could make investments themselves: various financial assets, such as sovereign debt, could be purchased by any willing buyer.[20] Some European states, such as France, offered their government debt in the form of life annuities.[21] They allowed individuals who had had the chance to accumulate some savings to maintain a certain status. Institution-based solutions depended quite clearly on financial, social or occupational resources which the aged had collected over the life cycle. For individuals who had always lived around the poverty

---

15 Held, 'Ausgedinge und ländliche Gesellschaft. Generationenverhältnisse im Österreich des 17. bis 19. Jahrhunderts.' In *Gerontologie und Sozialgeschichte*, 151–86.

16 In fact, single women not only as a demographic but socio-cultural phenomenon have been studied by Froide, *Never Married*.

17 Mitterauer, 'Familienwirtschaft und Altersversorgung', 191–92.

18 Stadtarchiv Würzburg, Archiv des Bürgerspitals, Abt. II Nr. 16, Fasz. II, fol. 98.

19 Conrad, *Vom Greis zum Rentner*, 185–97. Hudson, 'Disabled Veterans', 117–44.

20 A study exemplifying the diversified investment options open to willing buyers is Zuijderduijn, De Moor. 'Spending, Saving, or Investing', 38–56.

21 Spang, *Stuff and Money in the Time of the French Revolution*, chap. 1.

line old age was a daunting prospect. Generally, corrodies can be likened to "middle class welfare", i.e. instruments aiming at middling classes which had come under pressure in difficult circumstances, as they presupposed social and financial resources.[22]

The transactional aspect of corrodies made them stand out from other forms of early modern institutional provision. It runs counter to the classical idea of Christian charity which was conceived of as a one-way transfer from the rich to the poor. As is to be seen in the following, even contemporaries took issue with this aspect, both positively and negatively. However, between a thoroughly transactional and a fully charitable and gratuitous nature laid a large field of different shades of either of the two. Depending on various factors, such as chronology, geography, but even the very person of the applicant, compromises between an exchange of goods and the charitable mission of the hospital to care for the sick, poor and old, were struck. Balancing the two imperatives of financially sound policies which enabled the future operationality of the institution and the charitable mission for which it had been founded was baked into the very *modus operandi* of hospitals. Corrodies were simply an arrangement in which both imperatives came to light more clearly than elsewhere.

From a narrowly financial viewpoint, the complexity of a corrody lay in striking an equitable deal between both sides, one variable of which, however, was unknown to both parties: Corrodies were most often paid through a sum which had been established at the moment of admission of the elderly. It may have been paid in installments over time, yet its amount could not be changed *ex post*. The number of years which a corrodian would go on to live and the prices for foodstuffs several years in the future were almost impossible to gauge for hospital officials trying to set a price. Should the elderly die a few months into retirement, he or she would have massively overpaid the corrody. Likewise, should he or she live for another 25 years, the corrody price would pale in light of the costs of food, heating and housing accrued over all those years. The two parties thus incurred the risk of striking a very uneven deal. This problem seemed so serious to medieval lawyers that it even sparked a debate in the Middle Ages about whether corrodies were akin to usury, to which only a Papal decree in favor of corrodies put an end.[23]

---

22 Van Leeuwen, 'Guilds and Middle-Class Welfare', 61–90. McCants, 'The Role of the Charitable Institution'. Terpstra, *Abandoned Children of the Italian Renaissance*, chap. 6.

23 Hermann, 'Die Spitalpfründe', 16–17. Signori, 'Kontingenzbewältigung durch Zukunftshandeln', 117–42.

In practice, this financial logic was only one of an array of factors. Several textual sources from hospitals confirm that setting a price was not the outcome of a single formula or straightforward calculation but took the whole person of the applicant into account. Extreme cases, for example, in which a single individual received special conditions occurred when a powerful and high-ranking patron supported their application. In Würzburg, for example, an early seventeenth century inspection of the hospital, appointed by the bishop, described the common practice that an applicant's age as well as ability to pay were taken into account when setting a price. It detailed: "Rich corrodians, who all have to buy their corrody and apart from citizens also include foreigners admitted for a sum of money are considered for their age and weakness, i.e. whether they will enjoy the corrody for short or long."[24] The same report included the complaint by a poor corrodian who claimed that the hospital scribe "has reproached him for being *ex gratia* [highlighted by LP] in the hospital, that he had not been a citizen".[25] This shows the individual factors as well as the interplay financial and non-financial motives in admission decisions.

2 Emergence and Political Ramifications of Corrodies

Large-scale urban poverty was a structural feature of early modern European and thus German societies. Bad times marked by failed harvests, wars and/or economic depressions could add many more to the lines of those waiting for alms.[26] In this regard, early modern poor relief clearly addressed a social need. In light of this enormous demand, it must appear surprising that the elderly, as a quantitatively rather modest subsection, received so much attention. Demographic estimates of early modern populations caution modern readers neither to over- nor to underestimate their share: on the one hand they dispel the outdated myth that due to low average life expectancy elderly populations were minuscule. Depending on various contexts and chronologies, the elderly,

24 Stadtarchiv Würzburg, Archiv des Bürgerspitals, Abt. III, Nr. 190, fol. 224. "Reiche Pfründner welche ihre pfründ alle kauffen müssen, und neben den Bürgers Leuthen auch frembte umb ein summa gelts, nach gestalt ihres alters und schwachheit, in deren erwegung sie der Pfründt kurtz oder lang vehig zu sein, erachtet werden." This was part of a survey, conducted in 1620–1, of all hospitals and poorhouses in and around the city to assess their state and operations, giving advice on improvement.

25 Stadtarchiv Würzburg, Archiv des Bürgerspitals, Abt. III, Nr. 190, fol. 239. "Heinrich Hoffmann clagt, der schreiber habe ihm vorgeworffn, seye ex gratia im Spital, sey kein Bürger gewesen".

26 Jütte, *Poverty and Deviance in Early Modern Europe*, vol. 4.

defined as those aged 60 and older, made up roughly 10% of early modern urban populations.[27] Considering that physical decline could commence much earlier than that, the group of the "aging" might have been even bigger. The old and aging were thus a visible and lively presence in early modern cities, and Würzburg was surely no exception to that. On the other hand, the elderly obviously paled compared with the other demographic constituencies afflicted by poverty. The laboring poor, for example, defined as men and women of various age groups who could barely make a living in spite of working amounted to a much larger share of the population. Children, demographically much more numerous than the old, could as orphans be completely dependent on public or private charity[28] or as children of the lower classes harmed in their physical and cognitive development by poverty.[29] Unlike the old, policies aiming at care provision to them could claim to invest in future adults as potential contributors to the urban commonwealth.

From this vantage point, it is not self-evident that early modern aldermen or lords would want to dedicate a significant share of the always scarce resources for charity to a fairly small group. Also, corrodies, as other forms of all institutional provision, could only accommodate a small minority. A straightforward numeric explanation of the diffusion and the relative financial importance of this particular eldercare is thus not satisfactory. However, welfare allocation is rarely a direct function of quantitative importance and needs-testing, and even less so early modern forms of welfare. In fact, several factors characteristic of early modern welfare can be discerned in corrodies. In early modern institutional provision, the symbolic capital acquired by almsgiving could be central. There is a sizable historiography tying charitable foundations to the founder's desire for *memoria*, i.e. remembrance post-mortem and spiritual pay-off, which also found its expression in early modern law of foundations (*Stiftungsrecht*).[30] As the 1621–inspection summarized:

> Firstly, in the year of 1319 at the eve of St. John's day, Johann von Steren, citizen of Würzburg, has with the permission of bishop Gottfried von Hohenlohe built the Bürgerspital, endowed it with his patrimony, so that for all times twelve sick, old or frail people will be maintained in it.[31]

27 Ehmer, 'Altersstrukturen im Historischen Wandel', 408–10.

28 Safley, *Kinder, Karitas und Kapital*, 1. Meumann, *Findelkinder, Waisenhäuser, Kindsmord.*

29 Safley, *Children of the Labouring Poor.*

30 For an overview see Borgolte, *Stiftung Und Memoria*, vol. 10.

31 Stadtarchiv Würzburg, Archiv des Bürgerspitals, Abt. III, Nr. 190, fol. 191. "Erstlich Anno 1319 in Vigilia Sancti Johannis Baptistae, hatt mit verwilligung Bischoff Gottfriedens des geschlechts von hohenlohe, Herrn Johann vom Steren, Bürger zu Würzburg seeligen, das

The intentions and expectations of the "givers" mattered: Sandra Cavallo has emphasized this "supply-centered" perspective on early modern poor relief in her study on early modern Turin. Focusing on the benefactors' intentions and consideration much more than on urban poverty, she finds that funding charitable institutions and giving alms was an organic element in the power struggle between rival parties in the city. This was, however, not only instrumental: different actors chose various tools which they considered befitting to their political identity and their preferred form of government.[32]

The life cycle could play a particular role in making a symbolic argument about good governance. A popular series of prints depicting various social groups in the southern German city of Nuremberg also featured local corrodians. They were paired on the same leaflet, though, with a representation of local orphans.[33] The symbolic relationship between the two, as the adjacent description proves, is to be found in the life cycle: the urban authorities sought to make clear that urban welfare stretched across the whole human life cycle from infancy to old age. Not only the "givers" made use of this: the writers of supplication letters knew how to artfully combine the material needs of old age with arguments about years-long dutiful tax payments and obedient citizenship. Their position at the end of the life cycle enabled them to highlight their contribution to the urban commonwealth through the achievements of their lives.[34]

One of the most striking features of old-age poverty was that it was highly life cyclical. This meant that a considerable share of those who sought shelter at the hospitals' door had not been poor all their lives. In better times, when they were still in working shape, many had belonged to what can be called "urban middle classes". This anachronistic term defines social groups which were neither elites, such as patricians or rich merchants, nor part of the absolute have-nots. Unlike English historiography which has identified this "middling sort" in merchants and traders, in the cities of southern Germany artisans and craftspeople occupied these ranks.

These groups were far from being politically powerless, even though their channels of influence were most often informal. The most important piece of evidence for this hypothesis comes from the begin of "corrodization" in the late

---

Bürgerspital gebauth, und deselbig mit seinem vermög also fundiert und dotiert, dass zu ewigen Zeiten Zwölf Krancke, alte, oder presshafte Personen darin ernehrt …".

32 Cavallo, *Charity and Power in Early Modern Italy*.

33 Boener, *Nürnbergische Kleider-Trachten*, 40.

34 See other German-language studies on such supplications Scheutz, 'Supplikationen an den "ersamen" Rat', 157–206. Stanislaw-Kemenah, "An die Nechsterledigte Stelle", 85–104.

Middle Ages, i.e. the spread of corrodies. Siegfried Reicke has in his 1932–book identified a wave of "Verbürgerlichung" or, as it has been later called, "Kommunalisierung" in that period.[35] In many German towns, hospitals, which had been founded from the early thirteenth century onwards, were slowly taken over by expanding municipalities. Founders and former owners, such as bishops and princes, were pushed out of the leadership of the institution. In his still unrivalled thesis, Reicke linked this leadership change in favor of "Bürger", i.e. citizens, with the onset of "corrodization".[36] Urban governments felt more accountable towards the population and thus used welfare policies to bolster their legitimacy. Corrodies emerged – in this vision – as municipal governments diverted resources from the original purposes, as laid out in the institutional founding documents, towards social milieus on which their rule depended. In fact, guild riots were a recurring threat to municipal order in late medieval Germany, and welfare policies can be counted as one element of a larger social contract bolstering political stability.

Reicke's hypothesis has found much acclaim in subsequent German historiography. It is, however, ultimately difficult to prove or disprove. What is certain is that the origins of many large corrody schemes lie in the late Middle Ages. They have also been explained to stand in a tradition of devoted believers living at a hospital. For France, de Miramon has identified predecessors of corrodies in hospital confraternities. Those who had entered it were "semi-religious", in a grey zone between official ordination and lay piety.[37] To fervent believers it offered a way to give a more institutional form to their piety without formally entering a monastic order or being ordained as a priest. Single cases of noblemen who ceded an important part of their goods to the hospital in order to spend their last years in prayer and religious reflection there also preceded the rise of corrodies as a more coherent institutional provision.[38]

Even when corrodies became more institutionalized in the fifteenth century, pious and welfare motives for offering and buying corrodies are not easy to disentangle and were probably perceived as complementary by contemporaries. Along with larger societal tendencies of the early modern era, corrodies became more secularized and took the shape of an institutional provision. Religious services and hours of prayer were obviously still observed inside the institutions, however, the supplication letters in which applicants expounded

35 Reicke, *Das Deutsche Spital*, 196–277.

36 For a more critical note on Reicke's hypothesis see Pauly, 'Von der Fremdenherberge zum Seniorenheim', 110.

37 de Miramon, *Les 'Donnés' Au Moyen Âge*, chap. III.

38 Reddig, *Bürgerspital und Bischofsstadt*, chap. 4.2.1.

their motivations discussed much more often material than spiritual needs. Slowly and over time, religious motivations for institutional provision diminished, without ever fading completely. Rhetorically they always retained normative importance, such as a passage from a report on the Würzburg hospital shows: "After many laudable people in the intent to serve God have brought in thousand or more guilders and considerable vineyards, fields and meadows improving the hospital greatly".[39] What held them up after all was the legally binding status of the founding charter and hospital ordinances which, inspired by the former, set guidelines.

Out of these late Medieval origins, corrody schemes often continued to exist well over centuries, usually more long-lived than the political authorities that had created them. The many longitudinal studies of German hospitals give us a good sense of how these policies developed over time. Some, as in the cases of Tübingen and Regensburg, were dislodged in times of great turmoil, such as the Thirty Years' War (1618–48).[40] Facing crisis and devastation, hospital officials chose to abandon the for-pay scheme and focus on more indiscriminate poor relief for the large population that had fallen into poverty during wartime. In many cases, however, the sale of corrodies was left in place and its changes over time were more due to small adaptations or inadvertent changes stemming from the failure to adapt. Institutionalized control mechanisms were far and few. So-called "Visitationen", or visitations, of a hospital by its lord were anchored in the legal structure of hospitals, the so-called *Visitationsrecht*.[41] Yet it seems that these were only conducted when external political circumstances made this convenient, or a grave internal crisis, mostly financial, necessitated this.[42] Likewise, the visitations of the Würzburg hospital are a case in point, as the vetting of the sale of corrodies in the mid eighteenth century only resulted from a power struggle between the municipality and the local bishop over control of the institution.

Studying corrodies helps put the finger on several traits that were particularly characteristic of early modern welfare, and arguably partly due to them corrodies came under criticism in Würzburg. They showcase how some early modern welfare arrangement had organically grown over centuries and that,

---

39 Stadtarchiv Würzburg, Archiv des Bürgerspitals, Abt. III, Nr. 190. "Nachdem auch in diesem Spitl etliche vornehme Leuth aus andacht, Gott zu dienen hiebnvor kommen, und zu tausent und mehr gülden, auch Stadtliche Gütter an Weingärten, Äckhern, und wissen hinein gebracht und also den Spital herrlich gemehret."

40 Dirmeier, 'Das St. Katharinenspital zu Regensburg'. Aderbauer, *Das Tübinger Spital*. Sannwald, *Spitäler in Pest und Krieg*.

41 Begon, *De iure hospitalium*, pt. D.

42 Dirmeier, 'Das St. Katharinenspital zu Regensburg'.

in turn, they had rarely undergone systematic scrutiny and policy planning. Path-changing alterations came, if at all, in the form of external shocks dislodging the long-term policy drift. Long-term societal trends, such as secularization, very slowly shaped their form. The legal ramifications of hospital law (*Spitalsrecht*) and foundation law (*Stiftungsrecht*) remained stable for centuries. When discussing the sweeping reforms of the later eighteenth and early nineteenth century, we should bear in mind that such deliberate and purposeful interventions were rather the exception than the norm in early modern welfare governance. Small-scale adaptation and transmutations to contexts were as powerful a force in shaping welfare as political action.

Corrodies also prove to be a good example of how local political power dynamics could alter the directions of the stream of resources for welfare. Public institutional provision has obviously in no time and place been immune to power asymmetries, and political interventions of those who wanted a share of it. At the same time the frankness with which resources could be redirected to interest groups speaks to the inherently hierarchical and unequal structure of early modern societies. Whereas in later periods calls for rationalization and public utility as well as the modern state's quest for ever greater control of society shaped the way in which power and welfare were intertwined, corrodies exhibit characteristics distinctly early modern. They were a welfare scheme that emerged in the late Middle Ages due to the redistribution of the (scarce) available resources to middle classes. Being stable over centuries, their governance was more often than not rather permissive, showing that welfare governance had not yet assumed the commitment to wide-spread social intervention.

3 The Würzburg Bürgerspital and Hospital Sources

The *Bürgerspital zum Heiligen Geist* was the main civic hospital in a city which counted some 15,000 inhabitants in the late eighteenth century. Until the Napoleonic Wars, Würzburg was the residence city of an ecclesiastical principality, the prince-bishopric of Würzburg (Hochstift Würzburg), located in the northwest of modern-day Bavaria along the fertile valley of the river Main.[43] The local bishops thus also served as princes, ruling a mid-sized state in the highly fragmented Holy Roman Empire. Unlike some neighboring territories the state remained Catholic. Würzburg was by far the largest city in the state,

---

43 Schott, 'Fürstlicher Absolutismus und Barocke Stadt', 130–202.

serving as its residence and seat of government. Its history was characterized by clashes between the bishop and the municipality of the city, which was formally subordinate to the ruler, but had repeatedly tried to break free. This conflict impacted the local institutional provision, too: the Bürgerspital (literally civic hospital) bore its link to the municipality in its name and was conceived as an explicitly civic institution since its foundation in the early fourteenth century by an affluent local citizen. In 1580, one of the prince-bishops founded their "own" institution, the *Juliusspital*, to consolidate support among the local population. The Bürgerspital was controlled by the city council which in turn was *de facto* controlled by urban upper classes.[44] They nominated some of their peers to supervise the institution, even if they were hardly involved in day-to-day activities. When it came to the decision who to admit as a corrodian, it was up to these aldermen to vet the applications and grant admission.

The hospital was, however, not financed by the municipal budget, but was an independent, private and secular foundation. This meant that the rich citizens who had founded the hospital in the fourteenth century had also provided an endowment, the returns from which had to cover the costs of institutional provision, codified in the founding charter. As for many other medieval foundations, the substantial assets in the endowments consisted mostly of landed estates in the city's surroundings. Due to the mild climate of the river valley, many of its properties were and are still used for the cultivation of wine.[45] The viticulture thus provided the most important source of revenue for the hospital. To take the example of 1775: roughly a third of the hospital's cash revenue came from the sale of wine.[46] Another third came from the sale of other agricultural produce, mostly grain and wheat, but also lentils and livestock. Around one sixth came from banking services which the hospital provided to the local population, such as lending and collecting interests. This even understates this strong agricultural imprint. The bookkeeping was divided into two independent accounts, one in cash and one in kind. Some of the agricultural produce was never sold but instead used to make payments directly in kind and to feed the corrodians and distributed as alms. The economy of the institution was thus highly dependent on local agriculture and its performance,

44 For the two main books on the history of the Bürgerspital Würzburg see Bergerhausen, Wagner, *Quellen zur Geschichte des Bürgerspitals*. Franz, *Aus vier Jahrhunderten innerer Geschichte des Bürgerspitals*.

45 This had been the case for a long time, as a report from 1620–1 evidences: Stadtarchiv Würzburg, Archiv des Bürgerspitals, Abt. III, Nr. 190, fol. 193.

46 See the respective account book of 1775/6: Stadtarchiv Würzburg, Archiv des Bürgerspitals, Abt. IV, Rechnung Nr. 245.

resulting in a vulnerability to the ups and down of the former. (This continues to this date, as the foundation has weathered all winds of time and still exists. Having narrowed the scope of its activity, it mainly serves as a retirement home and winery.)

By the first half of the eighteenth century, the activities of the Würzburg hospital consisted in offering two typologies of corrodians, poor and rich ones (called *Unter-* resp. *Oberpfründner*). The number of rich corrodians hovered between 10 and 15 and that of the *Unterpfründer* was roughly twice as much. Poor corrodians were normally asked to lend a hand in daily maintenance works of the hospital and enjoyed a less abundant dietary plan. Consequently, they paid less for admission than their richer counterparts.[47]

Due to their longevity and institutional stability, most German hospitals conserve impressive archives which allow quite a thorough reconstruction of their activity. The same is the case for Würzburg. The source base for the study of corrodies relies mainly on the administrative records of the hospital. The administration consisted primarily of two parts: institutional provision and the management of the endowment. By owning land, the institution also assumed judicial functions for the dwellers which have left many administrative traces. Sources directly related to the sale of corrodies consist of the following source types: Account books record the payments corrodians made upon entering the institution.

Very importantly, sometimes the contracts between the institutions and the corrodians themselves have survived. They could be kept as loose papers or be registered in a respective book. This was the case in Würzburg where they were referred to as "Pfründbrieffe" and were registered in the "Pfründbuch".[48] In some institutions, especially where corrody sums were lower, it is not fully clear whether formal contracts were concluded at all. In some places the contracts were full of specific personal details which the single corrodians had negotiated with the directors. In Würzburg, they rather included very general terms of the deal as well as a lengthy declaration by the elderly to respect the hospital's ordinances and behave well.

The most revealing source about the socio-economic backgrounds of corrodians and their biographies are supplication letters which the corrodians submitted for their admission. In these letters they could make a detailed case for

47 For the work duties and diets see the hospital ordinance of 1711: Stadtarchiv Würzburg, Archiv des Bürgerspitals, Abt. III, Nr. 30. For the different entrance fees compare: Abt. II, Nr 19 Fasz. I & II and 18.

48 Stadtarchiv Würzburg, Archiv des Bürgerspitals, Abt. III, Nr. 36.

their admission, explaining how they had ended up in such precarious material circumstances and what motivated their request. Supplication letters offer unparalleled insights into the life stories of average people, for which they have been frequently used in studies.[49] At the same time, their veracity and reliability has repeatedly been doubted: the writers, either the poor themselves or scribes hired by them, possessed an obvious incentive to misrepresent the facts. They would, so the argument goes, subtly reframe inconvenient episodes in their lives or exaggerate convenient ones, based on what they expected would win them the director's favor. Interpreting these petitions involves careful balancing between those two poles.

Hospital officials drew up lists of inmates. In Würzburg, for example, a list of current corrodians was added to the yearly account book since the early 1700s.[50] One last, but equally important source type for the life and living standards of corrodians are hospital ordinances, or *Spitalordnungen*, which governed the rules of conduct and diets in the institution.[51] For Würzburg, the 1711–ordinance is especially revealing.[52] It stipulated the attendance of mass and regular prayers, but also very mundane questions, such as the prohibition of the resale of food rations or cleaning schedules; poor corrodians for example had to sweep their chambers at least two to three times each week. In addition, it contained a catalogue, divided by sex, of tasks which corrodians could be asked to lend a hand with, for elderly men watching the hospital's gates and trimming the plants in the hospital garden were foreseen, for elderly women, for example, many works related to cooking. These work duties should mislead no officials into recruiting "good workers": "Whatever work a poor corrodian has still force to perform, he should be called to do it. But the corrody should only go to those who for their high age and lack of force cannot make a living anymore."[53] Lastly, it described a weekly dietary plan (or at least an aspiration), a soup for lunch and a pretzel with wine for dinner on weekdays. To what extent ordinances strictly prescribed realities inside these institutions, or rather visions, is an ongoing debate.

---

49 For Würzburg see for example, Stadtarchiv Würzburg, Archiv des Bürgerspitals, Abt. II, Nr. 16.

50 Stadtarchiv Würzburg, Archiv des Bürgerspitals, Abt. IV, see the series of the *Rechnungsbücher*.

51 The source type has received increased attention in the last 15 years: Scheutz, Weiß, *Spital als Lebensform*; Scheutz, Weiß, 'Spitalordnungen als essentielle Grundlage der Organisation der Spitäler', in *Historia Hospitalium*, ed. Stollberg, Vanja, Kraas, 151–90.

52 Stadtarchiv Würzburg, Archiv des Bürgerspitals, Abt. III, Nr. 30.

53 Stadtarchiv Würzburg, Archiv des Bürgerspitals, Abt. III, Nr. 30.

4 Reforming Corrodies in Würzburg

Corrodies had never been without criticism, even if evidence of criticism is rather fragmented. It does not seem – or at least there is no written record of it – that the sale of corrodies was continuously reflected upon as a welfare policy by either directors, urban representatives, the corrodians themselves or outside observers. Often practiced for centuries, it was subsumed under habitual and time-proven practices. The critique mainly appears in two forms, one financial and one socio-political. The financial strand questioned whether corrodies were a good investment for hospitals. They argued that granting the elderly the right of free housing and food for an unforeseeable number of years was financially hazardous and could thus cost the institutions dearly. As the very idea of corrodies as retirement provision forbade to set a maximum number of years, the risk had to be reflected in pricing. Individual longevity being impossible to assess, the hospital directors would have had to come to an understanding of the average amount of time corrodians spent in the hospitals, in other words the average life expectancy. This line of critique often surfaced in time of financial uncertainty, or even crisis, when the hospital's finances were under pressure due to economic fluctuations or internal mismanagement (as we will see later).

The other line took a more principled stance about the basic scope and aim of institutional provision. It argued that elderly who could still afford a sometimes-handsome sum of entrance fees should not be the prime beneficiaries of urban welfare. In this vision, welfare was supposed to be means-based and first of all take aim at society's weakest groups in absolute terms. Corrodies thus emerged as a diversion of means from the really needy. This could also be linked to controversies within the hospital between different groups of inhabitants about prerogatives.[54] Likewise, they could be sparked by a rereading of the medieval founding charters of the institutions whose language normally made no explicit mention of corrodies, but rather generically of the "poor and sick", leaving ample space of interpretation to different readers.

In the financial and socio-political critique moralist undertones could be of conspicuous strength. Here, the elderly retiree was described as idle and lazy, which was morally reprehensible and should hence not be rewarded any public support. Both lines of criticism represented two different priorities of how corrodies should be handled and what they should ultimately be: one saw in them above all a financial tool to fill the hospital's coffers, while also providing

54 Pauly, *Peregrinorum, Pauperum et Aliorum Transeuntium Receptaculum*, 255–57.

welfare to the elderly. The other saw above all a welfare tool in them, while, luckily, earning a buck at the same time. Obviously, these two positions were not categorically incompatible, but they capture important prioritizations.[55] This juxtaposition inserts itself into a larger historiographic debate about the relationship between charity and economy inside welfare institutions.

The peculiar position of Würzburg's Bürgerspital at a political fault line between the municipality and the bishop helped bring discussion over the function of corrody schemes to light and produced a sizeable written documentation of them. At the same time, these discussions have to be always read through the prism of this conflict. Starting in the late seventeenth century, the government of the bishopric of Würzburg sought increasingly to centralize power.[56] This can be read as among the classical teachings of 'absolutist' political practice in which a state government ought to eliminate or sideline intermediate powers in its own realm. The city of Würzburg had a much longer history of clashes with the bishop, dating back to the late Middle Ages when it had repeatedly tried to shake off the bishop's yoke. This conflict was rekindled when a series of bishops attempted to reassert their power over the city, substantially weakening the municipal council. In this, the control over the large and wealthy foundation of the Bürgerspital became the bone of contention.

As explained above, the hospital itself was controlled by the municipal council. For a long time, however, the bishop had held the prerogative to conduct so-called "Visitationen", thus inspections, there. The last of such inspections before the conflict reignited, had been conducted in 1621, and was uneventful, describing the hospital's situation fairly positively, only raising attention to minor faults in the hospital's daily activities and spiritual order. Gathering testimonies from its inhabitants and employees and copying important documents such as the hospital ordinances it meant to assess the status quo in a factual way. As far as we know, remedying these was entrusted to the current directors without pressure from the bishop's government. In fact, at the same time several other welfare institutions in the city were vetted, suggesting that the inquiry belonged to a larger interest in institutional provision and the Bürgerspital had not been singled out. The visitation's report went so far to liken the considerable sums spent to buy corrodies by rich elderly people to

55 See how this juxtaposition is spelled out (and reconciled) for example in Sonderegger, 'Wirtschaften mit sozialem Auftrag. Stunz', 'Hospitäler im deutschsprachigen Raum', 129–59.

56 Schott, *Das Verhältnis*, 470–73.

the pious endowment which had set up the foundation in the first place.[57] Recounting the institutional history, it also still uncontroversially stated that

> the administration [of the institution] has been conferred by the founder to two members of the city council who should be the Spitalpfleger or Vormundt [directors] … the admission [of new corrodians] has undeniably been with the city council since the beginning of the foundation until now.[58]

The next visitation occurred only in 1691, indicating that for much of the seventeenth century the bishop's government probably saw little need in raising objections with the hospital's state of affairs. Following inspections were carried out at much greater frequency, such as in 1722 and 1749, each of them leaving behind paper trails, consisting of a report as well as a response from the municipal authorities, suggesting a completely different political climate.[59] Although chronologically separate, the three exchanges are in the following synthesized into a single debate. This is useful because apart from the details of each exchange it allows to access more general notions about how corrodies should be governed and how these notions were weaponized in the conflict.

In all three reports of 1691, 1722 and 1749, the bishop's officials essentially tried to prove and/or fabricate a case of misconduct against the city. By arguing that the institution was poorly run, they tried to have the municipal government, responsible for this, relieved of its duties. This partisan approach complicates the view on the actual situation at the institution, it allows, however, to study which arguments appeared credible and convincing to contemporaries. If there were any controversial policy decisions of the municipal stewards of the institution, the bishop's men would jump at them. In this, the handling of corrodies emerged as one line of attack, showing that there was potential of controversy to be exploited on this matter.

As a legal starting point the bishop's officials took the hospital's fourteenth century founding charters, which had only come down to contemporaries through several scattered and not fully reliable transcriptions. The latter stated that the founder had set up the hospital to feed twelve poor men. Corrodians, they argued, were not falling under this definition:

> Regarding upper or rich corrodies, as they are called by the directors, these have not been included in the foundational charter and they resemble more financial

57 Stadtarchiv Würzburg, Archiv des Bürgerspitals, Abt. III, Nr. 190, fol. 190 onwards.
58 Stadtarchiv Würzburg, Archiv des Bürgerspitals, Abt. III, Nr. 190, fol. 191–2.
59 Stadtarchiv Würzburg, Archiv des Bürgerspitals, Abt. III, Nr. 463.

> instruments [i.e. annuities, LP] which have been sold for 100 or more years by the city council.[60]

They imputed that under the government of the municipality the hospital had strayed too far from its original mission, prescribed by the unassailable authority of the founder some 300 years prior. "By whom and to what extent has the city council been granted permission to admit … poor and rich corrodians to this hospital?", they rhetorically asked in catalogue of questions sent to the city council.[61]

The municipality defended itself on several accounts: initially, the municipal officials reasoned that due to the poor state of transmission of the founding charter it was unclear what the founder's precise intention had been. They claimed to have searched the archive of the nearby monastery of Ebrach to possibly find further documents to elucidate the founder's mind, but to no avail. He might have intended a much broader idea of welfare, including the sale of corrodies. After all, the word "infirmus", the original Latin term used in the charter, could have various meanings ranging between poverty and sickness and might well include old and sick individuals. To strengthen their case, they quoted the Roman poet Terence who had equated old age with disease: "senectus ipsa morbus habeatur". In this state of uncertainty about the normative foundation, one should follow the established tradition, as previous generations of hospital directors had done. They wrote very abstractly in Latin,

> the respect and antiquity of all things … is the best interpreter and surest teacher, and also the most faithful and easy to follow, should not be changed, since the special conclusion is drawn from the venerable authority of antiquity, and thus is held to be in force by a special privilege.[62]

---

60 Stadtarchiv Würzburg, Archiv des Bürgerspitals, Abt. III, Nr. 463, fol. 28–9: "Wass nun aber die ober = oder reiche wie sie von den Pflegern gennant werden Pfründner angeht, da ist so zu wissen daß solche gar nicht fundiret oder gestifftet und dass solche mehr Leibgeding seyen, welche auch allschon vor 100 Jahren und mehr Jahren von allhiesigem Stadtrath …. verkauft".

61 Stadtarchiv Würzburg, Archiv des Bürgerspitals, Abt. III, Nr. 463, fol. 32 "Von wem und in wie weit dem Stadtrath das Jus erteilt worden … Ober- und Unterpfründner in dieses Bürgerspital auf und anzunehmen?".

62 Stadtarchiv Würzburg, Archiv des Bürgerspitals, Abt. III, Nr. 463, fol. 30–1 "Observantia atque antiquitas sunt omnium rerum optimae interpretes et certissimae magistræ; nec non mos fidelissimus adeoque facilis est, ut non mutandus sit. Dictum est enim, ex auctoritate vetustatis venerandæ, specialem conclusionem fieri posse; atque sic vim privilegii specialis habeat et tanquam constitutio reputetur." Also, for the following discussion, see this source.

The hospital officials underlined that the sale of corrodies was time-tested and had been in place long before anyone of the current members had taken office:

> since times immemorial [corrodies have been sold] and one does not know when this change [from the founder's intention] has taken place.[63]

In other words, they saw their actions as covered by precedent. In early modern Germany, tradition was imbued with normativity and the city officials put this social norm to their use. Alterations, which had over centuries been provoked by the vicissitudes of times, such as wars, were legitimate, especially as the original charter's language was ambiguous and its transmission dubious.

Likewise, the financial aspect of corrodies was mired in controversy. In the early eighteenth century, the hospital's finances were under considerable stress, as officials had admitted to themselves previously. In an internal memo, penned around 1740, officials bemoaned the "hard times" they had been in for many years", blaming poor wine harvests and the resulting default of the hospital's debtors and tenants for their misery.[64] The weight of maintaining several dozen people at the institution was clearly felt, as officials made an officials count of the hospital's inhabitants at this point finding 18 rich and 28 poor corrodians. Similar statements had already been made in the replies to the report of 1691 and 1722, suggesting they were undeniable.

The bishop's agents did not fail to seize on this, questioning various financial policies, from the directors' salaries to the sale of corrodies. They requested the disclosure of various internal financial documents. They portrayed the corrody as a very infelicitous investment for the hospital in which the directors had engaged. Even worse, the sale of a corrody which resulted in a loss for the institution (as the individual outlived the agreed-upon price) could imperil the charitable actions the hospital should actually carry out, such as almsgiving (which continued at a decreased rate). Here the financial and socio-political traditions of corrody criticism overlapped.

Had the hospital and municipal officials earlier tried to liken corrodians to any other welfare recipients, they later argued that they had put financial guardrails in place to ensure they kept making profit. Now, they described the

---

63 Stadtarchiv Würzburg, Archiv des Bürgerspitals, Abt. III, 190, fol. 195 "das der jetzige Stand schon seit Menschen Gedenken also und nicht wissend sei, wie und wann die Änderung geschehen".

64 Stadtarchiv Würzburg, Archiv des Bürgerspitals, Abt. II Nr. 16, Fasz. II, fol. 273–80. The same poor financial state had already openly been admitted in the reply to the report of 1722.

scheme as a savvy financial choice which they had utilized to collect extra funds for other poor relief activities. There had in no case been any wasteful spending on the rich corrodians: they had never ventured to cover their very expensive medical bills, simply providing food and shelter. To the contrary, reacting to recent price spikes they had set a minimum entrance fee of 500 guilders and had earned some 5000 guilders in the last years through the premature deaths of rich corrodians. This had allowed them to feed even more poor people through the extra income.[65] The hospital's account books show the claim of a minimum admission fee to be demonstrably false, however. It is unclear how they had calculated their revenue from corrodies. What they had in fact allowed for had been several gratuitous admissions of corrodians, which had been requested by eminent members of society and thus been irrefutable.

The bishop never managed to wrangle the hospital's control from the city. The discussion on corrodies had probably rather been a means to delegitimize the city's rule rather than a genuine interest in welfare policy. The shifting priorities through the three inspections indicate rather a search for a convenient attack line than a stable and strong position on the governance on corrodies. Regardless of this political background, the three reports of 1691, 1722 and 1749 and the respective replies between the bishop's government and the municipality shows what could reasonably be argued and how contemporaries believed they could attack or defend the sale of corrodies.

Ultimately, the controversy did have an impact on the institutional provision. In 1754 a decision was prepared to abolish rich corrodies, maintaining one single category of corrodians equal to what had earlier been called poor corrodies.[66] It is plausible to read this as a strategic sacrifice by the municipal officials to safeguard the main goal, the control of the hospital (which they succeeded to hold onto for another 50 years until the collapse of the bishopric amid the Napoleonic Wars). The accompanying documents put forward two lines of reasoning, omitting any direct mention to the preceding conflict. First, they argued that there had been for many years discord among poor corrodies claiming that they were "the true poor who the founding charter prescribed to be admitted to the hospital."[67] The reference to the founding charter was an unambiguous hint to the previous discussions, restating its importance.

It is unclear whether the poor corrodians had actually raised the issue or whether this served as a pretext to conceal the real motivations. Cases from other hospitals existed, where different types of welfare recipients had

65 Stadtarchiv Würzburg, Archiv des Bürgerspitals, Abt. III, Nr. 463.
66 Stadtarchiv Würzburg, Archiv des Bürgerspitals, Abt. II, Nr. 5.
67 Stadtarchiv Würzburg, Archiv des Bürgerspitals, Abt. II, Nr. 5.

contested each other's privileges, pushing the directors into action.[68] However, no mention had been made of any inmate's complaints before, although the bishop's agents had even questioned the hospital's inhabitants and could have very conveniently taken up the point. Possibly, poor corrodians served as a strawman for the municipal officials in whose mouth they could put words fitting their agenda. Thus, top-down reform was presented as bottom-up.

In a second note, undated but probably written somewhat later, the second line of reasoning motive became apparent. It cited the deficit the hospital had been running in the past ten years and then proposed the abolition of rich corrodies as a financial countermeasure. As has been shown, evidence for a financial malaise of the institution date back to the late seventeenth century and had been acknowledged by its directors. Discussing whether cutting rich corrodians off of their benefits was legally possible, it argued that some of them had been admitted for free and the others who had paid had been in the hospital for such a long time that they had consumed much more than they had paid. Unilateral modifications to the corrody contract were certainly not legal, but it seems that the corrodians caved in. A looming bankruptcy of the institution might have been threatening enough. Both lines of corrody criticism, one financial, the other socio-political, were combined in this attempt to corrody reform. From the documentation it appears that the reform was implemented in 1757 after a new diet plan for the corrodians had been agreed upon.

This was a fault line that had defined corrodies since their late Medieval origins. They sat in a grey zone between the classical definition of the needy and deserving poor and a more politically imbued and possibly self-interested understanding of the addressee which gave space to not-poor elderly. Both the bishop and the municipality could not escape discussing the liminal definition of charity, sometimes juxtaposing corrodians and "classical" welfare recipients, sometime explicitly denying any difference. "Middle class welfare", as such arrangements have been called, were certainly common and often tacitly approved of in the *ancien régime*, in case of public scrutiny, however, cracks started to show quickly. Whenever conflicts around the Bürgerspital erupted, its corrodies appeared an easy target for the detractors of the hospital's policies.

The second point concerns the weight of medieval founding charters: in the case of Würzburg, their unclear state of transmission created confusion around its content and allowed both sides to advance interpretations convenient to them. Nevertheless, the founding charter maintained its authority and referring to it lent credibility to arguments from either side. The main line of attack

68 Hermann, 'Die Spitalpfründe – Geistliche Wurzeln und bürgerliche Ausprägung'.

from the bishop's side argued that the directors appointed by the municipality had neglected it, which the hospital officials countered with a more generous interpretation of it. In addition, they had attempted to liken long-standing traditions, such as the sale of corrodies, to the founding mission. The maneuver ground of reform was thus still very much delineated by the medieval legal structure. Those pressing for change had to carefully detail its relation to the 400-years-old origins of the institutions.

What is noteworthy is that explicit arguments referring to public utility were missing, though they would be typical for later Enlightenment plans of welfare reform. One can read arguments in favor of redirecting welfare "more rationally" towards those in absolute need into calls for the abolition of corrodies. Abolishing the distinction between different classes of corrodians spoke to a notion of equality between welfare recipients, but the normative justification of such, at least explicitly, did not sit in more general thoughts about the value of equality and a rejection of unfounded social distinctions. The debate about corrodies in Würzburg thus shows that debates about welfare reform took place well before the age of great reforms set in in the later eighteenth and early nineteenth century.[69] Certain themes could be foreshadowed and hinted upon, while the playing field was still defined by the untouchable authority of tradition and venerable precedent. The foundations so many of which would be radically redesigned, their endowment reappropriated or simply dissolved and transformed in other judicial entities just decades later, constituted in Würzburg still the most important factor to deal with.

5 Conclusion

Even if more confined in their scope and vehemence, reforms of institutional provision were not restricted to the era of profound change between the later eighteenth and early nineteenth century. The exchange between the municipal and episcopal officials in the first half of the eighteenth century detailed here demonstrates that disagreements could flare up at moments of political tensions. Corrodies were contested and their legitimacy and functionality put into question by the bishop's officials in different lines of argument. Regardless of the overtly political pretext for these attacks they showcase that corrodies could provide fodder for arguments. Their transactional tendency which led to a preponderance of well-to-elderly as well as the financial risks associated

69 For respective overviews see Risse, *Mending Bodies, Saving Souls*, chap. 5; Frohman, *Poor Relief and Welfare*, chaps 2–3.

with this referred to normative conflicts over the distribution of public welfare and eldercare. These larger ideas of who should primarily benefit from public welfare were discussed, even if the practice of the sale of corrodies was centuries old and had tacitly been accepted by contemporaries for the longest time. These discussions avoided classic Enlightenment vocabulary, such as public utility, but did involve questions of justice. The normative source of this justice, however, remained firmly in the medieval charters of the hospitals, on which eighteenth-century contemporaries could project their ideas. They delineated the playing field for the argument. This locates the disputes at the Bürgerspital in Würzburg at the eve of modernization, a cautious harbinger of greater change to come.

CHAPTER 2

Building the City Hospital under State Control

Disputes between the Imperial and Communal Authorities in the Establishment of the St. Roch's Hospital in Pest

Ingrid Kušniráková

St. Roch's Hospital was the first hospital that was founded and operated independently of the Hospitaller Order of the Brothers of Saint John of God or the Sisters of St. Elizabeth in the Kingdom of Hungary, which was part of the Habsburg Monarchy. Due to its capacity, the number of its employees and its budget, it was the largest charitable institution in the country at the time of its opening and retained this status for many decades. The road to its foundation, from the initial plans to build a new municipal poorhouse in the early 1770s to its opening in 1798, took almost three decades. This example can be used to explain many things, such as how the idea to build a hospital in the town came about, who encouraged and supported it, who opposed it and why, and above all, how difficult it was to obtain funding for both establishment and operation of the hospital.

Neither Slovakian nor Hungarian historiography has yet produced a work that deals with these issues in a more substantial way. Hungarian historians who studied the foundation of St. Roch's Hospital in the past have mainly focused on the normative documentation related to the foundation, the architectural history of the building and the organization and financial endowment of the construction. Senior doctor Ignác Purjesz researched on the 1790s in his study of the foundation of the hospital, completely ignoring the earlier development when the original project of the municipal poorhouse was expanded to include the hospital. His explanations of the foundation and construction of the hospital were based almost exclusively on the interpretation of several official and normative documents from the period between 1793 and 1798.[1]

The architectural historian Alice Horváth examined the structural development of the hospital and the building project in relation to the changes in its use. She chronologically traced the decisions of the city and state

1 Purjesz, *Beiträge zur Geschichte der Gründung*.

 | HTTPS://DOI.ORG/10.1163/9789004755062-004

administration, which gradually expanded the original poorhouse project to include a hospital but also led to the construction lasting from 1781 to 1798. A large part of her study was devoted to the chapel of St. Roch next to which the hospital was built, as well as the structure and property ownership.[2] The historian Albert Gárdonyi examined the organizational and financial arrangement for the construction of the hospital and the progress of the construction work. However, he almost completely overlooked the addition of medical facilities to the hospital and prioritization of the healing function over the care-giving aspect.[3]

The only published monograph referring to the history of the hospital mentions, the laying of the foundation stone of the municipal poorhouse in 1781 in connection with its foundation and then goes on to discuss the project of the municipal hospital published in print in 1793 by the town physician Michal Haffner and its first statutes form 1798.[4] Given the time of publication, the authors of these works did not examine the construction of the hospital in the context of the reforms of the Viennese court, the influence of the theoretical concepts of the period, or in the context of the development of hospitals in other European cities.

In contrast to Slovak or Hungarian historiography, the "birth of the clinic" and the transition "from poorhouse to hospital" has been intensively discussed in the Western historiographies for several decades. The Michel Foucault's book *The Birth of a Clinic*, published in 1963, is an important impetus for the debate of the emergence of the modern hospital and its predecessors. According to Foucault, by abolishing medical schools in the 1790s, the French National Assembly enabled almshouses to become sites of medical research and training. He said there was a distinctive national style or way of France and referred to all earlier hospitals in other countries as "old clinics" or "proto clinics". Foucault's view that the birth of a clinic was a "rupture" or an "interruption" basically divided historians writing about the history of hospitals into two parties.[5] Some agreed with his thesis, others questioned the specificity of the French development, pointing to the existence of precursors to Foucault's proto-clinics and refusing to recognize a "break" from which the birth of the modern hospital could be dated. Historians have particularly criticized

2 Horváth, A Pesti Rókus-Kórház, 321–371.
3 Gárdonyi, A Rókus-kórház, 980–997.
4 Hollán, *Adatok és szemelvények a Szent Rókus Közkórház*, 18–19.
5 Mitchell, Politics in the Service of Knowledge, 192–193. Jones, Sonenscher, The Social Functions of the Hospital, 172–214.

Foucault's view of the emergence of the first clinics and the beginnings of clinical education for physicians in Europe.[6]

In the German-speaking world, a distinction between the terms poorhouses and hospital emerged in the second half of the eighteenth century, although the two were used synonymously for a long time, even in the nineteenth century. It was not until the twentieth century that the word hospital ("Krankenhaus") was generally used to describe a facility for the diagnosis and treatment of illnesses, or for obstetrics. Based on this brief interpretation of the origin and use of the term hospital, Foucault's thesis of the "birth of the clinic" at the end of the eighteenth century has been called into question. There is a consensus in historiography that a new institution in the provision of healthcare to the population had already emerged in the second half of the eighteenth century. The almshouses, which had previously been primarily care-giving facilities, gradually transformed into healthcare institutions. Even the proto-clinics had predecessors in which the basic principles of modern hospitals can be found. Facilities that were exclusively for sick people, such as leprosaria, plague infirmaries and hospitals for syphilitics, already existed in the Middle Ages.[7]

However, while the leprosaria and plague infirmaries were more concerned with isolating and providing care for the sick than treating them, the situation with syphilis was different. Syphilis was the first known chronic disease whose symptoms disappeared after a simple 6–8-week treatment.[8] Plague infirmaries and other similar facilities could also serve as a basis for the construction of general hospitals (as in Hamburg), but it was the facilities for the treatment of syphilis that played a special role in the history of hospitals. The architectural and spatial principles were decisive for the later development of facilities that focused on the treatment of the sick. Based on these principles, the hospitals were primarily intended to accommodate poor patients for whom, there was a chance of recovery or at least a significant improvement in their state of health under the given circumstances and known therapeutic options. Other features that distinguished hospitals from almshouses included the spatial division of the facilities into wards according to the type of illness, the categorization of patients based on the fee paid, the construction of appropriate facilities, the medicalization of treatment, more health personnel, and their inspections.[9]

6 Rosen, Hospitals, Medical Care and Social Policy, 142. Ackerknecht, *Medicine at the Paris Hospital,* 7–12. Risse, Before the Clinic Was "Born", 75–96. Greenbaum, Thomas Jefferson, the Paris Hospitals, and the University of Virginia, 609.

7 Greenbaum, "Measure of Civilization", 51. Jütte, Vom Hospital zum Krankenhaus, 31–38.

8 Sherwood, Treating Syphilis, 318.

9 Gelfand, A Clinical Ideal, 407–408. Jütte, Vom Hospital zum Krankenhaus, 40–49.

The idea of the direct or indirect development from poorhouse to hospital, from lifelong care to short-term treatment, is also questioned or rejected by historians who do not identify with Foucault's thesis on the birth of the clinic. Historians who have studied municipal hospitals in England and Germany between Enlightenment and Great War have worked on the premise that the link between a traditional poorhouse and a modern hospital is at best very indirect. Considering the scope and level of health care in both types of institutions and the people they admitted, they concluded that the most modern hospitals were founded independently of almshouses. A continuous transition from poorhouse to hospital was rare, and even if in some cases there was institutional or spatial continuity between the two institutions, this was not without conflict.[10]

The changes that took place in municipal hospitals in the late nineteenth century under the influence of modern medical discoveries such as antisepsis and asepsis represented a qualitative intervention in the development of hospitals. They changed from an instrument of general state-ordered protection against illness to a place where people could receive individual and predictable medical help in the event of illness.[11] One can speak of the emergence of modern hospitals in the last decades of the nineteenth century, when they finally freed themselves from their charitable mission and became medical-curative institutions that served all the inhabitants of a city. In the major cities, the transformation from traditional poorhouses to modern hospitals, at the turn of the twentieth century, was visible in the extensive constructions of the new hospital buildings.[12] These spatial and architectural changes were also the reason why some historians assumed that there was no continuity between poorhouses and hospitals, and a closer examination of this view could be more fruitful for further research than the opposite premise.[13]

Looking at the approaches, historians have taken to the emergence of hospitals, there are two basic perspectives. Historians who examine poorhouses and hospitals in terms of institutional or spatial continuity point to a gradual transformation of some poorhouses into hospitals, to an expansion of their nursing tasks to include the targeted treatment of the sick. And those historians who focus on examining the aims of both the institutions and their "clients" argue that the two basic attributes of both types of institution – lifelong

10 Reinarz, The transformation of medical education, 549–566. Labisch, Spree, Die Kommunalisierung des Krankenhauswesens, 9, 11–12.

11 Hickey, To Improve the Training of Nurses, 177–178.

12 Badertscher, A New Wishard Is On the Way, 348–351.

13 Labisch, Stadt und Krankenhaus, 253–296.

care vs. short-term treatment and a permanent socially dependent person vs. a curable patient are at the odds with the terminology of transition or gradual development. To solve this problem, it has been proposed to abandon the concept of a birth or transition and focus on hospital research over a time horizon of about one hundred years. Instead, one could take the middle of the eighteenth century as the starting point for this investigation, because at this time a discussion about the necessity of hospitals had begun, at least in medical circles. The end point could be seen as the middle of the following century, when the questions of 'how' and 'why' hospitals were founded were abandoned and attention turned to how they should be managed and financed.[14]

Despite their differences of opinion, historians from both camps agree that 'modern' hospitals were established in the last decades of the eighteenth century. Although they were already health institutions, they were set up and operated as part of the local poor relief, and many of them did not give up their traditional care-giving role until much later. This chapter focuses mainly on the first part of this period, from the 1770s to the 1790s. It aims to show the micro-history of this "transition" and to emphasize the discontinuity and uniqueness of the situation in Pest, where the urban elites attempted to establish a modern hospital. Similar to the case of the Würzburg hospital, the initiative came from the Enlightened ruler and aimed to control the local community and its economic resources. However, the community representatives resisted for a long time. It was only pressure and supervision from the Viennese court that made the construction of the hospital possible.

1 Municipal and General Hospitals

The first step towards a hospital of new type was the emergence of the so-called clinics or infirmaries which were founded in the second half of the eighteenth century by progressive professors from medical faculties in local poorhouses to create space for the systematic practical training of medics. The monarchs of the Enlightenment period supported their efforts, influenced by the professional discourse, as they shared the opinion that enough qualified doctors trained in theory and practice was the most important prerequisite for successful health reform and an improvement in the health of the masses. Many of these clinics later became part of the general hospitals that were established from the 1780s as part of the reforms in poor relief and welfare.

14 Rosenberg, And Heal the Sick, 428–447. Gillispie, *Science and Polity*, 198 nn. Dross, Krankenhaus und lokale Politik, 57.

General hospitals, created by merger and restructuring of several older charitable institutions and foundations, usually provided specialized care for the poor and health care under one roof. By creating large organizations under state supervision, monarchs sought to promote their idea of specialized and efficiently run care for the poor. The establishment of large capacity hospitals quickly proved to be counterproductive, particularly from the point of view of meeting established medical objectives. In many ways, however, these general hospitals became the model for smaller municipal hospitals. These were set up by the municipal authorities of the developing industrial and commercial cities from the end of the eighteenth century.[15]

Like the university clinics in Kraków or the general hospitals founded in Prague, Brno and Vilnius, the first municipal hospitals were usually established by converting or remodeling older municipal almshouses and facilities with institutional provision for corrodians, such as the Bürgerspital in Würzburg. However, the newly founded municipal hospitals were not intended to replace the poorhouses, but to expand the range of charitable institutions operating in the city. Although these hospitals were healthcare institutions intended for the short-term accommodation of patients with curable diseases, the motivation for their development was not purely medical. At that time, medicine was not yet able to heal the sick individually on a larger scale, so that the municipal hospital could offer most of its patients no more than comfort, basic care and a clean bed.[16]

Moreover, due to the increasing mass poverty in the first half of the nineteenth century, the charitable institutions were so overwhelmed that they could not even provide sufficient care for those people who met their usual admission criteria permanent incapacity to work and residence status in the respectively city.[17] The range of municipal charitable institutions was therefore extended to include hospitals, which were intended to care for the working poor suffering from an acute "curable" illness, regardless of their place of residence, and to restore their ability to work as soon as possible through the treatment available. Despite their medical and curative nature, municipal hospitals became part of the system of poor relief and the process of separating a poorhouse from a hospital, both physically and institutionally, continued in many cases until the end of the nineteenth century.[18]

15 Labisch, Spree, Die Kommunalisierung des Krankenhauswesens, 12–13.
16 Spree, Krankenhausentwicklung und Sozialpolitik, 85.
17 Labisch, Spree, Die Kommunalisierung des Krankenhauswesens, 16–17.
18 Spree, Sozialer Wandel im Krankenhaus, 245.

The healthcare reforms carried out by the Viennese court in the time of Maria Theresa focused primarily on the establishment of a state health administration and a functioning system of measures to combat epidemics – this was particularly evident in the example of the obstacles associated with the establishment of modern hospitals in the Kingdom of Hungary, Slavonia and Croatia, especially in the capital Zagreb. The training of individual categories of health personnel was regulated and their tasks redefined. The control of state authorities and town doctors over pharmacies was introduced. In 1770 the General Health Act (*Normativum generale in re sanitatis*) was issued. The court did not include the hospitals of the Brothers Hospitallers and the Sisters of St. Elisabeth, which at the time were active in some Hungarian towns, in their health reforms, as they were regarded as ecclesiastical and charitable institutions and not as healthcare facilities.[19]

The General Health Act, the basic legal framework for the organization and administration of health care in the Kingdom of Hungary, remained in force until the mid of the nineteenth century. During this period, hospitals, their establishment, administration, and financing did not fall within the jurisdiction and responsibility of the health authorities, as stated in the Act. Looking at the health legislation and the work of the health department of the Lieutenancy Council, the department of lieutenancy responsible for health agenda, the state occasionally regulated the activities of hospitals, usually as part of epidemiological measures to prevent the spread of cholera and other infectious diseases.[20]

The two basic impulses that contributed to the development of hospitals in the Habsburg Monarchy, Germany, Poland and other European countries in the second half of the eighteenth century – the university clinic and the general hospital – had almost no influence on the development of conditions in Hungary. In contrast to Galicia, where the hospital of the Kraków Academy had been operating since 1780, a regular university clinic for practical training of medics was not established in the Kingdom of Hungary until 1786. As it was financed from the public university fund, it was an institution with a very limited capacity, space and finances. A general hospital based on the Josephine model, as developed in Vienna in 1784, Brno in 1785 and Prague in 1790, was to comprise several specialized charitable and health institutions under the supervision of the state. This model was not introduced in Hungarian

19 Linzbauer, *Codex sanitario-medicinalis*, Tomus II, 535–571; Bokesová-Uherová. *Zdravotníctvo na Slovensku*, 143–146.

20 The selection of health legislation and regulations from years 1781–1845 was published by Linzbauer as a five-volumes work *Codex sanitario-medicinalis Hungariae III/1–III/5*.

capital Buda, and there were no real plans to set one up. The hospitals that had been established in Hungarian towns since the late eighteenth century as part of communal charity were founded by charitable foundations and contributions from the population and financed exclusively by them, but the ruler and the Council of Lieutenancy supervised their administration and the use of funds on the basis of their patronage rights.

According to the directive decree of 16 April 1781, the poorhouses, which were intended for all categories of socially dependent people, were to replace the specialized welfare and healthcare institutions. The social care was only to be provided for abandoned and orphaned children or sick and bedridden poor people. As in Würzburg, Prague, Brno, Kraków and other cities in continental Europe, orphans and abandoned children were to be cared for in orphanages and foundling homes, pregnant single mothers in maternity wards. Sick people who did not have the means to pay for a doctor or medication and could not be adequately cared for at home, were treated in a hospital. Almshouses (Armenhäuser, Siechenhäuser) were intended for people who were unable to work, disabled or terminally ill. At the same time, special institutions were to be built for the mentally ill.[21]

The current inmates of the existing charitable institutions were to be examined to determine whether they were socially dependent and in need of care. Those who did not belong to any of the above categories were to be released and receive a financial compensation. Authorized patrons could continue to decide on admission to their foundations but had to respect the character of the individual institutions, i.e. only admitting bedridden and disabled people to almshouses, sick people to hospitals and only abandoned or orphaned children to orphanages. Churches located next to charitable institutions were to be abolished. The votive offerings of the abolished churches were handed over to the Religious Fund; other assets were to be sold or leased, the proceeds of which were to be used to cover the needs of charitable institutions. In the late seventeenth and early eighteenth centuries, the bishops of Würzburg actually used a similar procedure in the civic hospital there.[22]

In the following years of his reign, Joseph II issued further new decrees that restricted the existing powers of the administrators of charitable institutions and foundations and increased the extent of state supervision over their administration. In order to meet the court's requirements, the administrators

21 Direktiv-regeln zur künftigen Einrichtung der hiesigen Spitäler und allgemeinen Versorgungshäuser (Guiding regulations on the establishment of local infirmaries and general care-providing houses).

22 Bayer, *Beschreibung der öffentlichen Armen-Versorgungsanstalten*, 31–32.

of foundations had to draw up a detailed inventory of their assets, hand over their bonds and promissory bills to the state and adapt their activities to the monarch's reformatory intentions.[23] Joseph II insisted that, as the supreme patron of the foundations in the country, he did not have to respect the provisions of their statutes or the will of their founders and could therefore change their aims and activities according to his current intentions and ideas.

After the death of Emperor Leopold II in 1792, the court practically withdrew from the responsibility of regulating or supervising care of the poor, apart from a few larger charitable organizations. In most cases, it merely examined the annual income and expenditure accounts and approved the founding charters of newly established institutions. The court decree of October 1818 defined the foundling wards and the asylums for the mentally ill as state facilities entitled to a state contribution, and the hospitals as municipal or private facilities not entitled to a contribution from the state.[24] As there was neither a foundling war nor an asylum for the mentally ill in the Kingdom of Hungary at this time, healthcare remained an exclusive matter for the local administrative units (towns, counties) or private charitable organizations.

2 The Decision to Found a Municipal Hospital in Pest and the Search for Its Optimal Form

The first ideas for the establishment of a charitable institution, called a hospital, emerged in Pest in the early 1770s. In 1772 an anonymous "*citizen and son of the city*" submitted a proposal to the Hungarian Chamber, the central authority entrusted with the administration of the royal estates and revenues in Hungary, to establish a municipal orphanage and build a new almshouse. In his opinion, the existing poorhouse, which had been built in the mid-eighteenth century by converting of an older house, was too small and had only a small income, so that a good proportion of the socially dependent people had to beg or die in poverty. If the property belonging to the poorhouse was sold and the proceeds pooled with the money from the sale of two other municipal properties from the previous year, the city council would have a total of thirty thousand gulden at its disposal. This would be enough to build a new hospital with a poorhouse in the suburbs, behind the Hatvani Gate, next to St. Roch's Chapel, "*without glamour and luxury.*" The author of the proposal did not have a "modern" hospital in mind, but rather a lazaretto or emergency

23 Linzbauer, Tomus III, 82–86, 192, 309–316.

24 Hlaváčková, Svobodný, *Pražské špitály a nemocnice*, 69–70.

shelter where sick poor people would receive care and treatment prescribed by a physician or surgeon and the necessary medication for a limited period of hospitalization.[25]

As the City Council stated in its response to the proposal, the idea of building a poorhouse next to St. Roch's Chapel was not new and had been resonating in the town for some time. From the early 1770s, the local burghers supported the plan with their endowments or bequests in their wills, no doubt due to the increasing pressure from the Viennese court to expand poor relief. A bequest of 20,531 gulden from Anna Maria Tausch for a new poorhouse, which the city received after her death in 1777, is cited as the main reason for the city administration's decision to begin construction. The foundation stone for the building, designed by the municipal master builder Josef Jung, was laid in a solemn ceremony on May 3, 1781; the planned capacity was 80 people.[26] The intention of the city administration, also with regard to Tausch's will, was to build a new municipal poorhouse that would be a traditional charitable institution. The city began building the poorhouse at the same time as Joseph II announced a fundamental reform of poor relief and charitable organizations in the monarchy.

Questioning the inviolability and immutability of foundations' charters opened the door, among other things, to the reorganization of local charitable institutions and the establishment of the General Hospital in Vienna and then in the capitals of the other provinces in the Monarchy and in Central Europe in general. In the early 1780s, not only the attitude of the court towards the care of the poor changed, but also the situation in Pest itself. Paradoxically, the status of capital city, which Buda received in 1783, had contributed to the development of neighboring Pest, which quickly became the administrative, commercial, and cultural center of the country. This led to an increase in the population, which was confronted with poverty and social dependence. As a result, there was pressure for the development of poor relief, the establishment of new charitable institutions and the expansion of their capacities.

As the city began building of the poorhouse next to St. Roch's Chapel without sufficient funding, construction progressed very slowly. This was also the reason why the court and the city authorities were able to intervene in the project time and again to change the character and capacity of the institution. The first step in this direction was taken by the city administration, which proposed in 1782 to establish a municipal elementary school in the building of the

25 Budapest Föváros Levéltára (Budapest city archives, hereinafter the BFL), IV. 1202 Pest város tanácsának iratai (Pest city council documents), Int. a. a. 4852.

26 Gárdonyi, A Rókus-kórház, 987.

existing poorhouse and to leave the dissolved Poor Clares convent to the city for the needs of the poorhouse. As the City Council explained in its justification, the convent building was not located in the city center, but in a suburb of the town, and unlike the poorhouse, it had a chapel where the sick and poor could seek spiritual comfort. Although it was small, the city had the necessary building materials to expand.[27]

Negotiations with the court officials regarding the acquisition of the monastery building dragged on for over a year. In May 1783, Joseph II decided that the abolished monastery could be given to the city on the condition that it would be used as a poorhouse where the old and the bedridden people would receive lifelong care at the city's expense.[28] Ultimately, the protracted negotiations over the transfer of the former Poor Clares convent to the municipal poorhouse were pointless, as a year later Joseph II decided that the building should be used for a different purpose. The city administration of Pest was informed by the Lieutenancy Council of the change in the Emperor's decision regarding the future use of the former monastery in a decree dated of October 26, 1784.[29]

According to of July 9, 1783, by the municipal authority for state power, two categories of people were admitted to the poorhouse at this period. The first were impoverished inhabitants of the city who were provided with lifelong care. The second, supposedly more numerous groups consisted of poor sick persons, including foreigners and beggars, who only stayed as long as was necessary for their treatment. In addition to the care of a physician or surgeon, they received the necessary medication, food and clothing. The poorhouse had an annual income of only 763 gulden, most of which came from renting out its assets. The remaining operating costs, 2,460 gulden, were paid from the city treasury. A considerable proportion of this, namely 959 gulden was accounted for by the cost of medicines. The city administration also stated in the report that a new poorhouse had been under construction for two years, in which the inmates of the existing poorhouse and other poor people were to be accommodated, and that a hospital was to be set up on the same site.[30]

The next report sent by city administration to the Council of Lieutenancy on January 26, 1785, was a response to its order of October 1784, stating that the poorhouse was increasingly being transformed into a hospital. In addition to

27 BFL, IV. 1202 Pest város tanácsának iratai (Pest city council documents). Int. a. a. 6392.

28 Ibid.

29 Magyar Nemzeti Levéltár Országos Levéltár (National archives of Hungary, National archive, hereinafter the MNL OL), C 80 Departamentum fundationum saecularium politicum (Department of secular endowments, hereinafter the C 80 politicum), 1784, f. 1.

30 BFL, IV. 1202 Pest város tanácsának iratai. (Pest city council documents). Int. a. a. 6312.

the doctor and surgeon, who were paid from the municipal treasury, the sick was also cared for by two orderlies employed and paid by the poorhouse. This report also contains the first reference of the proposal by the military surgeon Ferdinand Stipsics, who later became professor and dean of the medical faculty, to build a hospital with a capacity of 144 patients and 26 pregnant women next to St. Roch's Chapel. His proposal fundamentally changed the character of the entire project and from that point on, the new building was always considered first and foremost as a hospital. However, this change led to an increase in construction cost from the original 18,962 gulden to 31,376 gulden. As the city administration did not have the money to cover the additional costs or to pay for the running of the hospital, it took the opportunity to ask the Council of Lieutenancy and the monarch for help.[31]

The Viennese court had probably forgotten that the authorized use of the convent of the Poor Clares' had changed in 1784, and the monarch's mandate of 7 June 1786 ordered the construction of a medical and surgical clinic for medics and a municipal poorhouse in the former monastery. The costs for construction and operation of the clinic were to be covered from the fund of the poorhouse.[32] In this way, the practical training of medics in the Kingdom of Hungary was to be ensured in the same way as in the hereditary lands, where clinics were set up within the general hospitals by order of the monarch and were financed from their revenues.

After the discovery that the Poor Clares monastery had already been used for another purpose, the hospital was opened on a new mandate issued on August 16, 1786, which provided for the establishment of a clinic for medics in a university building, the construction and operating costs of which were to be covered by the university fund. Even if the poorhouse under construction at St. Roch's Chapel were completed, it would not be suitable for the practical training of doctors due to its great distance from the university and the low annual income. Another argument put forward by the court officials for the establishment two independent institutes was to increase the number of hospital beds for the city's poor inhabitants.[33]

Influenced by the discussions about the form of the university hospital in Pest, the issue of the completing the building under construction next to St. Roch's Chapel was once again a hot topic. On August 21, 1786, the city administration of Pest asked the court for permission to continue construction, and Emperor Joseph II, who was in Pest at the time, verbally instructed

31 Gárdonyi, A Rókus-kórház, 988.
32 Linzbauer, *Codex sanitario-medicinalis.* III/1, 253–254.
33 Linzbauer, *Codex sanitario-medicinalis.* III/1, 289–291.

the mayor to complete the "*half-finished building*" as a hospital. As a result, on August 29, 1786, the Lieutenancy Council instructed the city administration to submit the design and budget for the completion of the building as well as the method of adapting it to the needs of a hospital. The city prepared the required documents and submitted them to the Council of Lieutenancy on January 20, 1787.[34]

Before the Lieutenancy Council and its financial bureau could examine them, the monarch changed his decision again and ordered that the poorhouses in Pest and Buda be merged with the workhouse in Pest to form a single facility. The construction of the new poorhouse at St. Roch's Chapel was to be completely abandoned. As it was not expected that a new institution, similar to the general hospital in Vienna, would soon be established, the financial bureau of the Lieutenancy Council was instructed, on the basis a decree of November 18, 1788, to make a proposal for improving the care of poor patients in the Pest poorhouse.[35] On November 28, 1788, the Council of Lieutenancy proposed that all inmates of the institution who did not require medical care and all those who were not from the city should be discharged immediately.[36] This would finally transform the municipal poorhouse into a hospital and fulfil the emperor's intentions.

The planned restructuring of the Pest poorhouse or its merger with other institutions did not materialize. Joseph II died on February 20, 1790, and immediately after his death most of the foundation administrators in the Kingdom of Hungary demanded that the situation before his accession to the throne be restored. The city administration of Pest was no exception. As early as March 1790, it demanded that the construction of the poorhouse be allowed to continue, as it had been presented to the Council of Lieutenancy in 1787. They based their request on the fact that the building under construction was prone to damage and that the capacity of the existing poorhouse was insufficient for the constantly growing number of sick poor.

As the project to merge the Buda and Pest poorhouses with the workhouse was no longer relevant at that time, the Council of Lieutenancy instructed the financial bureau to evaluate the 1787 project and formulate an opinion. The officials of financial bureau took until March of the following year to respond. They stated that they had lost the 1787 project and that the Council would have to resubmit it, if they wished to consider it.[37] However, they provisionally took

---

34 MNL OL, Magyar kancelláriai levéltár, A 39 Acta generalia (hereinafter A 39), 7648/1794.
35 Ibid.
36 Gárdonyi, A Rókus-kórház, 989.
37 MNL OL, A 39, 7648/1794.

the view that it would be better to adapt the building next to the chapel of St. Roch for the needs of a hospital and continue with its construction. The conversion of the existing poorhouse, including the neighboring house of the Pintér Foundation, would be costly and the final premises would still not have sufficient capacity. The construction was to be financed from the sale of the old almshouse, the Pintér Foundation house and the capital from the exchange endowment fund originally earmarked for the construction of a poorhouse. The financial bureau also suggested that the city should submit a list of endowments that the founders wished could be used to build and equip the new facility.[38]

On February 11, 1792, the city sent a draft and a budget for the project, which was drawn up according to Stipsics' proposal. Based on the number of inhabitants and the number of hospital beds in Vienna, Stipsics believed Pest needed a hospital with at least 175 beds, intended for both paying and non-paying patients. One hundred beds were to be allocated to non-payers. A single-story building divided into three sections was proposed. Two sections were to serve as wards for men and women and the third was to be a poorhouse.[39] Along with the requested documents, the City Council sent the Lieutenancy Council responses to its questions regarding to the poorhouse under construction. These stated that the building, the construction of which had begun in 1781, was not intended as a hospital, but solely a poorhouse. The decision to combine the hospital with the poorhouse was made during construction to allow for more efficient administration. Both institutions were to have separate premises and their own sources of funding in the new building.[40]

The proposal submitted by the Pest City Council, was gradually examined by the financial and building bureaus, and based on their recommendations, the Council of Lieutenancy prepared a statement for the Hungarian Court Chancellery in Vienna. It stated that no decree had ever been issued for the Pest poorhouse, that it was located in the least suitable place in the city center, that it was small and poorly equipped and that the building could not be adapted to the needs of a proper hospital. Referring to these facts, as well as to Joseph II's of 1786, the Lieutenancy Council supported the city's request to proceed with the construction of the building next to St. Roch's Chapel, which was to serve as both a poorhouse and a hospital. The construction and its financing were to be fully supervised and controlled by the Lieutenancy Council and the organization of the hospital was to be discussed with the provincial

38 MNL OL, A 39, 7648/1794.

39 Gárdonyi, A Rókus-kórház, 991.

40 MNL OL, A 39, 7648/1794.

chief physician. On June 20, 1794, the Hungarian Court Chancellery approved the recommendation of the Lieutenancy Council and recommended that the monarch grant the request of the City Council.[41] Emperor Francis II accepted the recommendations of the offices on July 14, 1794. In the following months, he issued two further decrees that supplemented the first mandate and were more detailed.[42]

With his mandates, Francis II merely decided on the completion of the building next to St. Roch's Chapel and ordered which endowment funds administered by the city could be used for this purpose for the time being. His decrees in no way regulated the organizational structure of the new institution, its capacity or the necessary staff. The issue of financing the construction and operation of the facility also remained unresolved. The answers to these questions were left to a committee set up by the City Council in October 1794. The chairman of the committee was the Protomedicus (provincial chief physician), Gabriel de Veza, the other members were the senators, representatives of the elected community, and the town physician Michal Haffner.[43] Dr. Haffner's proposal, which was published in print, became the basis for discussions about the form of the new institution.

3 The Project for the Municipal Hospital in Pest

The City Council commissioned Michal Haffner, the municipal physician, to draw up a proposal comprising 359 articles, which he published in book form in German and Hungarian in 1793. A municipal hospital was a costly project that was previously unknown in Hungary. It was therefore necessary to convince both the City Council and the inhabitants of the city of the necessity and advantages of a hospital so that they would be willing to provide the financial support required for its establishment and operation. In the introduction to his proposal, Haffner attempted to support his arguments for the construction of a new hospital by describing the existing poorhouse. He characterized it as unhealthy, in a state that was ideal for the spread of so-called hospital fever, which resulted in a high mortality rate or at least a long treatment period even for minor illnesses. This increased the cost of the treating individual patients.[44]

41 Ibid.

42 MNL OL, C 80 Departamentum fundationum saecularium oeconomicum (hereinafter the C 80 oeconomicum), 1795, fontes (hereinafter f.) 1.

43 Ibid.

44 Haffner, *Versuch eines Vorschlages*, 2–4.

Haffner found the external appearance of the building repulsive and its location in the city seemed very dangerous to him, especially if an epidemic were to occur. The poorhouse had a capacity of 72 beds for all kinds of diseases, which in his opinion was too few given the ever-increasing number of workers in the city. The rooms were small, insufficient air circulation and daylight. When describing the interior, he said, among other things:

> It is cruel and sad to see the poor person forced to live on half-rotten straw, on a dirty floor in a narrow room. Often, especially in winter, so much human misery accumulates here that you have to step over one (person) to get to the next. How can a poor person heal when he lacks everything he needs?

The lack of natural light also made the work of doctors and surgeons more difficult. Complicated operations could not be carried out in the poorhouse due to the lack of healthy air, reasonably wholesome food, cleanliness and the necessary care, as they were dangerous and often fatal for the patients.[45]

After criticizing the situation in the existing poorhouse, Haffner presented his vision of a "well-equipped hospital that is needed and necessary." Like the medical principles promoted in the general hospitals of Prague, Brno, Kraków and Vilnius, the hospital building in Pest was to be built and furnished in such a way that it was easy to keep clean; the premises were to be easy to ventilate and heat. The intended operation of the hospital required an office for the doctor, an operating theatre with sufficient daylight, storage premises and service facilities for washing linen and bandages and cleaning medical equipment.[46]

As far as the patients were concerned, the basic principle was the separation of rooms for men and women. In addition to two larger wards – internal and surgical – two smaller independent wards were to be set up, one for healthy pregnant women and newborns, the second for deformed and mentally ill patients and for patients with rabies and venereal diseases – a fundamental feature that led to the emergence of modern-type hospitals not only in Pest, Prague, Zagreb and Vilnius, but in many other European care institutions. Two to three separate rooms should be available for convalescing patients so that they do not become infected with the acutely ill and catch hospital fever. Another three rooms were to be reserved for the city's sick prisoners and their guards. Not only the internal layout and equipment of the building was important, but also its location, an open area with healthy air, far away from swamps or muddy ground.[47] According to Haffner's calculations, Pest needed 220 beds

45 Ibid.
46 Ibid., 9–11.
47 Ibid.

for poor, non-paying patients – 100 for internal diseases (50 men, 50 women), 80 for surgery (40 men, 40 women), 24 for pregnant women and newborns and 16 for the mentally ill. But Haffner left the decision on the hospital's capacity to the City Council and the charity of the burghers.[48]

Haffner devoted a large part of his work to the conditions of admission and the way in which patients were to be accommodated. As the hospital was to meet criteria of humanity and tolerance, no social status or religious conviction was to be an obstacle to the admission of sick people in need. However, the declared religious tolerance only applied to Christian denominations. The city administration was to decide whether it would accept Jewish patients. In Haffner's opinion, the hospital was only intended for those who could be cured or for sick people whose state of health would improve because of the treatment so that they could return to their usual way of life. People who could not be cured by the medical science of the time were to be admitted to the poorhouse, so that they did not "take up" the space reserved for patients who could be cured or whose death could be prevented by early treatment.[49]

Similar to the statute of the General Hospital in Vienna, patients could only be admitted to the hospital on the recommendation of a doctor. Those who applied for free treatment had to present a certificate of poverty issued by the father of poor in their parish and the owner of the house in which they lived. Since "love your neighbor" was one of God's laws, Haffner took the view that admission to the hospital could not be refused even to a sick "destitute" foreigner who could not obtain such a certificate. In order to prevent the hospital from becoming overcrowded with "*wandering poor*" foreigners at the expense of "*domestic contributors*", the city was to defend itself against "*idle, lazy vagabonds*" by setting up a workhouse.[50]

Although the religious dimension was no longer as important for the hospital as it was for other charitable institutions of the time, Haffner still considered it very important. With regard to the religious needs of the patients, a Catholic chaplain was to be present in the hospital at all times and a spacious Catholic chapel, which was also suitable for public services, was to become an integral part of the hospital. In view of the expected denominational composition of the patients, clergymen of other Christian denominations were also to work in the hospital, but they were not to be paid from the hospital's income, but from the charity of their followers.[51]

48 Ibid., 21.
49 Ibid., 38–39.
50 Ibid., 40–42.
51 Ibid., 91.

Haffner prepared a complex and detailed proposal for the establishment and operation of the municipal hospital, which included the internal arrangement of the building, its interior design, admission criteria, requirements for staff and their duties and remuneration, the provision of meals, their portion size and quality, the organization of collections for the hospital and arguments in its favor. The proposal makes it clear that he was familiar with the General Hospital in Vienna, either from his own experience or from the press, the works of the Austrian cameralists Johann Heinrich Justi and Joseph Sonnenfels and the most important representative of the health police, Johann Peter Frank.[52]

In his work, Frank referred to the charitable institutions of the time as murder pits and the same expression was used by Haffner in his description of the situation in the Pest poorhouse.[53] The influence of the works written by representatives of both theoretical concepts can be traced back to the efforts to support single mothers, anonymous birth, the mother's right not to reveal the father's name and the arguments for the establishment of a foundling home and the protection of illegitimate children.[54] Haffner and his project were decisive in the founding of the hospital in Pest, the first municipal hospital in the Kingdom of Hungary, and it is likely that they also influenced the shape of hospitals in other Hungarian cities.

4 The Construction of the Hospital, Its Statute and the Conditions for the Admission of Patients

On 20 October 1794, a committee convened for the first time to oversee the completion and organization of the new charitable institution founded by the city administration in Pest. The minutes of the meeting show that the representatives of the city did not support the idea of a municipal hospital and instead tried to prevent its establishment. Although they presented Haffner's book to the court officials as a draft for the future form of the institution, two members were critical of it. One of them, Mayor Joannes Boráros, rejected the plan to complete the building next to the St. Roch's Chapel, contrary to the monarch's orders, and suggested adapting the existing poorhouse.

The other, Senator Valentin Hülff, agreed that the building should be completed, but in the form of a traditional poorhouse. He criticized Haffner's project on the grounds that it was expensive, and that the city did not have sufficient

52 Frank, *Ankündigung des klinischen Instituts*, 4.

53 Haffner, *Versuch eines Vorschlages*, 18.

54 Ibid., 45.

funds to implement it. The poorhouse, which was previously intended for the city's residents, would be two-thirds occupied by foreigners in its new form. In his opinion, Haffner was demanding a "charity" from his co-citizens that was beyond their means and that would attract even more socially disadvantaged people to the city. Hülff believed that a general hospital in the form proposed by the municipal physician, was necessary in the center of Hungary, but that the whole country should contribute to its construction and operation, not just the city of Pest.[55]

The court authorities supported Haffner's project, according to which the municipal hospital was to be built next to St. Roch's Chapel. It firmly rejected the objections raised by Boráros and ordered that the question of rebuilding the existing poorhouse should not be discussed further, as there was a general agreement that a new building was needed. He also considered Hülff's proposal to build the new hospital as a traditional charitable institution to be unacceptable and rejected it. However, his thoughts on limiting the construction costs were passed to Haffner, so that he could comment on them. In the meantime, Haffner had changed the design of the building in his project, which better suited the hospital's needs, and prepared a new calculation of the construction costs, which was slightly lower than the one originally approved. He also drew up a proposal for the capacity, staffing requirements and a calculation of the facility's annual income and expenditure.[56]

The monarch approved the proposal in the form submitted by Haffner on July 9, 1795, and the Court's Building Bureau only ordered a minor change to the construction plans. The order was published in the Kingdom of Hungary on July 28, 1795, as an edict of the Lieutenancy Council. Following the example of the Vienna General Hospital, where there was a two-tier hospital administration, the hospital was to be managed by a director – the head physician, who oversaw the professional aspects of healthcare – and an administrator – the house inspector, who was responsible for economic and financial matters. The head physician supervised the surgeon, his two assistants, the pharmacist, the midwife and eight orderlies – four men and four women. The hospital also employed a chaplain, a clerk, two servants and a porter. They would all be housed at the institution in addition to their salaries. Meals, laundry and cleaning were to be provided by selected suppliers. As for the hospital's capacity, it was to have 88 free hospital beds – 80 for the sick, 6 for newborns and 2 for the mentally ill. A further 16 beds were earmarked for the poor of the Pintér Foundation, 48 beds for the poorhouse and 58 for fee–paying patients, 12 of which

55 MNL OL, C 80. oeconom, 1795, f. 1.

56 Ibid.

were for new mothers and 6 for mentally ill. The daily fee was set at 12 kreutzer (*grajczár*), of which 2 kreutzer represented the hospital's profit. The use of the remaining 27 beds of the total capacity of 237 beds was at the discretion of the hospital management or they could be used for patients who wished to pay for premium accommodation.[57]

The annual operating costs of the institute amounted to a total of 9,407 gulden, but the expected annual income was only 7,468 gulden, out of which 3,000 gulden were to come from the city treasury. This left a deficit of 1,938 gulden, which was to be covered by collections from the town's inhabitants or by tapping into other sources of funding. The cost of the building and furnishing of the hospital was estimated at 49,213 gulden, of which the city only had 46,134 gulden at its disposal. Both Haffner and the court officials believed that this deficit could be bridged through the procurement of cheaper building materials or through a discount on transportation or construction work by the burghers. The construction was to be carried out under the supervision of a royal commissioner and in close cooperation with the municipal physician Haffner.[58]

The secretary of the Lieutenancy Council, Anton Zirty, was appointed the royal commissioner for the construction of the hospital and performed his role very energetically and responsibly. He convened a joint meeting of the City Council on August 10, 1795, and the elected Council on August 10, 1795, which he attended in person, to announce the publication of the monarch's mandate regarding the form of the new facility. On this occasion he gave a speech in which he declared, among other things:

> Hitherto, you have had an institution which was a poorhouse in name only. There was little room for the needy and they could only be cared for very inadequately. Now a well-equipped and adequate poorhouse with a capacity of 237 beds for the bedridden, new mothers and mentally ill is being built next to the St. Roch's Chapel, and all illnesses will receive the necessary treatment there.[59]

At this meeting, Zirty initiated the establishment of a committee to organize the construction and required finances. The members of the committee, with him as chairman, were the municipal physician Haffner, three representatives of the city administration and four representatives of the elected municipality council. Zirty set up the committee with the aim of eliminating the influence

57 Ibid.
58 Ibid.
59 Purjesz, *Beiträge zur Geschichte der Gründung*, 20.

of the burghers who, in his opinion, had constantly delayed and postponed the construction of the new building up to that point. Zirty charged that the City Council had never been in favor of the new facility and had thwarted the efforts of those who had done all they could to promote its construction. He feared that the council would deliberately use the lack of money to start construction as another excuse to postpone or scrap the project altogether.[60]

Therefore, the Council of Lieutenancy had to order the city administration to provide the necessary funds under threat of sanctions. The committee was to become the supreme authority that would make the final decision on all matters relating to the construction and furnishings of the new building, including the capital and interest from the endowments that was to be used to finance the hospital. To ensure that the City Council could not further complicate its activities, contravene its decisions or limit its power, Zirty proposed that the city administration be stripped of all decision-making powers. It should not be allowed to make any decisions, and all related issues should be discussed in committee. The city administration was only allowed to give an opinion on its proposals and submit them to the Council of Lieutenancy for a decision. The Lieutenancy Council approved Zirty's proposals for the management of the construction of the new facility without objection.[61]

The committee, chaired by Zirty, met for the first time on August 12, 1795. The minutes of the meeting show that it dealt with all the matters relating to the construction and internal organization of the hospital – financing, provision of building materials and management of the construction work, but the main part of the agenda was devoted to the charitable foundations that were to support the hospital. Despite prioritizing the will of the donors, the court officials gradually decided to use all known charitable endowment foundations, administered by the city to fund the construction and operation of the new facility.[62]

Although both the committee and the city administration were supposed to pursue the same goal, cooperation between them was complicated and problematic. Regardless of the authority or jurisdiction of the City Council, Zirty was uncompromising in promoting his proposals with the objective of obtaining the missing funds for the construction and the permanent financial provision of the new non-profit facility in the city. The City Council was against a gradual concentration of all available funds to finance local poor relief, as the hospital and the poorhouse could only care for a small proportion of the

60 MNL OL, C 80, oeconom, 1795, f. 1.
61 MNL OL, C 80, oeconom, 1795, f. 1.
62 MNL OL, C 80, oeconom, 1795, f. 1; 1796, f. 27; 1797, f. 13; 1798, f. 8.

socially dependent. Most of the poor remained dependent on extra-institutional aid, which also had to be financed. Zirty accused the city administration of failing to organize and, above all to the effectiveness of the weekly collections, which were intended to raise the missing funds for the construction and operation of the hospital.[63]

The City Council replied that the inhabitants of city were already financially drained by their support of the ever-increasing number of wandering beggars, whom they could not refuse to help and therefore the contributions to the workhouse and hospital were constantly falling. The representatives of the city considered the care for this category of socially dependent people to be more urgent than the completion of the hospital and therefore proposed in March 1796, contrary to the orders of the monarch and the Council of Lieutenancy to use part of the new building (temporarily) as a workhouse. The city administration's argument was that the sick poor were being cared for in the existing municipal poorhouse, but that there were no other suitable premises for the workhouse that would eliminate begging in the city.[64]

The establishment of the workhouse on the grounds of the hospital was not intended to jeopardize its completion, but rather to support it. The inhabitants of the city no longer needed to give money to beggars and could instead financially support an organized form of institutional and extra-institutional aid.[65] With the support of the court, Zirty succeeded in rejecting the city administration's proposals and objections and pushing ahead with his own, so that the building preparations could finally be completed and the foundation stone was laid again in a solemn ceremony on August 30, 1796. The inauguration of the new hospital and poorhouse took place on May 28, 1798.[66]

After the construction work was completed, the city administration issued a printed announcement informing the public about the opening of the new facility and the conditions for admitting patients to the hospital, similar to those in Prague, Brno and Zagreb. The institution was to have a total capacity of 237 beds, 16 of which were designated for poor of the Pintér Foundation, 43 for the poorhouse, 88 for non-paying patients and 80 for paying patients and new mothers. The standard rooms cost 12 kreutzer per day, the premium rooms were 30 kreutzer (two to three people per room) or one gulden if there was

63 MNL OL, C 80, oeconom, 1796, f. 27.
64 Ibid.
65 Ibid.
66 Ibid.

only one person in the room. Both paying and non-paying patients were only admitted if they had a curable illness.[67]

The hospital was primarily set up for the inhabitants of the town. Therefore, the city administration took it for granted that priority in the admission of paying and non-paying patients was given to people from Pest or those who had acquired the right of live in the city after 10 years of residence. However, the number of people without the right to live in the city who had come to Pest, the economic and commercial center, for trade, work or other reasons was growing. In order to maintain public order and health and out of "love thy neighbor", the hospital could admit paying or non-paying "foreigners", on condition that it had free beds, and were not terminally ill. In order to keep the number of non-paying foreigners admitted to a minimum, the hospital only admitted sick and pregnant women who were completely destitute and without help and whose lives were in danger.[68]

The local poor who were unable to pay for their treatment had to present a certificate of poverty and the city administrator could then decide whether to admit the sick person or in case of doubt, order an investigation into their assets. Apprentices could only be admitted if their guild confirmed that they would pay the daily fee of 12 kreutzer for them. Servants of the Hungarian nobility who lived and worked in Pest and did not have the right of residence in the city, had to be admitted at their employer's expense, while holders of the right of residence were admitted free of charge. If the noble employer "forgot" his unwritten obligation and refused to take care of his sick servants, the hospital had to provide treatment free of charge.[69]

The basic framework for the existence and activities of St. Roch's Hospital was outlined in the statutes drafted by Dr. Haffner and approved by the municipality and the Council of Lieutenancy. Referring to the monarch's decree of July 8, 1795, the document defined the requirements for the management of the hospital, the composition of the hospital staff and the detailed duties of all employees. The municipality, as the hospital's sponsor, had to control the management of the hospital and ensure its financing (investment of capital, collection of interest and the register of estates). As the monarch and, through him, the Council of Lieutenancy held the highest patronage rights over the foundations in the country, they reserved the right to supervise the administration of the hospital. The municipality was obliged to provide the Lieutenancy

67 Purjesz, *Beiträge zur Geschichte der Gründung*, 25–29.
68 Ibid.
69 Ibid.

Council with all important information about the hospital, its operations, its finances and the management of its assets.[70]

In view of the scope of the required activities, the municipality established a special committee for the administration of the hospital, chaired by the hospital director and composed of the municipal accountant, the chief surgeon, the administrator, the tribune of the people and two burghers. The conditions and circumstances for the admission of patients, which were listed in the above-mentioned notice, published in print, were supplemented and defined more precisely by the statutes. Only the head physician could decide on the admission of a patient. He was obliged to ensure that the hospital and its wards were not overcrowded, that the number of non-paying patients remained stable and that a sufficient number of beds were available for the admission of paying patients. The sick poor who were found on the street by the city guards were first to be taken to an authorized official of the city and, if he agreed to take them in, to the head physician for examination.[71]

The hospital building was handed over to the city in April 1798 and the committee chaired by Zirty completed its work as planned. On April 17, 1798, however, the emperor appointed Zirty as royal commissioner for the ceremonial opening of the new facility. In this role, he was involved in recruitment of the new staff and organized the transfer of the old poorhouse to the new premises. The patients moved into the new hospital on May 24 and 25, 1798, and new patients were admitted from 1st July.[72] In the first year, the hospital admitted 873 people, around half of whom (447) were treated free of charge. Most of them (773) were Roman Catholics.[73]

5 Conclusion

St. Roch's Hospital is an example of a municipal hospital that was spatially and institutionally linked to the existence of the municipal poorhouse. At least from the mid of eighteenth century, the Pest poorhouse partly fulfilled the role of a hospital for the sick poor, who were generally not from the city. Although the sick patients were cared for and treated by a doctor or surgeon in the institution and received the necessary medication, it was not really a real hospital at that time. The permanent residents and the sick patients were neither physically nor organizationally separated, there were no wards or orderlies.

70 *Topographia Nesocomii et Ptochotrophii.*

71 Ibid.

72 Hollán, Adatok és szemelvények, 29.

73 Purjesz, *Beiträge zur Geschichte der Gründung*, 34.

Although the institution continued to operate in an unchanged form, under pressure from circumstances and the court authorities, it was increasingly expected to fulfil the role of a hospital from 1783 onwards. The doctor Ferdinand Stipsics was the first to propose the extension of the poorhouse with a modern hospital in the mid of 1780s, but it was the municipal physician Michal Haffner who managed to push this through a decade later.

The proposals of the two doctors took into account the professional opinions of the time on the form of a modern hospital, but unfortunately, they were not based on a realistic financial foundation. The municipal poorhouse, which had been established at the end of the seventeenth century, after the liberation of the city from the Ottomans, had very limited assets and an annual income that was not sufficient to finance the construction of a new building and the more financially demanding operation of the hospital. The attitude of the city's elites, without whose support it was impossible to realize such a project, was ambivalent. Some of the city representatives considered the establishment of a hospital to be necessary and supported it. However, those who considered such a facility to be useless and financially very demanding had greater influence. In line with the typical discourse of the time, they feared that the hospital, which would also be open to non-resident patients, would attract even more socially dependent people to the town.

Crucial to the success of Haffner's was the support of the state authorities, who approved the foundation and construction of the hospital despite a lack of funds. In the Josephinian tradition, which also applied to the hospitals in other cities of Habsburg Monarchy, care for the poor was to be financed exclusively from the charity of the burghers, but the court officials had the right to administer and control the use of funds received. As a result, the city administration became responsible for providing the necessary funds for the construction of the hospital, but the state power assumed responsibility for the administration and use of the available financial resources. It was not possible to ensure that sufficient funds were available to finance the construction without drawing on the funds of all the city's known charitable foundations, regardless of the will of their benefactors, although after the death of Joseph II, the primary objectives of the foundations once again became sacrosanct.

As part of his plan, Haffner informed the City Council that the long-term operation of the hospital would be financially demanding and that it would therefore be necessary to continuously advertise the hospital to the city's residents.[74] The municipality accepted his proposal and from the beginning published all important documents related to the establishment and operation of

74 Haffner, *Versuch eines Vorschlages*, 97.

the hospital in printed form, mostly in German and Hungarian. The first documents to be published were requests for support from the townspeople for the new hospital through donations or participation in charity collections.

Once the building was completed, a notice was published announcing the opening of the hospital and the conditions of admission for patients, which also included a copy of the hospital's statutes. The city administration continued this tradition in the following years. Through printed matter or newspapers, it informed the populace about the number of hospitalized, cured, or deceased patients, their origin and their faith; the annual statement of income and expenditure was also published. From an "unwanted burden", the hospital became for a symbol of the town as a community and of the charity of its inhabitants.

In his proposal published in 1793, Haffner stated that Pest needed a hospital with at least 220 free beds for the number of its people. The newly opened institution had 237 beds, 55 of which were for the inmates of the municipal and Pintér poorhouses and only 88 were reserved for all categories of non-paying patients, including young mothers and the mentally ill. By the late 1820s, the hospital's lack of capacity had become a much-discussed problem in the city. Leopold Windisch, who became chief physician of the hospital in 1829, issued a detailed report on the condition of the hospital and its patients, income and expenditure, shortly after his appointment, which appeared in print.

The main aim of the published report was to make the public aware that the hospital's capacity was too small due to the ever-growing population and the impoverishment of the city.[75] As space within the hospital was limited, the shortage of beds was solved in the early 1830s by the establishment of additional centers or new branches of the hospital. At the beginning of 1840, the hospital had three such branches. The oldest had 60 beds, another, founded the year before, had 140 beds and the third, opened temporarily in the winter of 1839/1840, had 106 beds. Each branch had its own doctor and was economically and administratively subordinate to St. Roch's main hospital.

The problem was that St. Roch Hospital had limited capacity and only an interim building. Thanks to two large testamentary bequests worth more than 100,000 gulden, the completion of the hospital's main building and the expansion of its capacity had been under consideration since 1831. Construction work began with delays in the spring of 1838 but was interrupted after a few months due to a devastating flood and only resumed in 1840.[76] A year later, it

75 Windisch, *Gründliche Darstellung der Einrichtung des bürgerlichen Krankenhauses*, passim.

76 Sámuel, Das Pesther Krankenhaus zu St. Rochus, 30.

was completed and new statutes for the hospital were adopted, which were no different from those of 1798. The new statutes reflected in particular the increased number of health and nursing staff and the increased fees for the treatment and stay of paying patients.[77] St. Roch's Hospital became an institution focused solely on medical care and treatment in the mid-1850s, when the original almshouse and the Pintér Foundation moved to the new municipal poorhouse building.[78]

Acknowledgement

The study is part of the project APVV-21-0371 Glamour and Fall of the Nobility. Strategies of aristocratic representation in the history of Slovakia and the VEGA project No. 2/0025/25 Transformations of the Hungarian aristocracy in the 18th and 19th centuries. Social and economic power, changes in cultural values and lifestyle.

77 Instruction für das bürgerliche Kranken-Spital, in Szabad Királyi Pest Város "Szent Rókus" polgári kórháza részére 1842. és 1868.

78 Rozsay, Das Pester städtische Versorgungshaus Elisabethineum, 12–13.

CHAPTER 3

Under the Patronage of the Viennese Court: the Medicalization of Hospitals in the Croatian Lands, 1760–1804

Ivana Horbec

Situated on the south-eastern borders of the Habsburg Monarchy, the Croatian lands served mainly as a defense zone and border area with the Ottoman Empire throughout the early modern period and beyond. Due to the constant threat of war, they were legally and administratively divided into two different regions: one military and one civilian. When the term the 'Croatian lands' under Habsburg rule is used, it explicitly refers to these two administratively separate parts within the monarchy. The first part, known as Civil Croatia-Slavonia, formed the core of the Croatian-Slavonian Kingdom.[1] This region belonged to the Hungarian part of the monarchy, known as the Lands of St. Stephen's Crown. It was administrated and financed by the Hungarian and Croatian-Slavonian provincial authorities predominantly led by the estates, mostly the nobility, and adhered to Hungarian law. Prominent towns in this region that are important for the history of hospitals were Zagreb (also known as *Agram* in German documents), Varaždin, Križevci (*Kreutz*), Koprivnica, Rijeka (*Fiume*) and Osijek (*Essegg*).

The second part of the Croatian lands under Habsburg rule belonged to the Military Frontier, or Military Border. This extensive area was built along the border with the Ottoman Empire from the sixteenth to the nineteenth century.[2] It was administrated directly by the court authorities in Vienna (in

1 The official name of the Kingdom was "the Kingdoms of Croatia, Dalmatia and Slavonia" (*Regna Croatiae, Dalmatiae et Sclavoniae*). However, Dalmatia was ruled by Venetian Republic, and its name has only been used as an expression of legal claims. In this chapter, the term "Civil Croatia" or "civilian part" for this political entity is used in order to avoid more complex title. The name refers to the three to four Croatian counties (Zagreb, Križevci, Varaždin and Severin from 1776 to 1786) and three Slavonian counties (Požega, Virovitica, Srijem). This region was organized in counties based on the Hungarian law that were led and financed by the local estates.

2 Military Frontier established on the southeast borders of the Habsburg Monarchy with the Ottoman Empire was divided into Slavonian Generalate, Varaždin Generalate, Ban's Generalate and Karlovac Generalate, and was incorporated into the Croatian-Slavonian Kingdom in the late 19th century, thus forming 'Croatian lands' under the Habsburg rule. North-eastern part of the Military Frontier was not part of this research.

 HTTPS://DOI.ORG/10.1163/9789004755062-005

particular by the War Council) and consisted of several headquarters that functioned as administrative units. The most important towns in this region included Bjelovar, Brod, Kostajnica, Gradiška, Vinkovci, and Karlovac, which also served as central hubs for military administration (see Map 3.1). Although they were smaller in comparison to the towns in the civilian part, some of these towns were of great importance in the connection with the history of hospitals in chapter 2 of this paper.

More extensive research was carried out on the quarantine stations on the Military Frontier on the borders of the monarchy in the eighteenth century, which were of crucial importance in combating epidemics, but were not hospitals in the true sense of the word. Their organized structure and

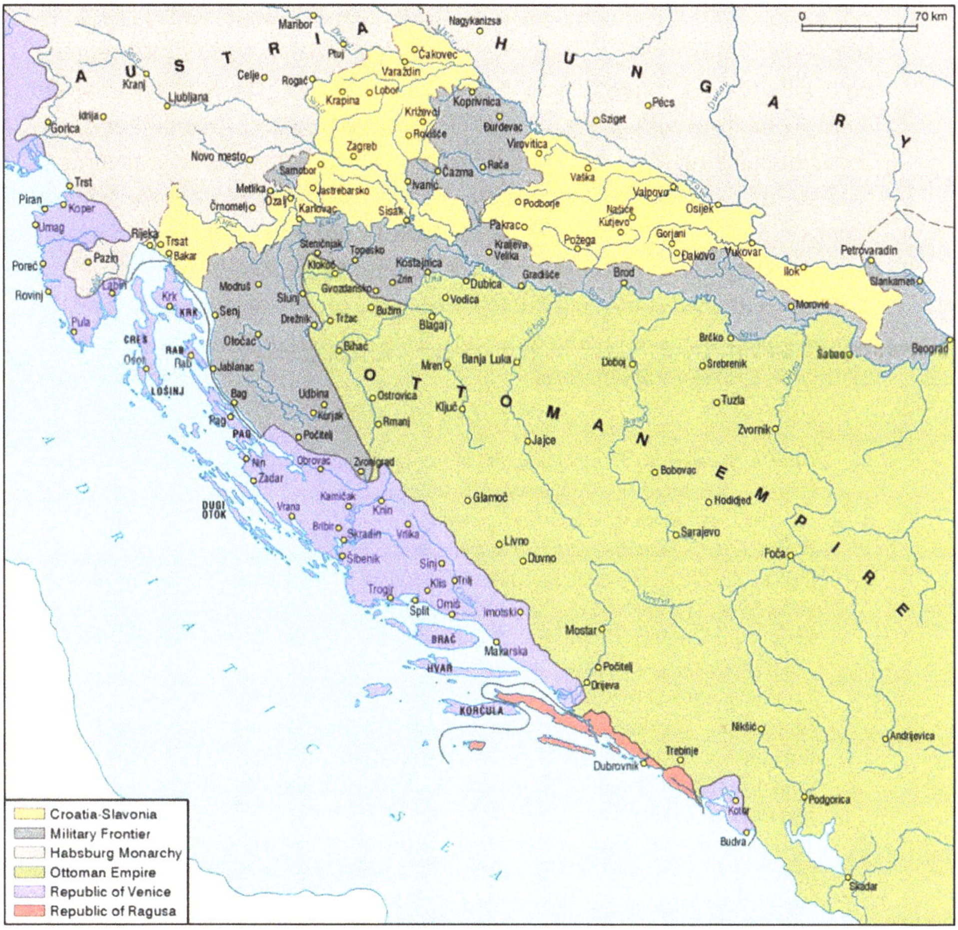

MAP 3.1 Croatian Lands in the eighteenth century. In Ivana Horbec, Maja Matasović, "Voices in a country divided: Linguistic choices in early modern Croatia", Eds. Willem Frijhoff, Vladislav Rjéoutski, *Language Choice in Enlightenment Europe. Education, Sociability, and Governance*. Amsterdam, Amsterdam University Press, 2018, 111–142, here 115

the employment of medical professionals laid foundations for later hospital facilities in the region.[3] In this context, the hospital in Osijek occupied a special position, as it was strategically located near the Ottoman borders, where military hospitals were indispensable due to the presence of the Habsburg army.[4] No less important at the time was the hospital in Bjelovar, where the headquarters of the Varaždin Generalate was stationed on the military border.[5] Hospitals in Civil Croatia in the eighteenth century, primarily hospices that functioned as charitable institutions, have received less attention from historians.[6] The attempts to establish the first modern hospital in Zagreb in Civil Croatia are also still relatively unexplored.[7]

Scholarly publications on the history of Croatian hospitals in the second half of the eighteenth century are remarkably scare, dealing mainly with individual cases and drawing on fewer available historical sources. This could be largely attributed to the scattering of archival material, with many documents, especially medical reports, having been discarded. For the Military Frontier, there are archival collections for each Generalate. However, the number of surviving documents is smaller than originally available.[8] The official records in German are particularly important for the history of healthcare in the Military Frontier in eighteenth century.[9] As for Civil Croatia, most of the documents written in Latin covered the practices of the provincial administration.[10] Many of them concerned communication between the provincial authorities and the central government in Vienna and Buda. This official communication focused mainly on the financial matters.[11]

---

3 Horbec, Skenderović, 'The Quarantines', 190–230. Buczynski, 'Kuga, kontumaci i karantena', 191–208. Bogavčić, 'Od kontumca to bolnice', 263–294.

4 Firinger, Utvić, *Povijest bolničkih ustanova*.

5 Habek, *Iz povijesti zdravstva*. 'O prvoj bjelovarskoj bolnici', 21–30.

6 Piasek, 'Tradicija hospitala', 459–468. An overview on the history of hospitals until the 18th century is available in Horbec, *Zdravlje naroda*, 205–225.

7 Mazzura, *Javna bolnica*. See Hirc, 'Bolnica milosrdne braće', 541–550. See also Dugački, 'Zagrebačka Zakladna bolnica', 74–79.

8 Croatian State Archives (hereinafter: HDA), holdings no. 426 and 429 to 444.

9 Some of the important collections are: Austrian State Archives (hereinafter: ÖStA), Kriegsarchiv (hereinafter: KA), Zentralstellen/Wiener Hofkriegsrat; Militärhofkommissionen/Sanitätshofkommission; Finanz- und Hofkammerarchiv (hereinafter: FHKA), Ungarisches Kamerale.

10 HDA-1 (Croatian-Slavonian Parliament) and HDA-10 (Croatian-Slavonian Ban) for the period up to 1760s; HDA-12 (Croatian Royal Council) for the period 1767–1779, especially its Health Department. For the second part of the 18th century, holdings HDA-28 to HDA-34 keep sources of county governments that often refer to health issues.

11 The most important collection of central bodies is kept in the State Archives of the Hungarian National Archives (hereinafter: MNL OL), section C (Archives of the Locotenential

Given the fact that historical sources on the history of healthcare institutions in Croatia are scattered in archives in three present-day countries and in different languages, it is understandable that historical research on this topic has been relatively limited. Most studies have focused on the history of Croatian hospitals from the nineteenth century onwards, especially the second half, when many permanent military and civilian hospitals were established. This chapter thus shows that there were already intensive discussions and planning for the first hospitals in the decades before. Similar to Würzburg in Lower Franconia, Prague in Bohemia, Kraków in Galicia or Vilnius in Lithuania, the Age of the Enlightenment was a time when health and illness became an important political issue, although not exclusively so.

During that period, hospitals in Croatian lands underwent a process of medicalization. They evolved from purely charitable houses to recognized public facilities dedicated to medical treatment. Medical care was provided in charitable and other hospital institutions, which became focused on treatment and the employment of professional medical staff. While this change was still far from the standards of the General Hospital in Vienna, it laid the foundations for the establishment of hospitals in a more modern sense and reflected trends in the development of the state administration. Their efforts were aimed at creating permanent institutions that focused on organized medical care for the population. As in Pest, Prague and Brno, the ideas that shaped the new type of hospital came primarily from the Viennese court, which was concerned with health policy and gradually implemented it in most provinces.

The administration of the civil and military parts in the Croatian lands differed fundamentally from Würzburg, where the city lord – the bishop – exerted pressure on the corrodians of the burgers' hospital in a power struggle with the municipal self-government. The foundation of the provincial hospital in Zagreb was also different from that of the hospital in Pest, whose establishment was initiated by townspeople. The civil and military parts of the Croatian lands – geographically adjacent, governed by the same ruler and with a similar economic order – reacted in different ways to the growing realization that medical facilities were necessary. The adoption of Habsburg health policy was influenced by the level of funding, administrative capacity and the availability of medical professionals. While both parts faced obstacles, this study argues that the medicalization of hospitals posed a greater challenge in Civil Croatia

Council), especially its Health department (C66). For the period before 1779, section A (Hungarian Court Chancellery) is the most important, especially holdings A1 and A39. Financial documents are kept in FHKA in Vienna, Ungarisches Kamerale.

than in the Austrian hereditary lands. This challenge arose from the lack of financial resources and the fixed structure of the estate administration.

The first part of the chapter presents the Habsburg policies that shaped the development of health facilities in the Croatian lands. While the overarching ideas were similar, their implementation varied considerably between the military and civilian parts of the Croatian lands. Given the stronger political and financial influence of the Viennese court in the Military Frontier, the second part examines developments in this region. The third part of the chapter explains how the Croatian estates adapted to the Enlightenment challenges of hospital medicalization in the civil sector after the General Hospital in Vienna was established as a model for the entire monarchy.

1 Enlightenment Hospital Policy

The Croatian lands had mainly charitable facilities until the second half of the eighteenth century, which relied heavily on Christian charity and practices such as isolating the infected rather than providing comprehensive medical care. This was limited and simple, confined to the essentials. In the urban centers, there were primarily hospices that cared for the homeless, travelers and terminally ill people who did not have the means to heal themselves. These facilities provided vital services such as shelter, food and clothing.[12]

Health care in hospices was not provided by medical professionals. Instead, these institutions were often run by monks, especially in the eighteenth century, particularly by Franciscans, and the Brothers Hospitallers of Saint John of God who were also heavily involved in care institutions existing in Prague, Brno and Vilnius. The convent hospices were part of their charitable mission and were mostly financed by alms and private donations. In contrast, in the Military Frontier – a region where Habsburg rule was only established in the eighteenth century and where there was no tradition of hospices in the urban centers and market towns – only the provisional military hospitals operated (*Feldspitals*). These hospitals were specifically intended for the treatment of wounded soldiers and had a distinct medical

12 For general overview see Risse, *Mending Bodies, Saving Souls*, 73ff. See also Lindemann, *Medicine and Society*, 132ff; for Croatian lands Horbec, *Zdravlje naroda*, 205ff.

purpose. They were staffed by surgeons from the Habsburg army and were run by regimental physicians.[13]

With the growing awareness of the importance of organized health care, which manifested itself in the founding of the hospitals in Vienna and Pest, the first modern hospitals with a medical focus also emerged in other Central European cities. Poverty and illness were increasingly linked and seen as detrimental to the economy and the general welfare. This view formed the basis for the secularization and medicalization of hospitals, which profoundly influenced Franconia, Austria, Hungary and the Croatian lands as well. The increased concern for public health in Central Europe originally arose as a reaction to the frequent plague epidemics in the early eighteenth century, which often came from the Ottoman territories and necessitated organized measures to combat epidemics.[14] From the 1720s, the establishment of the so-called *cordon sanitaire* along the eastern borders of the Habsburg Monarchy was an example of this response – an elaborate network of guardhouses and quarantine stations that developed and remained in place until the late nineteenth century. This system included the permanent deployment of physicians and surgeons, the establishment of protocols for isolation of the infected under medical supervision and the involvement of medical professionals in health matters.[15]

The reform of the Medical School of the University of Vienna in the mid-eighteenth century played a pivotal role in the organization of the public health care and served as a model for other medical faculties in Pest, Prague or Vilnius. The principles of intensive involvement of court authorities and medical professionals, as exemplified in the *cordon sanitaire* were gradually applied more throughout the Central Europe's healthcare system. This development culminated in the enactment of the General Norm for Public Health in early 1770, which not only standardized measures at the borders but also imposed strict regulations on all practicing physicians throughout the Habsburg Monarchy.[16]

---

13 Bazala, *Poviestni razvoj*, 90–91.

14 Horbec, Skenderović, 'The Quarantines', 191ff.

15 Emperor Charles VI mandated a permanent cordon sanitaire in 1728. See Lesky, *Österreichisches Gesundheitswesen*, 16–17.

16 'Sanitäts- und Gesundheitsordnung', published in *Supplementum Codicis Austriaci*, 1247–1298. For the version of this Ordinance issued for the Hungarian part of the monarchy cf. 'Generale Normativum in Re Sanitatis', published by Balázs, *Generale Normativum in Re Sanitatis 1770*.

The establishment of the General Hospital in Vienna had an influence on many German states and other provincial capitals of the monarchy. The Viennese model, which included the consolidation of hospital foundations, the centralization of hospital capacities, and introduction of continuous medical care for patients, shaped the subsequent development of the hospital system in the region. Of particular importance for the Croatian lands was the establishment of the hospital in Pest, which served as a major center for healthcare administration and education. In 1784, the only medical faculty in the eastern part of the monarchy, which had previously been located in Trnava and Buda, was moved to Pest. At that time, the medical-surgical clinic (*Clinicum medico-chirurgicum*) was set up to make it easier for students to practice.[17] As already described in detail in the previous chapter on the history of the municipal hospital in Pest, an institute for the sick and care of the poor (*Kranken- und Versorgungsinstitut*) was opened in 1798. The municipality of Pest took a significant step towards comprehensive medical care in the hinterland.[18]

2 The Military Frontier: a Necessity as a Predecessor of Organized Medical Institutions?

As already mentioned, the organized health system in many Central European cities arose from the measures taken to combat the frequent plague epidemics. With advances in medicine and a better understanding of the transmission of infectious diseases, coupled with an increasingly extensive network of executive institutions – initially in Vienna as the administrative center, later in the provincial capitals – the Enlightenment monarchs took over the definition of measures to combat epidemics in constant consultation with the university experts and controlled their implementation. In terms of funding, communication with local authorities, the establishment of rooms for medical and preventive care and the involvement of medical professionals, such an organization was a precursor to the later development of continuous general healthcare, which was first applied on the Military Frontier in the eastern part of the Habsburg Monarchy.[19]

After the establishment of a fixed border with the Ottoman Empire by the Treaty of Karlowitz in 1699, the area along the eastern borders of the monarchy

---

17 The provision on the University Hospital in Pest see in Linzbauer, *Codex sanitario-medicinalis*, 253–254, 289–291.

18 See *Neue Courier aus Ungarn* 9 (19 January 1799) 41–42.

19 Lesky, *Österreichisches Gesundheitswesen*, 41–44.

became a testing ground for the experimental reforms of the Viennese court. A permanent military administration was established in the region, independent of the local estates, which supplied the Habsburg army with trained soldiers. Medical care in this area was important not only for the treatment of military wounded and disabled people, but also for monitoring the health of travelers (mostly merchants) who came to the monarchy, as the Treaty of Karlowitz established free trade between the two states. Based on the experience of the previous decades, the Habsburg authorities wanted to harmonize these new economic measures with the necessary health measures. From the late 1720s, permanent quarantine sites were organized at border crossings near major frontier towns.[20] In the 1730s and 1740s, the initially simple wooden stations for receiving travelers developed into a complex, carefully organized system for isolating for 14 to 40 days, depending on the epidemiological situation in the neighboring districts. All their goods, both commercial and personal, were disinfected according to precise procedures and checked daily by medical staff to ensure they were safe.[21]

A turning point in this area can be seen in 1770 with the enactment of the General Norm for Public Health, as the first comprehensive standardization of the public health service and general measures to combat epidemics. All regulations up to the middle of the nineteenth century were based on this standard.[22] The quarantine station in Brod (today: Slavonski Brod) is an example of the complex system that such institutions developed into after the adoption of the General Norm.[23] The Brod quarantine station was built along the Sava River and consisted of two separate parts (see plan 1). One wing was unexposed (left on the plan) and contained accommodation with courtyards and sanitary facilities for the quarantine officials. The other wing exposed to infection (on the right of the plan) was separated from the unexposed part by palisades.

There were two huts for travelers, each divided into four separate compartments and each containing a living area, a kitchen with a stove, a courtyard with a rack for airing clothes and a toilet in the courtyard. The exposed part also housed the quarantine staff, who carried out the disinfection measures and monitored travelers (wardens, servants, guards), and were therefore considered to be at risk

20 In this part of the Military Frontier there were permanent quarantine sites in Slunj, Kostajnica, Brod, Gradiška, Mitovica and Zemun.

21 See plans of quarantine sites in Slankamen (1738) and Kostajnica (1743) in HDA-430, box 4, 1738/4-32 and HDA-904, no. 137. For early provisions on isolation and disinfection cf. HDA-430, box 4, 12–17/1738.

22 'Sanitäts- und Gesundheitsordnung', *Supplementum Codicis Austriaci*, 1247–1298. Balázs, *Generale Normativum in Re Sanitatis 1770*. Lesky, *Österreichisches Gesundheitswesen*, 41–44.

23 HDA-430, box 12, 1770/12-120.

of infection. There were also stables and warehouses for housing horses, livestock for sale and other commercial goods that were disinfected, as well as a special closed room for fumigation (of letters and similar products). The largest area of this part consisted of a ventilated courtyard for airing objects. In a completely remote part of the quarantine station there was a so-called hospital with two patient rooms, a separate kitchen, and a morgue. The connection between the two wings of the quarantine station consisted of three rooms for the inspection and examination of travelers, separated by a partition with an opening that was used for health checks by doctors or surgeons at a safe distance.

The idea of building military hospitals on the border also developed from the quarantine stations. Certain principles of their functioning had a considerable influence on the later operation of the hospitals. Among the most important principles that can be highlighted here are the separation of hospital institutions from the care of the poor, the constant presence of medical personnel and daily health checks, and the establishment of special sites designated for medical purposes. The Habsburg military organization generally required medical professionals who were able to provide medical assistance to wounded soldiers and people with disabilities. These professionals were provided with accommodation, food and regular salaries. Consequently, health protection at the Military Frontier was organized earlier than in Civil Croatia, and medical personnel were ensured to carry it out. The *Regulamentum militare* of 1747 already stipulated that each Generalate (there were four in this part of the Military Frontier) had to have a military protomedical officer as chief physician, a second physician, a surgeon with apprentices and a military surgeon in each department of the army.[24] In the following decades, medical headquarters with military pharmacies and infirmaries with several beds were set up in the centers of the frontier regiments. In the second half of the eighteenth century, the number of medical professionals increased. Now each regiment usually employed two doctors and a trained midwife as well as 12 surgeons who were deployed across companies.[25]

Although previous research suggests that hospitals in the modern sense were not established on the Military Frontier until the 1830s, when special buildings were erected for this purpose, there is evidence in the sources that military hospitals existed even earlier. By researching archive plans and sources related to the city of Bjelovar, Dubravko Habek was recently able to prove that a permanent hospital was established there as early as 1760, and not in 1845 as

24 Linzbauer, *Codex*, vol. II, 229–230.

25 On medical experts in the Military Frontier see Bazala, *Poviestni razvoj*, 89–96. There were 2–4 regiments per generalate, all acting as administrative and military units.

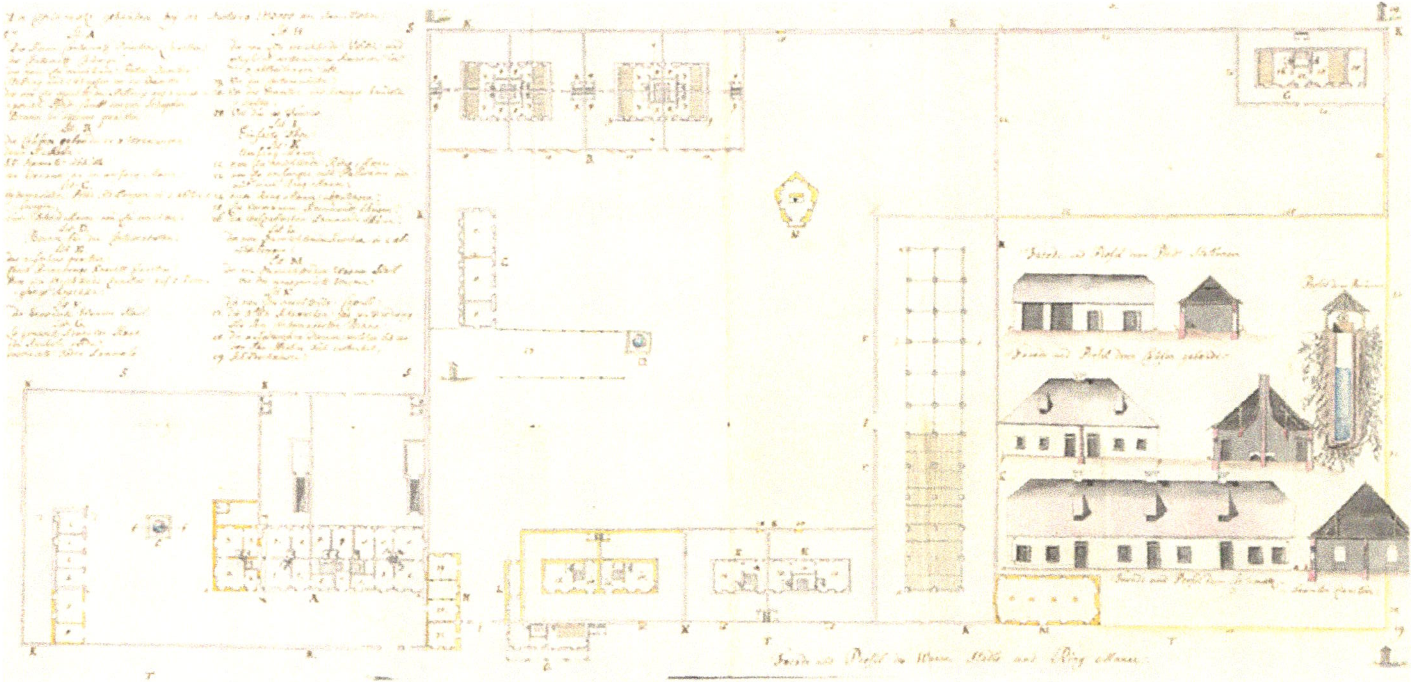

FIGURE 3.1 Plan of the quarantine station in Brod, 1770 (source: HDA-430, box 12, no. 12-120/1770)

Unexposed part: (A) Living quarters for officials, 1. Quarantine director's quarter, 2. Surgeon's quarter, 3. Priest's quarter, 4. – 5. Stables and storerooms, 6. Well; (H) Rooms for visits and examinations, 19. For travelers, 20. For officials and Habsburg merchants, 21. For Ottoman subjects

Exposed part: (B) Huts for travelers, 7. Living space, 8. Small kitchen, 9. Toilet, 10. Wall; (C) Stables for horses with three sections; (D) Well for travelers; (E) Residences for staff, 13. Residence for the supervisor, 14. 15. Residences for servants; (F) Warehouse for goods exposed to infection; (L) Room for fumigation / steam cleaning; (N) Chapel

previously mentioned in the literature.[26] In 1800, the hospital employed 17 surgeons and had 24 beds. It functioned both as a military and civilian hospital and was financed with both military and civilian funds. According to information from 1811, the hospital was supported from military funds by the Đurđevac Regiment, from military funds by the decision of the Court War Council, and from a special hospital fund. The civilian funds came from the Bjelovar City Magistrate from a special hospital fund, which was intended for the equipping and financing the hospitalization of poor, but exclusively acutely ill citizens.[27]

As it was important to maintain similar hospitals for the Habsburg army and the demographic structure of the imperial borderlands, in the 1770s Maria Theresa ordered the construction of military hospitals with a medical purpose at the headquarters of the Military Frontier. A plan for three military hospitals in the Slavonian Generalate has been preserved from 1777 – in Nova Gradiška, Vinkovci, and Mitrovica (see Plan 2).[28] This plan is one of the earliest hospital plans in this area and was intended to serve as a universal model for the construction of hospitals throughout the monarchy. The hospital was designed as a single-story building with a hospital garden and a fountain. It had a special wing with two rooms each for male and female patients and a ventilation corridor, which was "considered necessary for such a hospital." It also contained separate apartments for the hospital director and a surgeon, a kitchen and a pantry.

It seems that these plans were not realized, probably due to the involvement of the Habsburg army in the War of the Bavarian Succession (1778–1779) and a lack of funds. The hospital in Bjelovar remained the only one until 1787, when Emperor Joseph II continued the efforts to establish hospitals on the Military Frontier by issuing the Cantonal Ordinance for the Military Frontier.[29] In this decree, the Emperor Joseph II clearly outlined the main tasks of military hospitals and emphasized both their medical and educational functions: "Hospitals and institutions for the treatment of diseases must not only take measures to treat them with the help of medical personnel, but also investigate the causes of the occurrence of these diseases and propose appropriate measures to contain them."[30]

26 Habek, *Iz povijesti zdravstva,* esp. 143–151; Habek, 'O prvoj bjelovarskoj bolnici'. My recent research proved Habek's claims. One of the documents from January 1787 states that the hospital in Bjelovar exists "from long ago" and that it has "only 24 beds". Cf. HDA-430, box 24, 37-5/1787.

27 Habek, *Iz povijesti zdravstva,* 144–145. HDA-430, box 24, 37-5/1787.

28 'Reambulirter Normal Project Plan Lit. C, in Betreff der drey Slavonischen Graenitz Militaire Spitaler, wovon einer zu Neugradisca, Winkovcze und Mitrovitz zu stehen kommet; und von hohen Orten einstweilig den dato 8. Novembris 1777 begnehmiget worden', HDA-430, box 24, 37-54/1787 (enclosed with other plans of the year 1787).

29 HDA-430, box 26, 37-5/1787.

30 As cited in Habek, *Iz povijesti zdravstva,* 69. On the Regulation see Buczynski, *Pa to su samo Hrvati,* 175–181.

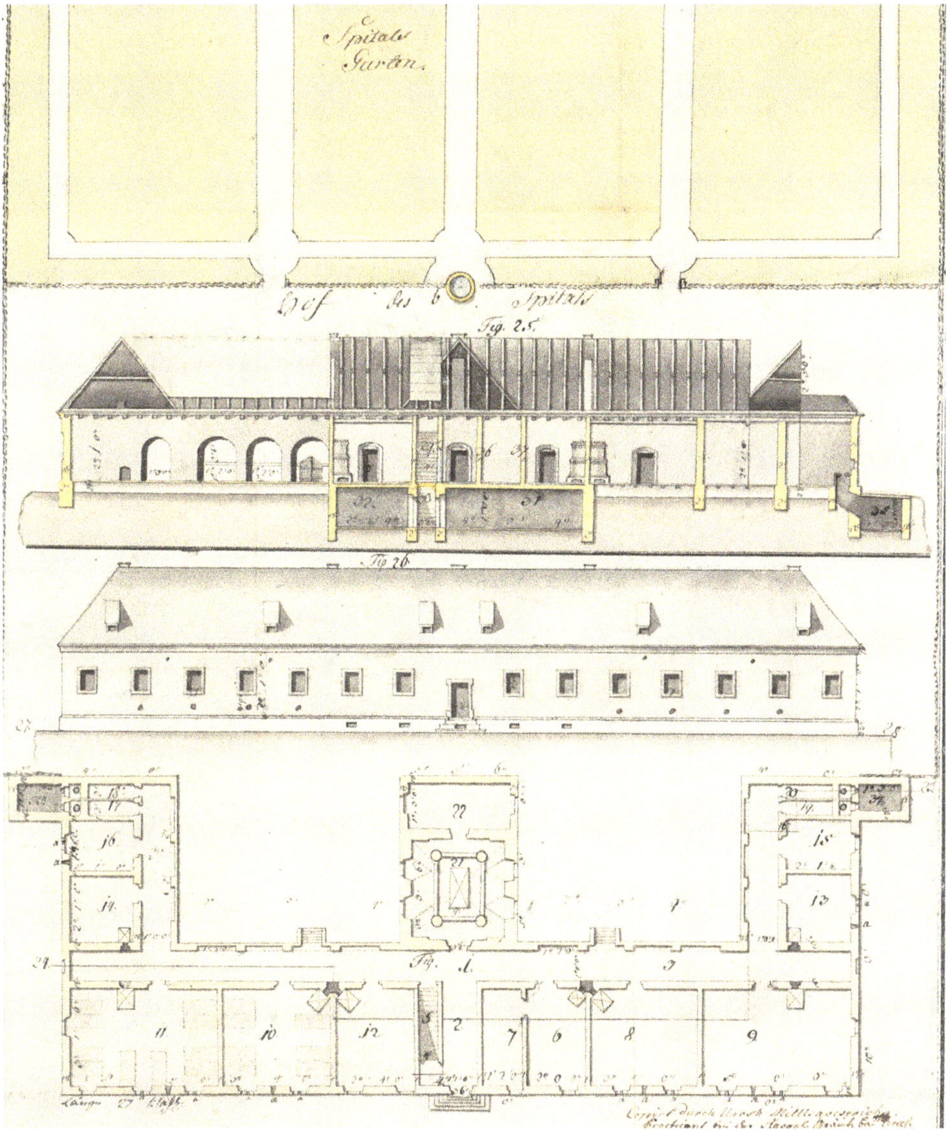

FIGURE 3.2 Plan for military hospitals in Nova Gradiška, Vinkovci and Mitrovica;, HDA-430, box 24, 37–54/1787

Legend: 1. Floor plan, 2. Entrance, 3. Corridor, 4. Staircase door, 5. Staircase to the basement, 6. Quarter to the hospital director with a bedroom, 7., 8., 9. Rooms for women, 10., 11. Rooms for men, 12. Surgeon's quarter, 13., 14. Convalescent room (separate for women and men), 15., 16. Rooms for the deceased and equipment storage, 17., 18., 19., 20. Toilets for men and women, 21. Kitchen, 22. Pantry

As a result of this regulation, several hospitals were set up on the Military Frontier.[31] In order to save money, now new hospital buildings were not erected, but existing military buildings were repurposed. An example of this approach the plan for conversion of the brigade commander's quarters in Vinkovci (see plan 3).[32] The building was a single-story structure with an L-shaped floor

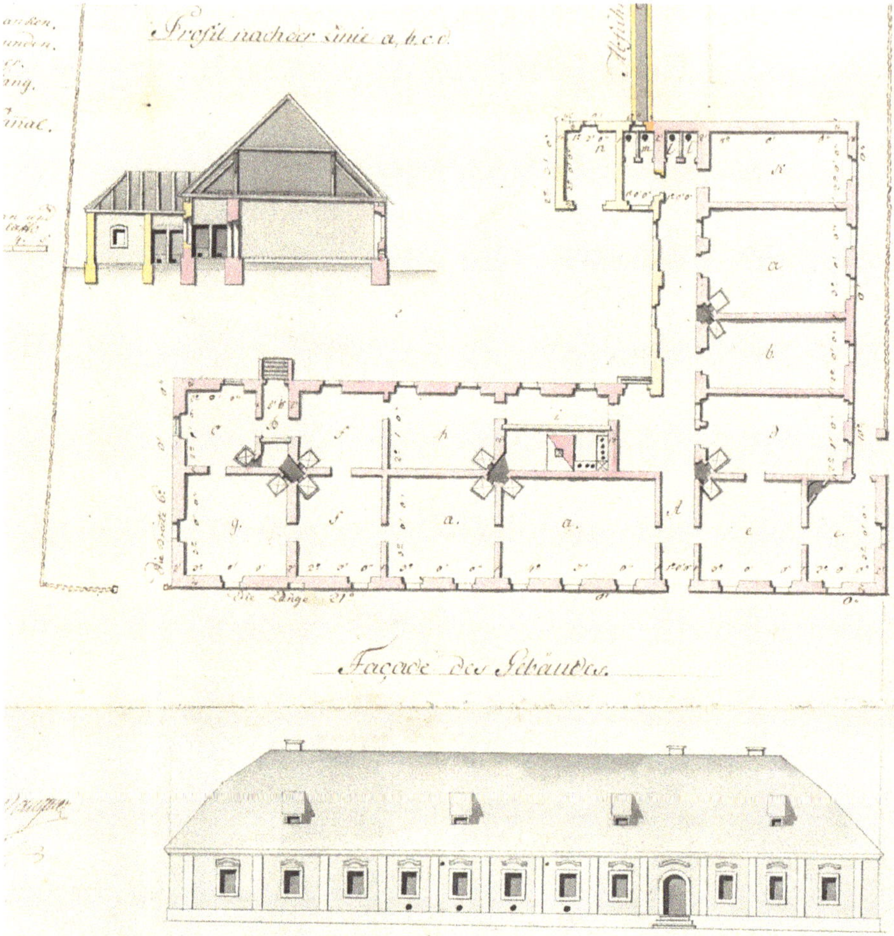

FIGURE 3.3 Plan for the conversion of the brigadier's quarters in Vinkovci into a military hospital, , 430, box 24, 37-54/1787

Legend: a. Three rooms for patients, b. Bathroom, c. Room for the mentally ill, d. Waiting room, e. Room and chamber for the director, f. Two rooms for surgeons, g. Pharmacy, h., k. Dining rooms, i. Kitchen, l. Toilet for patients, m. Toilet for healthy individuals

31 Habek, *Iz povijesti zdravstva*, 72–77.

32 'Plan Lit. A des in dem Brooder Regiments Staabsort zu Vinkovcze Militaire Spitals betreffendt, wie solches aus der alldort vacant befindlichen Brigadierswohnung zu adaptieren wäre', HDA-430, box 24, 37-22/1787.

plan, which was converted into a military hospital without any additional construction work. The hospital consisted of three rooms for patients and one for the mentally ill, as well as rooms for the hospital director and surgeons. It also contained a pharmacy, a kitchen, two dining rooms a waiting room, a bathroom and separate toilets for patients and healthy people. Like other hospitals, it also had a well-ventilated corridor and a sewage system.

3 First Hospitals of New Type in Civil Croatia

In contrast to the Military Frontier, the cities of Civil Croatia had a tradition of caregiving facilities, which were mostly run as charitable institutions without financial support from the Viennese court or the employment of medical professionals.[33] With the increasing interest of the court officials in the organization of public healthcare from the 1760s onwards, court decrees to local authorities regarding the investigation of conditions in town hospices were issued with higher frequency. These were primarily concerned with reviewing their capacities and finances. In 1760, Maria Theresa instructed the Hungarian Lieutenancy Council to examine the state of all hospitals in the Hungarian cities and to report back to the central health institutions. Obviously, there were no adequate results, as the same order was repeated in 1766, indicating that administrative structures in the Hungarian lands were not yet linked to institutionalized treatment and that the facilities were still predominantly depended on the charitable activities of the church and religious orders.[34]

In addition to the lack of financial resources, there was also a general shortage of trained medical personnel in Croatia. According to the General Norm of 1770, each county had to employ a physician and 3–5 surgeons to provide administered general health care in their area. They were often the only medical experts in the region. They were in short supply and were sent from Vienna.[35] A certain change occurred in Croatia with the establishment of the Croatian Royal Council, which had a special health commission tasked with monitoring the state of health institutions. Only a few months after taking up its work, the Council began to inquire about the state of these institutions in the counties and towns. The results were so sobering that in 1771 Maria Theresa

33 Croatian cities had a population ranging from two to, at most, five thousand inhabitants. The majority of the population (97%) was still rural.

34 ÖStA, FHKA, Kamerale Ungarn, Fasc. r. Nr. 787, Subd. 2.: Spitäler, 43 ex Feb 1766, fol. 4.

35 HDA-1, box. 211, no. 532; for the reports on medical experts in the counties cf. MNL OL, C66, box 123.

ordered all hospices and orphanages to be put into operation and properly maintained.[36]

A report on the inspection of hospices in Croatian towns three years after this decision reveals the actual condition of the individual hospices. In 1774, the Zagreb hospice had assets in the form of land and cash amounting to 7,240 gulden, with annual income from interest and rent of just over 500 gulden. This annual income was comparable to the average annual salary of a middle-level civil servant official. Twenty men and two women was accommodated, albeit in very poor conditions and in cramped rooms. Due to a lack of money and space, the hospice could not house any more poor people. The hospice in Križevci only had a total capital of 140 gulden and nine people who had to feed themselves by begging were placed there. The building was made of wood and was so dilapidated that it was estimated that it would not last no more than two or three years.

The town of Varaždin had two hospitals, one next to the other. The smaller one cared for six women and provided a shelter. It was financed exclusively by donations collected by the women staying there. The larger hospital had an annual income from property and capital of less than 150 gulden, enough to employ just one person. The premises was also very cramped and consisted of a single room with a roof in need of repair. The wooden hospital in Koprivnica had a total capital of just over 600 gulden, which resulted in a negligible annual income. It had room for six women, who were only given accommodation and had to collect donations for the hospital. Most of the money was spent on maintain the building and funeral expenses. The hospital's facilities were better than those in other towns, and with minor repairs could accommodate about twenty people.[37]

In the eastern part of the civil territory, the situation was not much better. In 1773, the municipal hospice in Osijek had only three beds for women and two for men, and the hospice in Požega had only three beds.[38] It is obvious that the main problem of municipal hospitals in Civil Croatia in the eighteenth century was the lack of funding, not only from private sources, but also from public funds. However, there was no effective answer to this problem. In response to

36 HDA-12, series 12.1 (Protocolla sessionum), book VIII/1, 281, book VIII/2, 580–581; ÖStA, FHKA, Kamerale Ungarn, Fasc. r. Nr. 787, Subd. 1.: Stiftungen 1771–1772, 153 ex Oct 1771, 6 ex Jul 1772, 108 ex Nov 1772.

37 ÖStA, FHKA, Kamerale Ungarn, Fasc. r. Nr. 788, Subd. 2: Spitäler, 50 ex Oct 1774, fols. 17.–39.

38 Habek, *Iz povijesti zdravstva*, 85.

the above-mentioned report, the court in Vienna could only encourage the city magistrates to pool endowments so that the interest could generate additional funds. Citizens were also urged to donate more to hospices and to bequeath part of their assets in their wills.[39] Similar to the Austrian lands, it was decreed that no foreign beggars were to be admitted anywhere in the kingdom, in any village or town, but were to ordered to return to their home country. Native beggars who were in the cities were to be sent back to their place of birth, and finally, all available places in hospices were to be filled exclusively by the poor or disadvantaged.[40]

Parallel to these measures, the court in Vienna made considerable efforts to promote care facilities and advocated their establishment at local level, with a clear focus on their medical purpose. A crucial aspect of this initiative was the conversion of funding mechanisms from private sources to public funds, combined with the introduction of state supervision over the operation of the healthcare facilities. The transformation of healthcare provision into new type hospitals required a primary focus on medical treatment. The structure of healthcare facilities was inspired by advances in practical, exemplary teaching methodology in medical education, particularly through the establishment of university clinics. This marked a significant shift, although this idea also met with criticism from leading experts of the time, who considered hospitals to be "factories of death" due to the high mortality rates in confined spaces.[41]

The new type of hospital was intended exclusively for the acutely ill, pregnant women and the mentally ill; people with chronic or incurable diseases were not admitted. Daily visits to the doctor were also offered to the impoverished population who could prove their poverty with certificates from parishes or poorhouses. The patients treated were divided into four classes according to their financial status, which determined the cost of accommodation. They ranged from patients who were accommodated in private rooms with full care to patients who received social assistance and were transferred to the hospital's account during their stay. In this way, they became accessible to wealthier people who needed medical care. This concept differed from that of the municipal hospital in Pest, which had originally been built as both a charitable

39 Piasek, 'Varaždinsko zdravstvo', 27.

40 Bernard, The Limits of Absolutism, 209–210.

41 On hospitals in Vienna see Puschmann, *Die Medizin in Wien*, 56ff. Risse, *Mending Bodies, Saving Souls*, 257ff. On clinics in German speaking lands see Broman, *The Transformation of German Academic Medicine*, 59–66.

and medical institution. In Pest, the hospital as a mere almshouse had been overcome, but had not yet a fully developed into a modern healthcare facility.

Emperor Joseph II attempted to bring additional order to the financing and maintenance of health facilities. In 1787, all magistrates were instructed to maintain hospitals, and the care of the sick and infirm was made to the duty of every authority. Existing funds for hospitals had to be placed under the ultimate control of the Endowment Commission (*Stiftungskommission*), which was responsible for ensuring that the funds were used wisely. Surplus funds had to be used for other health facilities in the monarchy, in particular for the remaining hospitals in the counties and towns.[42] Toward the end of Joseph II's reign, responsibility for the hospitals was transferred to the secular authorities, and the clergy and religious orders were completely deprived of the right to inspect or administer such institutions. This regulation did not catch on and was soon revised.[43]

The health policy of the Habsburg court and the founding of the General Hospital in Vienna resonated throughout the monarchy. The Croatian estates were aware of the importance of a hospital with a medical purpose. The attempt to build the first modern hospital in Zagreb shows how challenging such an undertaking was in the individual provinces. In 1785, the provincial administration initiated the establishment of a hospital with a medical purpose in Zagreb. It was triggered by the outbreak of a serious infectious disease (probably influenza), in which "the sick died in the streets for lack of a hospital, more without any help than due to the severity of the disease."[44] However, the hospital was not founded.

In 1792, when the county's medical reports indicated the appearance of a new "terrible fever", the initiative was renewed.[45] The Supreme Count of Zagreb County, Nikola Škrlec Lomnički, proposed the construction of a general hospital in Zagreb with the help of "all Zagreb authorities".[46] This "help" referred to the consolidation of all available funds for the construction and maintenance of the hospital, which were administered by the City of Zagreb, Zagreb County, the Diocese of Zagreb and the Chapter of Zagreb. The city offered a plot of land for the hospital at the foot of the city walls, on the site of the customs house, where a place for a hospital garden was also planned, similar to the plans for the construction of the hospital on the Military Frontier (see Map 3.2, red line).

42 Linzbauer, *Codex* III-I, 431–432.
43 Linzbauer, *Codex* III-I, 549–551.
44 Cited according to Mazzura, *Javna bolnica*, 3.
45 See reports on health state in the Zagreb County, HDA-34, box 56, 105/1792.
46 Mazzura, *Javna bolnica*, 3.

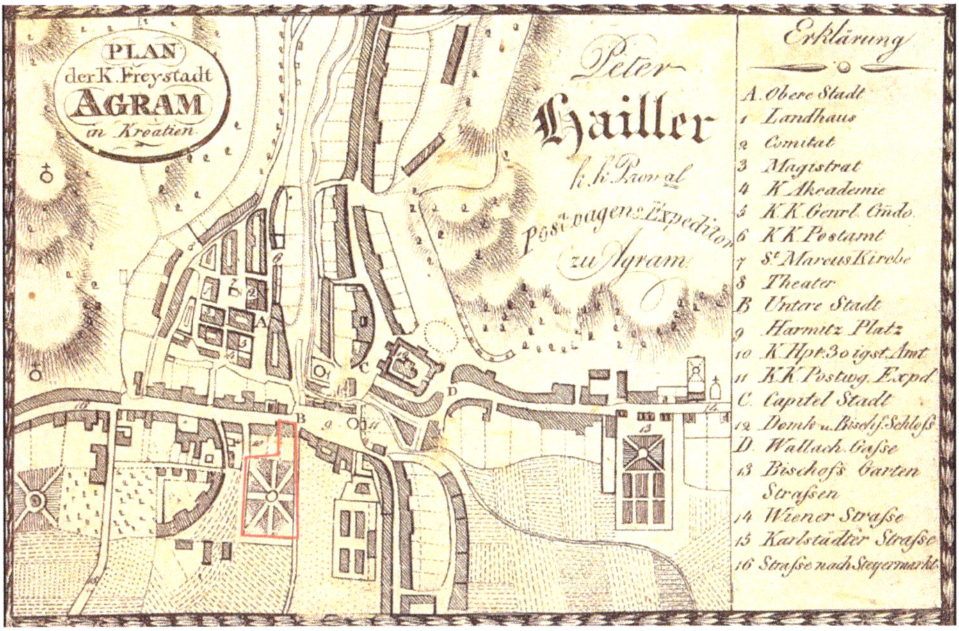

MAP 3.2 Map of the Imperial free city of Zagreb in Croatia. Peter Hailler, *Imperial and Royal Provincial Mail Coach Expeditor of Zagreb*, ca. 1825. City of Zagreb Museum; https://laszowski.com/wp-content/uploads/2024/03/14.4.4-Plan-Zagreba.pdf

The proposal was accepted, and a special committee was set up with the task of planning the establishment of the new so-called civil hospital. This committee consisted of representatives from all the authorities involved, who prepared the layout of the hospital very meticulously: A detailed plan for the operation of the hospital was drawn up, with specific instructions for the hospital director and medical staff. In December 1793, cost estimates were obtained for the construction of the hospital building, which amounted to 28,753 gulden, which was an enormous sum for Zagreb at the time.[47] Construction of the new hospital began one year later but was halted in 1795 due to a lack of funds. In the following years, according to available records, a campaign was conducted among the nobility and the wealthier citizens of Zagreb and Zagreb County to donate for the construction of the hospital.[48] Some funds were raised in this way, but still not enough to start operating the hospital as originally planned.

At the turn of the century, when the Napoleonic Wars in Zagreb were expected to result in large number of military casualties and the hospital

---

47 HDA-34, box 166 (sine fol., chronologically ordered).

48 List of donations cf. in HDA-34, box 167 (sine fol; chronologically ordered).

building was still not completed, the Bishop of Zagreb, Maksimilijan Vrhovac, invested funds from the Zagreb diocese to complete the building and set up a temporary military hospital.[49] This renovated military hospital served as basis for the establishment of the new healthcare facility. In 1803, the Zagreb County, in cooperation with Bishop Vrhovac, formed a new committee with the task of immediately transforming this building into a civil hospital and providing medical staff and finances. Based on the work of the committee, a new plan for the operation of the hospital was developed and approved by the letter of endowment from the court of Emperor Franz II in Vienna.[50]

The financial framework for the operation of the hospital had already been established in the 1790s. Similar to many hospitals in other Central European cities, the available funds were pooled by various authorities (ecclesiastical, municipal, testamentary). Each authority retained the right to a certain number of beds in specific wards, as will be described later. From the Public fund for Civil Croatia, the Viennese court approved funds amounting to 3,648 gulden for the construction costs. This approval was based on the fact that the building had already been completed but was additionally damaged during its previous use by the military. The original plan for the hospital could not be realized due to a lack of medically trained staff in the region and insufficient funds to hire them.

It was therefore decided to entrust the professional management of the hospital to the Order of the Hospitaller Brothers of Saint John of God, who had the rights to care for the sick in Hungary since 1723 as part of their charitable work. After an agreement was reached with the Hospitaller Brothers, it was stated that the authorities – in contrast to previous instructions – would not interfere with the medical care provided by the Brothers. Instead, the agreement focused solely on the financial feasibility of maintaining the hospital. This agreement ensured that the Hospitaller Brothers, which was already authorized to provide this medical care, would oversee the operation of the hospital.[51]

In the beginning, the Zagreb hospital combined charitable and medical purposes. The hospital was a two-story building with a pharmacy, a chapel

49 Mazzura, *Javna bolnica*, 3–4.

50 The foundation document dated March 16, 1804, written in Latin, can be found in HDA-34, box 167; MNL OL, A 57, 2671/1804 (Libri Regii), book 61, pp 297–304 (available online at https://archives.hungaricana.hu/en/libriregii); and in Mazzura, *Javna bolnica*, 29ff. (translated into Croatian). When not indicated otherwise, subsequent information regarding the functioning of the hospital has been derived from this document.

51 The original contract from 1803 was signed by the representatives of all Zagreb authorities and the Order. HDA-34, box 167 (sine fol.).

dedicated to the Suffering Jesus, and a hospital garden (see Plan 5). According to the foundation charter, it consisted of three main wards: Shelter for the poor and disabled (*Nosocomium*), infirmary (*Xenodochium*), and shelter for the mentally ill (*Gyrgatum*). Although the founding charter itself mentioned the existing practice of housing these wards in different buildings with separate administrations, they were merged due to lack of funds. Patients were admitted to the *Xenodochium* for treatment "only while the illness lasted," meaning that chronic patients were not admitted.[52] The task of this ward was to help patients and convalescents "in a comfortable and useful way." No rules were prescribed for the care of patients in the Xenodochium, as the rules of the Hospitaller Brothers already regulated this aspect.[53]

There were three types of accommodations in this ward: free, donated, and paid. Free accommodation was granted to any sick "true pauper" who, as confirmed by the authorities, had no one who could care for them at home "according to human judgment" or who lacked the means for such care. A bed in medical care cost the authority sending the patient 100 gulden per year, with 16 beds originally set aside for this purpose. An initial fund of 33,483 gulden was secured for these patients, which was pooled from various funds of the City of Zagreb, Zagreb County, church foundations, and private bequests. Endowed places in the infirmary could be established by any private individual with a capital of at least 2,000 gulden per bed, with the possibility of combining donations from various sources. In this case, the donor had the right to choose who should be admitted to the hospital and could also finance better food supplies (provided it was approved by the doctor).

Like the hospitals in Pest, Prague and Brno, the facility in Zagreb, based on the Viennese model, had several paid beds, which were divided into two categories. Patients in shared rooms paid 24 kreutzer per day for accommodation, food and medical care, while those in private rooms paid 1 gulden per day. Hospital places were designated for all patients equally, regardless of their status,

52 The term "Xenodochium" traditionally marked a shelter for foreigners in cities, and this is how the term has been translated in Croatian historiography so far. However, from the description of the Zagreb hospital, it is clear that this department was dedicated to acutely ill individuals and therefore had a medical purpose.

53 During the preparation for the establishment of the hospital, the committee proposed a detailed procedure for handling patients, including three types of menus for the "severely," "moderately," and "mildly" ill. However, since it was agreed that the hospital would be run by the Brothers Hospitallers of Saint John of God, no further instructions for medical care of the patients are found among the sources, only financial reports. Cf. HDA-34, box 166 (sine fol.).

religion, or gender. Bishop Maksimilijan Vrhovac set up a special endowment of 13,100 gulden for the admission of women and stipulated that

> A suitable, virtuous woman, inspired by the true spirit of charity, was to be entrusted with the care of the women, together with a maid. Their task was to supervise and manage the cleanliness and proper care of the female patients with food, medicine, and other necessities.[54]

In addition to the funds already allocated, 4,374 gulden and 10 kreutzer were initially provided for equipment (furniture, medical instruments) and 3,000 gulden for the pharmacy from the County of Zagreb.[55]

The second ward, the shelter for the poor and disabled (*Nosocomium*), was a continuation of the functions of earlier caregiving facilities in the Zagreb area and provided a better organized environment and supply of food and clothing. The annual cost of maintaining a poor person was estimated at 50 gulden, with the hope that this amount could be increased. The city administration pledged to pay 15,000 gulden for 15 paupers, the Zagreb Chapter pledged to pay 12,000 gulden for 12 paupers, and the Zagreb Diocese had no allocated principal, so the bishop pledged to pay 50 gulden annually for one pauper. The poor were admitted to the *Nosocomium* for life and could only be sent to the Senior of the Hospitaller Brothers with a written notice by the authority that had undertaken to pay for them.

The Hospitaller Brothers took care of the institutional provision for the poor, who received clothing "made of cloth or linen, of the quality, color, and cut available at the lowest price." The foundation laid down the desired menu: the food was to consist of "good bread," two "well-prepared" hot meals for lunch and bread and a hot meal for dinner. A meat dish (beef) was served at least once a week. When the hospital opened, the poor who were housed in the existing facilities were to be transferred along with their possessions, the new hospital only provided two bowls per person. The poor housed in the hospital were accountable to the Senior of the Hospitaller Brothers and had to obey him under the threat of expulsion. They had to look after patients in other wards and were not allowed to leave the building without permission "to put an end to their mischief." They also had to hand over any income they earned outside the hospital to their proper superior.

---

54 Mazzura, *Javna bolnica*, 11.

55 For a list of the necessary equipment, cf. the assessment from November 23, 1796, in HDA-34, box 166 (sine fol.).

The third ward, the shelter for the mentally ill (*Gyrgatum*), had no funds of its own. However, the above-mentioned agreement stipulated that the order was obliged to admit mentally ill patients to the institution and that the admitting authority paid an annual lump sum for their care. The lump sum was estimated at 100 gulden for "quit lunatics" and 150 gulden for "raving lunatics". The founding charter stated that the Superior of the Hospitaller Brothers agreed to these amounts out of a strong desire to establish this institution, even if it meant losses for the Order, in the hope that "funds would increase over time".

The Hospitaller Brothers received no additional renumeration for the administration of the hospital and medical care. It was expected that additional funds would come from the pharmacy revenues and donations from the incorporated chapel of the Suffering Jesus, as well as the possibility that the participating institutions would increase their endowments over time.[56] The administration of the hospital was not left to the Hospitaller Brothers alone. It was agreed that a special committee, consisting of representatives from all the authorities involved, would manage the hospital. This committee was to take care of all necessary matters with the Order. The hospital in Zagreb was ceremonially inaugurated on August 23, 1804, with many prominent public figures in Civil Croatia giving speeches, which indicated the importance of such a project.

4 Conclusion

The experience of establishing medical facilities on the Military Frontier – a region on the borders of the Habsburg Monarchy, administered by the Viennese court and was crucial for the defense against epidemics associated with campaigns and invasions – illustrated how the support of imperial administration significantly influenced the establishment of new health facilities. Despite financial and personnel challenges comparable to those faced by Civil Croatia, the Military Frontier had previously succeeded in organizing continuous medical care solely through secular authorities. From the 1720s onward, medical practices significantly shaped health regulations and contributed to the spread of knowledge about how to deal with infectious diseases. In addition, the quarantine stations and military administrations attracted medical experts from other parts of the monarchy, who were essential for the establishment of hospitals in the imperial border regions, as the example of the

56 Over time, the city of Zagreb allocated a significant area of land near the city for the hospital. Cf. Mazzura, *Javna bolnica*, 38ff.

Civil Croatia shows. With more secure funding and medical expertise, the hospitals on the Military Frontier took on a distinct curative and medical function.

The development of healthcare facilities in the second half of the eighteenth century throughout the monarchy demonstrated what was needed to adapt a hospital of new type. Initially, secular authorities began to play a central role in promoting local hospitals that focused on medical functions. There was a significant shift in the funding of these facilities from private to public sources, accompanied by centralized government oversight. The central government actively promoted the training and employment of qualified medical professionals and emphasized the importance of medical expertise in hospitals. This led to a distinction between the charitable and medical roles of hospitals. In the late eighteenth century, two concepts of hospital institutions emerged in the Croatian lands: those that primarily catered to social needs and those that focused on medical care. They contributed to public health measures and became integral parts of public health system, recognized for their broader societal impact.

However, the path from the concept discussed to its promotion and implementation was extremely tortuous. It was by no means a straightforward that was completed once-and-for-all. Apart from initial, unrealized initiatives, it took a full twelve years from the decision to build and to open the hospital in Zagreb. A much more complex hospital was completed in Vienna in eighteen months. While the construction of hospitals in other cities of the monarchy (e.g., Prague, Brno, Pest) also faced significant legal, financial and organizational challenges, the experience of building the hospital in Zagreb underlined the immense difficulties that provincial towns faced despite a strong political will and carefully prepared plans.

The biggest challenge was undoubtedly the financial aspect, as the funds accumulated over the years proved to be insufficient for the construction and maintenance of such a facility. To make matters worse, Zagreb did not have a medical faculty until the second half of the nineteenth century, and the Viennese court was reluctant to invest in a hospital that did not serve as a university clinic, even though it was the only hospital in the entire province. In Zagreb, the construction of a new hospital depended on the provincial authorities. Another major problem was organizational nature: the severe shortage of medical professionals in Civil Croatia eventually led to medical treatment being entrusted to the Hospitaller Brothers.

This represented a significant departure from the imperial efforts, when rulers such as Maria Theresa and Joseph II sought to secularize healthcare and emphasized state control over institutional provision. The completion of the hospital in Zagreb was only secured by the need to accommodate the Habsburg army during the Napoleonic Wars and by the financial support of the Bishop of Zagreb. Despite its expansion to 460 beds in the second half of the nineteenth century, the Zagreb Civil Hospital was not a great success; towards the end of the nineteenth century, the city administration found itself embroiled in disputes with the Hospitaller Brothers over hospital capital. Financial losses were frequent due to disorganization and poor hygiene. In 1931, the hospital was demolished and relocated to St. Spirit's facility, which was then on the outskirts of the city and still stands today.[57]

Acknowledgement

This research was conducted within the project SANITAD funded by the Next-Generation EU fund.

57 On the subsequent fate of the hospital see Dugački, 'Zagrebačka Zakladna bolnica'; on the dispute with the Order of the Hospitaller Brothers cf. Mazzura, *Javna bolnica*.

CHAPTER 4

Neither State nor Private: the Care of Body and Soul in the Prague Hospitals of the Brothers of Mercy and the Sisters of St. Elisabeth, 1780–1850

Eva Hajdinová

Historical research on the Hospitaller Order of the Brothers of St. John of God and the Sisters of St. Elizabeth tends to focus on the care they provided in the early modern period. By the seventeenth and eighteenth centuries, the orders had established an impressive network of convents and hospitals around the world.[1] In Europe, America and Asia, they created almost indispensable caregiving institutions for many patients who were admitted regardless of their origin. In the Habsburg Monarchy before the Enlightenment, the two religious orders, commonly known as the Brothers and Sisters of Mercy, were the main providers of outpatient and short-term hospital care. Apart from some older works that have dealt with the history of the Hospitaller convents in the Bohemian lands from the perspective of institutional history, the internal life of the orders and the careers of their individual members, as well as deeper analysis of the patients there has recently been a strong interest in the history of medical care.[2]

In this context, historians systematically analyzed the methods of diagnosis, the occurrence of various diseases and the development of mortality of male and female patients. They had shown that the two convent hospitals in Prague applied gradually improving diagnostics, reflecting a growing knowledge of anatomy, pathology, therapeutics, and pharmacy among their staff.[3]

1 McMahon, *The story of the Hospitallers*, passim. Russotto, *Origine ed evoluzione storica*, passim.

2 Brothers of Mercy is a name commonly used in Central Europe for the Brothers Hospitallers of Saint John of God, officially the Hospitaller Order of the Brothers of Saint John of God. The term 'Brothers of Mercy' is thus perhaps not quite accurate, but it is commonly used. Aside from older publications, mainly recent publications such as Strohmayer, *Der Hospitalorden des Hl. Johannes von Gott*. Watzka, *Vom Hospital zum Krankenhaus*. Watzka, *Arme, Kranke, Verrückte*. Watzka, 'Die Krankenprotokolle der Barmherzigen Brüder.' Kušniráková, 'Pacienti a zdravotnícky personal.' Blessing, *Katholische Krankenpflege im Spannungsfeld*.

3 Ebelová, 'Die Entstehung der ersten Krankenhäuser.' Ebelová, 'Úroveň diagnostiky.' For pharmaceutical knowledge, see Kolda, 'Zárodky zdravotnických knihoven.'

 | HTTPS://DOI.ORG/10.1163/9789004755062-006

They also examined the history of convent hospitals outside Prague, for example caregiving facilities of the Brothers of Mercy in Brno/Brünn and Valtice/Feldsberg.[4] The historians covered the usual categories researched as part of the hospital history: the occurrence and relative representation of certain diseases, the age and social structure of the patients, the absolute and average length of their hospital stay, and the success rate of treatment. Less attention was paid to medical staff in these studies.[5] None of them focused specifically on mentally ill patients.

Although both the Order of the Brothers of Mercy and the Order of the Sisters of St. Elizabeth had escaped the Josephinian dissolution of the monasteries thanks to their practical mission, their reputation had suffered from the anti-clerical policies promoted by some of the reform-minded representatives of the Enlightenment. The merits of scientific progress and specialized diagnostics were increasingly taken over by newly founded secular hospitals, which were set up on the initiative of the central and provincial civil authorities and combined medical care with clinical teaching and applied medical research.

However, the institutionalization of the new secular hospitals took some time, and despite a gradual increase, their capacity could not fully meet the needs of the provincial capitals.[6] The convent hospitals, especially those of the Brothers and Sisters of Mercy, therefore held an irreplaceable position until well into the middle of nineteenth century. At the height of the Josephinist religious and medical reforms, the two aforementioned orders were also tasked with the systematic care of mentally ill religious, diocesan priests and members of ecclesiastical orders in various provinces of the Habsburg Monarchy. The convent hospitals were to set up new specialized wards in order to provide adequate social and medical care for the religious, the lowest ranking part of the social elite. In the initial phase of their existence, patients from the general population were also temporarily treated in these wards, as the public mental asylum was only established in Prague in 1790.[7]

---

4 Watzka, Jelínek, 'Krankenhäuser in Mitteleuropa vor der Aufklärung.' Jelínek, 'Klášterní nemocnice řádu Milosrdných bratří.'

5 Jelínek was in 2015 the main organiser and guarantor of congress 'The Brothers Hospitallers of St. John of God in the Germanic province to 1780's/Provincia Germania de Orde Hospitalario Sancti Johannis de Deo per annum 1780', which took place in Brno, in the former convent of the Brothers of Mercy on 27–28 March 2015; for its programme, see https://www.biskupstvi.cz/storage/akt/9922.pdf [accessed 12 December 2023].

6 Foucault, *The Birth of the Clinic*. Keel, *L'avènement de la médecine clinique*.

7 Hlaváčková, Svobodný, *Pražské špitály a nemocnice*, 47ff. Vencovský, *Počátky české psychiatrie*, 52–56.

In contrast to Czech historians, who paid almost no attention to the development of those convent hospitals after 1780 and did not address the issue of care for the mentally ill, Austrian colleagues have studied the care of the mentally ill in the hospitals of the Brothers of Mercy in Graz and Linz. They examined mentally ill patients who were admitted to the hospitals of the merciful brothers from the sixteenth to middle of the eighteenth century and investigated the official records of the convent hospitals. In addition to a quantitative and qualitative analysis of the patient registers, they also examined inventories of the physical equipment in the hospital rooms and operating theatres. They described the treatment in these hospitals, including the prescriptions for the medicines used there, and the financial aspect of the treatment, such as the question of endowments and patrons.[8]

According to Carl Watzka, as early as the sixteenth and seventeenth centuries, the "insane" were considered to be genuinely ill and therefore curable at least in some institutions – including the hospitals run by the Brothers of Mercy. They were therefore not only regarded as criminals, outcasts, asocial individuals, or people who had lost their minds. Therefore, the mentally ill were not excluded from society and isolated but received treatment. Watzka dispelled the myth of the 'liberation of the mentally ill from their shackles around 1800' and showed that this only applied to some of today's institutions for the mentally ill. The core of his work, however, concerns the period before 1750.[9]

The aim of this chapter is to fill a gap in existing research by addressing the history of Prague's convents after 1780. The chapter presents findings pertaining on the topics researched in hospital history, focusing on the hitherto unexplored origins of the special ward for mentally ill clergy and laity, which was established in the Prague Hospital of the Brothers of Mercy in 1783. Until the establishment of the Prague Mental Asylum (*Prags k. k. Irrenanstalt*), the Hospital of the Brothers of Mercy operated a new ward for mentally ill religious (*geistliches Irrenhaus*), which was generally known as the Priest's House (*Priesterhaus*). It was the only place in Bohemia that systematically cared for the mentally ill religious. For more than 120 years, it functioned as a specialized and independent medical institution in Bohemia. It also served priests from outside the Prague archdiocese.[10] In Moravia, during the same period, the care

8 Watzka, *Vom Hospital zum Krankenhaus*, passim.

9 Watzka, *Vom Hospital zum Krankenhaus*, passim.

10 Especially dioceses of Leitmeritz, Budweis, and Königgratz. In Moravia, a ward for mentally ill clerics was created in the convent of the Brothers of Mercy in Staré Brno (Alt Brünn) in 1785; Hajdinová, 'Péče o choromyslné duchovní v brněnském špitále.'

of the mentally ill clergy was entrusted to the Brothers Hospitallers in Brno/Brünn.

There was no comparable special institution for nuns in Bohemia, but in the 1780s and 1790's the Prague Hospital of the Sisters of St. Elizabeth admitted and treated mentally ill women. The treatment at the hospital deserves special attention, as it followed on from the Sisters of Mercy's earlier care for the mentally ill, which was not systematic but was part of their mission. In fact, the Sisters of St. Elizabeth in Prague suffered from long-term underfunding; they were entirely dependent on aristocratic patronage and appear to have received only limited financial support from the state-administered Religious Fund, which was established in February 1782 as part of the Josephinist reforms to provide financial assistance to both secular and regular clergy. Viennese state administration clearly prioritized financial support for priests needed in pastoral service over support for nuns.

This chapter explores how the interplay of charity, modern medicine, and church administration operated under the imperial rule in Prague at the end of the eighteenth and first half of the nineteenth century. It traces how the two most important convent hospitals approached the criteria of a "modern health care institution" and in which aspects they differed. Based on the analysis of patient registers that survived the damage suffered by the convent during a devastating flood and the Napoleonic Wars, the chapter presents the medical conditions of the mentally ill and the partial knowledge of their treatment.[11] The first part of the chapter presents the establishment of convent hospitals in Prague. The second part deals with the institutionalization of the care of the mentally ill in the convent hospitals. The third part deals with the treatment of mentally ill patients and their individual testimonies in a broader historical context.

1 Brothers and Sisters of Mercy: the Establishment of Convent Hospitals in Prague

The order, officially known as Ordo Hospitalarius Sancti Joannis de Deo, was originally founded as a pious confraternity in Granada in 1539. Three decades later, the Pope Pius V established the fraternity as a religious congregation with the bull *Licet ex debito*, which referred to the biblical story of the merciful Samaritan. Soon after the order was founded, the hospitals of the Brothers

11 See more Hajdinová, 'Léčba nebo náprava?', passim.

of Mercy took over the care and treatment of the acutely ill, partly because the brothers received special training in therapy and nursing.[12] Most members of the order were lay brothers: only some were ordained as priests and were able to administer the sacraments to patients and other brothers. According to the order's statutes, the brothers cared for male patients regardless of their race, religion and, above all, their social status. Women and children were only treated in emergencies and only as outpatients. The effectiveness of the convent hospitals of the Brothers of Mercy was because they concentrated on the temporary, short-term medical care of a large number of sick people, while social care was left to other institutions.

The Convent of the Brothers of Mercy in Prague was founded in December 1620 on the site of a former mediaeval hospital next to the small Old Town church of St. Simon and Judas Thaddeus (Na Františku), which was owned by local Protestants at the beginning of the seventeenth century.[13] The land was given to the order by Emperor Ferdinand II as an expression of gratitude for the care of the wounded from the famous Battle of White Mountain. In 1629, the friars began building a convent hospital for the poor.[14] The hospital grew considerably over the following decades. In the eighteenth century, the convent hospital of the Brothers of Mercy in Prague was the second largest in the Habsburg Monarchy in terms of the number of beds after the hospital in Leopoldstadt in Vienna.[15]

Since 1622, the care of sick women has been the task of the Order of St. Elisabeth, whose founder, Apolonia Radermecher, was the superior of the Aachen hospital. In Prague, their convent hospital was founded at the beginning of 1719, when the sisters settled in Prague's New Town on a hill called 'Na Slupi', on land that had previously belonged to the Servite Order, and soon set up an infirmary there.[16] The first two sisters of the Order of St. Elisabeth came to Prague from Graz, but the convent was founded as a daughter house of the

12 Strohmayer, *Krankenpflegeschulen im Hospitalorden*, passim.

13 Buben, *Encyklopedie řádů, kongregací a řeholních společenství*, 376. Bogar, *Milosrdní bratři*, 178–180.

14 The oldest convent of the Brothers of Mercy in Central Europe was founded in 1605 in Valtice (Feldsberg) in Moravia by Karl, Count Liechtenstein. See Bogar, *Milosrdní bratři*, passim. Buben, *Encyklopedie řádů, kongregací a řeholních společenství*, 368–406.

15 Bogar, *Milosrdní bratři*, 103.

16 For more on the Sisters of St Elizabeth, see Schäffner, *Geschichte des Ordens und der Heilanstalt*. See also Křečková, Kuchařová, *Dějiny konventu alžbětinek v Praze*. The idea of establishing another convent hospital in Prague was largely driven by the tragic experience of a new plague epidemic that hit Prague in 1713 and took the lives of 10,000 to 12,000 of its inhabitants; see Hlaváčková, Svobodný, *Pražské špitály a nemocnice*, 25.

Vienna House of St. Elisabeth. Emperor Charles VI was initially reluctant to provide the necessary funds for the foundation of a convent and hospital, but the sisters managed to raise money from numerous noble patrons. As with the Brothers of Mercy, the running of the convent and hospital was then financed from the interest on endowments, alms and donations. However, while the merciful brothers were able to maintain twelve beds from the start of their hospital, the Sisters began almost a hundred years later with just six beds.[17]

The Sisters of St. Elisabeth's premises became a fully-fledged hospital in 1726, when a new large patient hall was built according to contemporary plans for convent hospitals.[18] Throughout the eighteenth century, the Sisters struggled with inadequate funding and a growing number of patients seeking their help. One of the reasons for the unsatisfactory financial situation was the fact that they were a cloistered order: Unlike the Brothers of Mercy, they were therefore unable to go around the city asking for direct donations. In times of war, they cared for wounded soldiers, both as outpatients and inpatients. Until the early 1840s, their hospital was the only institution apart from the General Hospital in Prague that took in women in need of medical help.[19]

To give a general sense of the quantitative importance of these convent hospital networks within the Habsburg Monarchy, it may be noted that in 1806, 16,800 patients, were admitted to the 25 hospitals of the Brothers of Mercy including 1,100 non-Catholics and 21 Israelites. In Galicia alone, the Sisters of Mercy owned 5 religious houses with healthcare facilities and treated almost 7,000 people in their hospital in Lviv/Lemberg within two years.[20] The number of patients in the Hospital of the Brothers of Mercy in Prague was considerable and comparable to other provincial hospitals. In the middle of the eighteenth century, with a capacity of seventy beds, it treated around one thousand patients per year. In the following decades, the number of patients and beds grew, increasing by half within a hundred years.[21]

---

17 Buben, *Encyklopedie řádů, kongregací a řeholních společenství*, 369. Křečková, Kuchařová, *Dějiny konventu alžbětinek v Praze*, 26.

18 This hospital ward was built thanks to the support of Maria Margarethe, Countess of Wallenstein, an important patron of the convent. Empress Maria Theresa bequeathed in her testament to this convent a considerable sum of 30,000 gulden. See Postřihač, *Dějiny kláštera a nemocnice*, 8.

19 Hlaváčková, Svobodný, *Pražské špitály a nemocnice*, 85.

20 Kopetz, *Österreichische politische Gesetzkunde*, 271–272.

21 Held, *Kurze Geschichte der Heilanstalt der Barmherzigen Brüder*, 100. The physician Jan Theobald Held calculated that in the two centuries of existence of the hospital of the Brothers of Mercy, a total of 182,566 patients were hospitalized there. According to Hermann Haas, the numbers were even higher; Hass, *Das Krankenmaterial des Spitals*, Tabelle I–VI.

The Sisters of St Elizabeth initially cared for around four hundred women per year as inpatients, who were looked after by forty nurses at this time. Over the course of a hundred years, the number of patients treated rose to almost one thousand. These figures do not include the care of the numerous outpatients.[22] In the 1790s, there were around 90 newly admitted female patients per month; in the years 1800–1820, their number dropped to 30–50 women per a month. This trend probably reflects the fact that some Prague women preferred care in the women's ward of the General Hospital and especially in the maternity hospital. Within the Austrian Province, the Prague Hospital of the Sisters of St. Elisabeth was a rather modest institution, while the Hospital of the Merciful Brothers was, the largest next to the in Vienna–Leopoldstadt.[23]

Both convents were founded on the outskirts of the city, but not far from the center, which increased their attractiveness. The reasons for choosing a semi-peripheral location were traditional: the lower population density and easy access to water sources provided better hygienic conditions. This location also made it possible to create large gardens and build various service buildings. The Brothers of Mercy not only had a kitchen garden and a medicinal herb garden, but also an ornamental garden, stables for horses and cattle and a chicken coop. The gardens not only provided fresh food but also enabled the patients to go for walks. This was an advantage that the ever-growing new public hospitals in densely built-up urban environments could not always offer. Although they initially had landscaped courtyards, the number of green spaces decreased in the first half of the nineteenth century. *Elisabethinerinnen* had less land at their disposal, but their gardens were also sufficient, especially given the generally lower capacity of the hospital (except during the war years).[24]

Both convents with their hospital edifices were built in an early modern layout typical of such institutions, as square, multi-story buildings arranged around a corridor and with an enclosed area on the first floor around a central courtyard. The Hospital of the Brothers of Mercy was continuously extended by adding further wings to the original building. A large-scale, unifying reconstruction of the convent was completed in 1753 after the acquisition of new neighboring properties. The new building complex had a total capacity of 108

22 Until 1840s, the number of female patients hospitalized annually ranged between 700 and 1,000, whereby exceptional were only years 1817–1820, when the number dropped to 400–530 patients a year. For exact numbers of hospitalized women year by year, see Schäffner, *Geschichte des Ordens und der Heilanstalt*, 195–197.

23 Křečková, Kuchařová, *Dějiny konventu alžbětinek v Praze*, 62.

24 Bogar, *Milosrdní bratři*, 192. Hlaváčková, Svobodný, *Pražské špitály a nemocnice*, 32.

permanent beds, to which number of temporary beds were added. With this reconstruction, the hospital became not only the largest in Prague, but in the whole of Bohemia. It also operated a pharmacy that supplied both inpatients and public. After the reconstruction in the mid-eighteenth century, the hospital's patients even had access to a library for convalescents.[25]

The architecture of the Prague's convent hospitals corresponded to contemporary standards. The main buildings of the hospitals, which were built in the early phase of their existence, retained their form and function throughout the eighteenth and basically the nineteenth century. From 1753, the Hospital at St. Simon and Judas (as the Prague Hospital of the Brothers of Mercy was also called) had three hospital halls for different types of diseases with a capacity of 47 (infectious diseases), 32 (chronic patients and injuries), and 24 beds (clinical teaching). The hospital also had a convalescence room with five beds, an operating theatre and two baths.[26] In the nineteenth century, the number of hospital beds stabilized, and new baths were added. Since the founding of their hospitals, both the brothers and the sisters separated infectious patients, which reduced mortality, especially during outbreaks of virulent infectious diseases (plague, typhus, smallpox, cholera).[27] In the seventeenth and eighteenth centuries, the average mortality rate was 12%, which was quite satisfactory for the time. It remained stable in the first half of the nineteenth century but rose to 22% in times of war or epidemics.[28]

In both convent hospitals, only the furnishings of the rooms changed during the period under investigation here. The main rooms were dominated by an altar, which stood in a clearly visible position at the top of the room. The beds, which stood under high windows on the long walls of the wards, had straw mattresses and curtains or canopies for a long time.[29] At the Hospital of the Brothers of Mercy, these textiles were removed in the 1840s for hygienic reasons and covered commode chairs were added.[30] In 1870, the hospital's facilities were expanded to include a surgery and an infirmary for outpatients. Joannes de Deo Sobel, the chief physician and prior at the time, began a general modernization of surgical equipment. His efforts were inspired by the modern

25 Hlaváčková, Svobodný, *Pražské špitály a nemocnice*, 34.

26 Held, *Kurze Geschichte der Heilanstalt der Barmherzigen Brüder*, 93, 96.

27 Bogar, *Milosrdní bratři*, 200.

28 Ebelová, 'Úroveň diagnostiky,' 193. Cf. Watzka, 'Die Krankenprotokolle der Barmherzigen Brüder,' 319. See also Watzka, Jelínek, 'Krankenhäuser in Mitteleuropa vor der Aufklärung', 235.

29 Národní archiv [National Archive, henceforth NA], fond [files, f.] KMB Praha, Signature [Sign.] A I., books 104–136.

30 Hlaváčková, Svobodný, *Pražské špitály a nemocnice*, 34.

methods of sterilizing instruments with iodine proposed by the Edinburgh surgeon Joseph Lister.[31]

The hospital of the Sisters of St. Elisabeth also extended over two floors and had several rooms for the sick with a capacity of 33 (main hall), 17 (minor diseases) and 12 beds (convalescents).[32] On the second floor there was a pharmacy and a smaller ward for patients with severe infectious diseases. Most of the patients were on the first floor. There was also a smaller operating theatre on the same floor, the walls of which were painted with oil paint. During epidemics, the patients could also be accommodated in a smaller adjoining room.[33] The total capacity of the hospital during the period under investigation was up to 70 beds. At some point in the second half of the nineteenth century, a small autopsy room was set up.

Both hospitals also treated outpatients with less serious injuries or complaints. Outpatients could receive bleeding, medication and ointment and have their wounds cleaned and dressed. They also maintained a dental emergency room, which was in operation at the Convent of St. Elisabeth until 1904. According to the rules of the two orders, the hospitals were for the acutely ill, and while short hospital stays were indeed the norm, some long-term patients can also be found.[34]

This brief description of the external appearance and furnishings of the Prague convent hospitals shows that both institutions were equipped in a way that corresponded to the requirements of the time. It is fair to say that they were very similar to the recently founded civil hospitals such as those in Pest and Zagreb which had to contend with the curse of charity and treatment under one roof. The main advantage of those new secular hospitals in Central European cities, was the comfort provided by their functional facilities. New type hospitals were already equipped with water pipes, sewage systems, and high-quality heating. The need to adequately heat hospital wards was, of course, also considered in church-run institutions. Staying in a heated cell came the reason, or perhaps rather the excuse, for an incident that occurred between patients being treated in the special ward for the mentally ill priests in the Prague hospital of the merciful brothers.[35] On the last day of October 1786, the mentally ill merciful brother Aventin Excelli verbally and physically attacked his confrere, seriously injured him in the head. The subject of the

31 Deo Sobel, *Geschichte und Festschrift*, 122–123.
32 Šámal, *Klášter a nemocnice*, 19.
33 Weitenweber, *Die medicinischen Anstalten*, 148.
34 Postřihač, *Dějiny kláštera a nemocnice*, 21–22.
35 NA, f. KMB Praha, box 156.

argument was allegedly a colleague's refusal to hand Excelli the key to the warming room.[36]

2 Institutionalization of Care for the Mentally Ill in the Convent Hospitals

The Prague Hospitals of the Brothers and Sisters of Charity of St. Elisabeth, like other hospitals run by this orders in Graz, Pest and Zagreb, already admitted some mentally ill patients in the early modern period.[37] In May 1769, the then Archbishop of Prague donated 10,000 gulden to the Hospital of the Brothers of Mercy to finance five beds for mentally ill priests.[38] One of the first patients to benefit from this donation was Daniel Nawik, a native of Klatovy (Klattau) and fourth-year theology student, who was admitted to the hospital for an unknown period of time from February 1773. He was assigned one of the foundation beds, probably because he was an orphan and his mother was destitute. The young man lost his mind (*Sinnverwirrung*) and was unable to continue his studies at the seminary.[39]

Unlike the Brothers of Mercy, the Sisters of St. Elisabeth received no special financial support for the care of the mentally ill. However, as early as the 1770s, the Sisters of Mercy received petitions for the hospitalization of lay women from the city councils of towns around Prague pointing out the danger that the mental disability of these unfortunate women posed to their children and husbands. In two cases, the applications were successful, and the women were committed.[40]

The status of the convent hospitals changed radically with the Josephinist reforms. In line with the older ecclesiastical initiatives, the so-called 'directive rules' (*Direktivregeln*) formed only the first part of the emerging institutional care for the mentally ill. This legislation, which reorganized medical care in the Habsburg Monarchy, was promulgated by Joseph II in the form of an edict that came into force on 24 May 1781. The regulations laid down how healthcare facilities were to be built. General hospitals were to care for poor patients and maternity hospitals were to help impoverished mothers give birth. Like other

36 NA, f. KMB, box 156. Testimony of Pater Othmar Knížek.

37 Ebelová, 'Úroveň diagnostiky,' 195. See also Watzka, 'Die Krankenprotokolle der Barmherzigen Brüder,' 329.

38 Buben, *Encyklopedie řádů, kongregací a řeholních společenství*, 368.

39 NA, f. KMB Praha, box 156.

40 NA, f. AKA Praha 1719–1948 (1949), box 4.

cities on the European continent including Pest and Zagreb, the general hospitals were also to build wards for foundlings, orphanages, infirmaries for the poor, facilities for the chronically ill, and asylums.

In addition, new imperial decrees in the spring and summer of 1783 decided that the special wards for the treatment of mentally ill priests, monks, brothers, and nuns should be set up in the convent hospitals. These decrees should be seen in the context of the emperor's broader intentions regarding reform of the Church and the clergy. In a decree dated March 3, 1783, it was stipulated that the emperor's decision should prevent ecclesiastical superiors from abusing their considerable autonomy and depriving them of any possibility of imprisoning members of their community for years under the pretext of "insanity, obstinacy or simply out of a spirit of persecution" (*aus bloßem Verfolgungsgeiste*). Should the abbots or abbesses learn of an outbreak of "insanity" in one of their subjects, they must immediately report this to the district offices (*Kreisamte*).[41]

Like the Brothers of Mercy, the Sisters of St. Elisabeth were also ordered by imperial decree in 1783 to care for the mentally ill sisters of different congregations. The Prague convent Na Slupi originally had four beds for sick nuns.[42] As more and more convents were dissolved, the situation of the older nuns worsened because there was no one to help them. The Mother Superior of the convent repeatedly wrote letters to the Provincial Government in Bohemia (*Böhmisches Gubernium*) and to the City Council of Prague's New Town, in which she refused their requests to admit mentally ill women. In the 1790s, the sisters rarely hospitalized mentally ill women from poor background from the towns of Prague and the surrounding to their convent hospitals for the reason of capacity.[43]

Both the Brothers of Mercy and the Sisters of St. Elisabeth treated patients free of charge, although the cost of caring for the religious was higher than the cost of caring for ordinary patients in other wards, especially when it came to hygiene, such as mattresses and bedding.[44] Various convent hospitals of the monarchy made use of a legally independent fund (*Religionsfond*), established by the Viennese court, which was administered by the court authorities and

41 John, *Lexikon der K. K. Medizinalgese[t]ze*, 271–272.

42 NA, f. AKA Praha 1719–1948(1949), book 4. Letter of the Mother Superior to the town hall, dated 12 March 1790: '*Sie [die Elisabethinerinnen] auch nicht in Stande Vorhand sind solche Krankheiten zu Curriren, so wäre es auch nicht wohl thunlich vier Geist Person in das allgemeine Kranken Zimmer zu unterbringen, wo die Überhäufung deren überaus schweren Kranken täglich anwachst.*'

43 NA, f. AKA Praha 1719–1948 (1949), registry of patients, book 25.

44 Some of the mentally ill patients due to their state of health and laxative effects of medications required increased care for hygiene. NA, f. KMB, box 155. *Bennenung den Gegenstände [für] das Filialirrenhaus bey den Barmherzigen Brüdern*, August–October 1815.

whose main capital consisted of the sold and auctioned assets of the dissolved monasteries. The funds to cover the costs of the Hospital of the Brothers of Mercy came as well from donations and pensions to support these so-called 'deficient priest', no longer able to perform their duties. Such regular pensions, which usually amounted to 200 gulden per year, were granted to infirm, old, or mentally ill priests by the decision of the Prague archbishop's consistory.[45]

The stay of mentally ill or troubled priests continued to be supported by nobles or town councils, who were the benefactors of the individual priests from the time of their ordination (the principle of the so-called *titulus mensea*). During this period, the church and landed nobility remained irreplaceable providers of charitable care for sick, elderly, and mentally ill religious as well as for the general population. In the late eighteenth century, the most important patrons of both hospitals were the Clam-Gallas family, led by Countess Josefa Caroline and her father Christian, Count Clam-Gallas. They regularly organized theatre performances in their Prague palace, the proceeds of which were divided between the Sisters and the Brothers of Mercy.[46] Following the principles of the Vienna General Hospital, which attempted to take over the administration of the hospitals in Pest and Zagreb, the two convent hospitals in Prague also admitted paying patients, who received better meals if they were prepared to pay for their stay.[47]

The Austrian monarchs sometimes made extraordinary donations through the provincial government. In addition, the hospitals occasionally organized fundraising campaigns, especially in times when Prague was in economic distress. During the deterioration of material conditions associated with the Napoleonic Wars, both hospitals received the attention of the ruler himself. Emperor Francis I visited the hospital of St. Elisabeth in September 1804 and donated a relatively modest sum of 500 gulden for its operation. After the convent went bankrupt in 1811, the emperor helped the sisters by covering their debts from the war years.[48] In September 1819, the Hospital of the Brothers of Mercy also received significant financial support from the ruler, who visited the Prague hospital with his wife and Crown Prince Ferdinand.[49]

45 NA, f. KMB Praha, book 529 – Kostgänger Register, 1801.

46 NA, f. KMB Praha, book 529. See also Deo Sobel, *Geschichte und Festschrift*, 116.

47 Payments were always made at the end of hospitalization and one can speak of relatively large amounts: 36 kreuzers a day in class I, 20 in class II, and 10 kreuzers in class III (the classes were defined according to patient's wealth).

48 Křečková, Kuchařová, *Dějiny konventu alžbětinek v Praze*, 64.

49 De Deo Sobel, *Geschichte und Festschrift*, 118. The dilapidated parts of the building were renovated and departments newly equipped according to various specializations (surgery, ophthalmology, internal medicine, etc.).

3 The Mentally Ill Patients in the Convent Hospitals

As for the number of patients in the Priest's House, between January 1784 and 1852, the Brothers of Mercy cared for at least 152 persons (with 181 registered hospitalizations), mostly clerics.[50] In the years 1783–1811, the ward for the mentally ill admitted 94 other secular patients. Many of them came from the lower social classes. Thanks to the foundation set up by Countess Theresa von Goltz, patients who had lost their parents (*Elternloß*) could also be admitted. However, the number of persons from the general population had decreased over time, probably due to a lack of ward capacity and their allocation to the mental asylum established at the General Hospital. The number of people admitted was certainly higher than one can found in the registers, as only partial records have been preserved for the first years of the ward's existence. Two thirds of the mentally ill priests in the care of the ward came from the Prague archdiocese, the remaining third from other three dioceses in Bohemia. The number of suspended priests was twice as high as the number of monks and religious brothers. Many Brothers of Mercy were inmates themselves because their mental state required additional care, and they were therefore unable to remain in their usual cells.[51]

In the 1780s, many members of the dissolved monasteries were transferred to pastoral ministry with lower degrees of ordination. Some adapted better than others; older and infirm members of religious orders often ended up in the care of the Brothers of Mercy. In principle, the placement of the religious in the care of the Brothers of Mercy was decided by their superiors, the responsible consistory and the order. The ward accommodated patients of all ages, from two novices to old, retired priests. Of the total number of patients (152) recorded during the reporting period, only two patients apparently volunteered for admission to the ward (due to physical infirmity and advanced age).[52]

The insufficient capacity of the foundation beds and the inadequate infrastructure were factors that the Hospital of the Sisters of Mercy in Prague had to contend with practically since its foundation. They probably also contributed to the fact that the management of convent was not prepared to admit mentally ill nuns. A vivid example of this is the case of Theresa von Eck, a Carmelite nun from the convent in Pohled/Frauentahl in Eastern Moravia. In March 1790, Sister Theresa was admitted due to melancholy, but

50 NA, f. KMB Praha, book 533.
51 NA, f. KMB, Praha, box 156.
52 NA, f. KMB Praha, book 533.

the Mother Superior of the Sisters of Mercy soon asked for consent with her release. The patient's condition was described in correspondence with the Bohemian provincial government as an unfortunate state that offered little hope of improvement due to apathy and lack of cooperation on the part of the patient.[53]

There is no information about the nun's age, her family situation before the vows or the cause of the melancholy and its manifestations. A surviving document reports that Sister Theresa originally came from the convent of the Carmelite nuns of the Lesser Town in Prague. In 1782, the convent was dissolved and most of the sisters were temporarily transferred to Frauenthal, 140 kilometers away. This involuntary move (nuns traditionally moved less between different convents than monks and friars) may have affected the patient's psyche. Theresa's presence was not welcomed, as the Hospital of the Sisters of Mercy had no room available at the time, and Sister Theresa had to be accommodated in a ward for secular patients. This was considered undesirable by the administration of the convent.[54]

In the end, the convent did not open a special ward for mentally ill nuns. However, it continued to accept mentally ill women from the general population, albeit only for a short-term treatment. The sisters also refused to care for incurable and long-term mentally ill women who would literally 'occupy' the space for other sick persons. The Mother Superior explained her refusal in the case of the hospitalized Josefa Sedlin de Vienau in her letter to the Böhmisches Gubernium of 29 October 1785. Sedlin, a presumably impoverished noblewoman, was suffering from paralysis because of a stroke. She was hospitalized in the convent hospital for over a year and her condition did not improve. Apparently, she got drunk and did not follow the hospital rules. The Mother Superior wrote that she was a drinker, slept like the healthiest of people, and everything indicated that she could live for a few years.[55]

Apart from the lack of suitable facilities for the hospitalization of mentally ill women, the negative attitude of the convent administration was probably also influenced by an ongoing conflict between the court authorities (represented by the Church Commission) and the Sisters of St. Elisabeth in the 1780s. At that time, the sisters were restricted in their traditional piety and monastic life by a decision of the emperor. The fact that the Sisters of Mercy had to repeatedly ask the provincial government for permission to accept new novices was considered particularly annoying. It was not until 1789 that an

53 NA, f. AKA Praha 1719–1948 (1949), box 4.
54 NA, f. AKA Praha 1719–1948 (1949), box 4.
55 NA, f. AKA Praha 1719–1948 (1949), box 4.

emperor's decree allowed the Prague convent to accept new novices without restriction. By this time, however, the difficult legacy of the Josephinist reforms had already given way to two decades of war against revolutionary France and Napoleon, because of which the convent had to care for many military convalescents and suffered from a lack of funds. These factors meant that the admission of mentally ill was reduced to a minimum.[56]

During the five decades covered by the research, the medical care of the mentally ill hospitalized by the Brothers of Mercy was supervised by the *ordinarius* of the hospital, i.e., a specialist in internal medicine. One of them, the Prague physician Jan Theobald Held (1770–1851), deserves special attention because he insisted that each patient should be treated according to his temperament and character. He therefore advocated individually tailored treatment. In the years 1815–1822 Held was head of the Mental asylum, which was established as part of the General Hospital in Prague. This gave him the opportunity to expand his experience in the treatment of people with mental disabilities. He played a crucial role in the beginnings of psychiatry as an independent field of medicine in the Bohemian lands.[57]

The financial and administrative operation of the ward was controlled by an "*inspector domus Presbyteri*" who was primarily responsible for the discharge of patients.[58] In the mid-1810s, the ward's average annual capacity stabilized at fifteen patients.[59] Since the foundation, the ward of the Brothers of Mercy had eighteen rooms and a large common anteroom, which was used by the patients during day.[60] It usually accommodated between fifteen and twenty patients, which meant that all beds were occupied. In the 1820s, the number of patients rose to over thirty, which probably implied that more than one person was staying in the original one-person cells. By 1823, a room for eight 'madmen' (*Zimmer für 8 Irrsinnige*) and a room for 'disruptive' patients (*Zimmer für ruhestörende Kranke*) had been in place.[61] Apparently, patients could be locked up and isolated for up to several days during their "mania". In October 1809, for example the 25-year-old secular priest Josef Kramář, who had been admitted to the ward due to mental confusion of mind and excessive alcohol consumption, wrote in his complaint to the Prague Archbishop's Consistory

56 Schäffner, *Geschichte des Ordens und der Heilanstalt*, 81.

57 Jan Theobald Held, *Fakta a poznámky k mému budoucímu nekrologu*.

58 NA, f. KMB Praha, book 115. Inventory of 3.7.1825.

59 NA, f. KMB Praha, box 155: *Rapport über den Stand der Irrsinnigen in dem Fillialen Haus bey der Barmherzigen Brüder, Juli 1815*. This number of 15 remains constant in reports for the following months.

60 Vencovský, *Počátky české psychiatrie*, 66.

61 NA, f. KMB, book 115. See also Held, 'Ausgedinge und ländliche Gesellschaft,' 94.

that he had been confined in a locked room for 17 days in the summer, because he had spent a night outside of the monastery without permission.[62]

As there was not enough space in the ward of the Brothers of Mercy, it is not clear whether religious and lay patients had separate rooms. Patients seemed to share rooms and were divided according to the severity of their symptoms. The general population was admitted thanks to additional endowments. The pressure to admit lay patients was certainly considerable, as often a high-ranking person would request it. For example, a 21-year-old 'maniac' Paulus von Dory, court clerk (*k. k. Hof Concipist*), who came from the Hungarian town of Szomba, was first admitted as an inpatient for seven months from June 1814 to January 1815 on the recommendation of Count [Michael Maximilian Franz] von Althann.[63]

Most of the patients recorded in the registers spent less than a year there. Many stayed in hospital between two and four weeks. Fewer patients remained up to three months, indicating the urgent need to admit new patients.[64] For a few persons, it is explicitly stated that they were 'cured', while several others were discharged without further details. Gottlieb Ignatius Mayer, for example, a 42-year-old merchant from Liberec, was hospitalized for mania for three and a half months, from November 1813 to February 1814, at his wife's request. He was one of the few patients who left the ward 'completely healed'.

Although the reintegration of the religious into their ministry was a clear priority of both the Court and the Church, only about twenty percent of the patients were able to return to their religious duties. Almost half of the patients died on the ward of the merciful brothers, which was quite high number in the context of the time.[65] Stephanus Brauer, for example a Benedictine monk from the Emmaus monastery, a native of Trier who suffered from dementia, was in the hospital care for 44 years, from April 1819 to May 1863. This length of stay

62 NA, f. APAII, box 1364. *Species Facti über meine Behandlung bei die Barmherzigen Brüder*, presented to consistory on 16 October 1809.

63 NA, f. KMB Praha, book 533.

64 66 of the 181 cases captured by the registers spent at most three months in the hospital of the merciful brothers and 104 patients spent here less than a year. All in all, 36% of patients admitted to the hospital of Merciful Brothers in Valtice (Feldsberg) during the second half of the seventeenth century stayed for at most 4 weeks, about 22% stayed for 2–4 weeks, and about 13% stayed 4–6 weeks; see Watzka, Jelínek, 'Krankenhäuser in Mitteleuropa vor der Aufklärung', 254.

65 Due to the high age of many of the patients, it is not surprising that 45% (69 individuals) of them eventually died at the ward. Only for 16 persons from the entire register it is explicitly stated that they were 'cured'. See Hajdinová, 'Léčba nebo náprava?', 27.

was made possible in part by the aforementioned religious pensions, which covered at least part of the costs of food and treatment.

Some patients were cared for by the Brothers of Mercy over for a long period of time; in particular, patients for whom there was no hope of recovery apparently remained in hospital until their death. The layman Johannes Hutter, who had been unable to work since childhood and suffered from 'madness', spent 58 years on the ward. He died of old age in March 1858 at the venerable age of 84.[66]

Female patients only stayed in the Sisters of Mercy Hospital for a few weeks, two to three months at most. The five-month long stay of 44-year-old Anna Tchatchkin from the Prague district of Kotzen (V Kotcích), who was hospitalized for 'hysteria' (*hysterisch*), was completely exception. During the period covered by the study, there were only two brief remarks indicating that the patient's health had improved, but details of the treatment unfortunately remained unknown.

As for the Hospital of the Sisters of Mercy, some elderly 'feeble-minded' women also died there. The sample of mentally ill female patients is unfortunately too small to be representative, but it seems that most of them were middle-aged women.[67] But there were also exceptions. For example, in early 1790, 17-year-old Anna Linderin, 'feeble-minded' woman, was admitted here for less than a month. In December 1810, 70-year-old Ludmila Kostjatin, a widow diagnosed with weakness and "*debilitas*" died 15 days after her admission.[68] Despite their primary focus, the sisters obviously not only took in sick women, but also old and poor women who had no family to care for them.

The Priesterhaus – ward in the convent of Prague's bothers served primarily as a place for medical and psychiatric-therapeutic care. During the period described here, priests characterized as 'undisciplined' were nevertheless repeatedly admitted to the ward. Their hospitalization was the result of inappropriate behavior, in particular the failure of priests to fulfil their obligations and to lead an 'exemplary moral life'. Looking at the entirety of the Prague patients examined, the more general statement can be confirmed that the care of the mentally/psychically ill in the convent hospitals of the merciful brothers was

66 Another 12 persons stayed in the hospital for over 30 years, mostly until their death. As for the following examples. See NA, f. KMB Praha, book 533.

67 Period 1790–1793: Katarina Maškin, 44 years, weak nerves (*Nerven Schwachheit*); Mariana Krankenbein, 27 years, mad (*blödsinnig*); Mariana Dlawasin, 39 years, cramps in the head (*Kopf Krämfungen*), while Barbara Seychertin (34), Eleonora Slamin (28 years), and Anna Lutzin (45 years) were all admitted for 'melancholy' (*melancholisch* or *Melancholey*).

68 NA, f. AKA Praha, book 26.

not 'mere isolation of these persons.'[69] The mental ward combined the older practice of admitting persons with inappropriate behavior with a new approach that promoted early clinical psychiatric treatment of mental disorders.

Of interest are the cases of priests who were admitted four or five times, mostly for mental health problems, but sometimes as a form of disciplinary punishment. In addition, some patients were repeatedly committed and even had to be housed in the so-called 'Georgianum', a reformatory established in 1826 in former St. George's Monastery at Prague Castle and intended for recalcitrant priests of the Prague archdiocese.[70] This was also the case of the aforementioned "recidivist" Josef Kramář, who assisted at a mass on November 29, 1821 in a drunken state and caused a scandal in a Prague church when he overturned the liturgical vessels and tried to flee from the city.[71] Kramář nevertheless returned to the *Priesterhaus*. He was hospitalized a total of four times (1809, 1815–1819, 1821–1826, 1830) and thus spend around nine and a half years in hospital.[72] His mental and physical condition deteriorated and attempts to reinstate him as a priest failed repeatedly. He was hard of hearing in one ear and rather unsteady on his feet. In the end, the doctor diagnosed him with debility.[73]

Since the nineteenth century, the ward for the mentally ill had a high turnover of patients. Several patients tried to escape from the convent hospital, which could have been due to their mental illness. In some cases, it was only a temporary desertion, in others it was a permanent departure: a 45-year-old candy seller from Kralupy, Joseph Mocker who was also diagnosed with 'mania', left the hospital in January 1815 after less than three month 'without permission'.[74] An interesting case of a joint escape of two hospitalized patients occurred in April 1823: Leopold Veselý, a 26-year-old brewer from Prague, was apparently an incorrigible runaway (*ein unverbesserlicher Auswürfling*). His accomplice, Ivan Tuček, was one of the merciful brothers who were *in correctione* at the time.[75] Another recidivist, Josef Křepelka, who was described as undisciplined and plagued by mania, complained to the consistory in August

69 18 priests (almost 10% of all patients) hospitalized in the ward for mentally ill were characterised as undisciplined. Cf. to the general statement of Watzka, *Vom Hospital zum Krankenhaus*, 68.

70 NA, f. APA II, box 1428.

71 NA, f. APA II, box. 1364.

72 NA, f. KMB, book 533 – Register of insane ecclesiastical patients.

73 Ibid. See also NA, f. APA II, box 1364.

74 NA, f. KMB Praha, book 533.

75 NA, f. APA II, box 59.

1835 about his placement in a room arrest, where 'he was condemned to inactivity and had to take care not to be beaten'.[76]

4 Treatment of Patients in Convent Hospitals

The Hospital of the Brothers of Mercy differed from the hospitals in Pest and Zagreb not only in its capacity and experienced staff, but also in the fact that it offered medical students practical training. The first autopsy demonstration was performed here in 1685 by Sebastian Christian Zeidler (1620–1689), professor at the medical faculty of the Prague University. Zeidler had set up an 'anatomy hall' in the convent hospital in 1649, allegedly at his own expense, and donated it to the medical faculty. During the Enlightenment reforms, which emphasized the need for better theoretical and clinical training, the hospital regularly collaborated with the medical faculty. In this respect, it occupied a special position among Prague's healthcare facilities.[77]

In 1761, the convent remodeled the auditorium where students performed autopsies. In the same year, the hospital began reporting all deaths from infectious diseases that occurred on its premises to the Faculty of Medicine.[78] Later, the hospital provided eight beds for students of anatomy and internal medicine. This was followed five years later by the introduction of clinical teaching in surgery: thanks to the prior willingness, clinical training could now take place in 50 beds. In 1791, however, all teaching was moved to the new General Hospital, mainly because this new facility had wards for both male and female patients. Later, the Hospital of the Brothers of Mercy had an operating theatre rebuilt, which was used exclusively for internal needs.[79]

In both hospitals, patients were cared for by trained staff. The Hospital of the Brothers of Mercy made use of the expertise of both paid secular professionals and the brothers themselves, who worked as orderlies, attendants, pharmacists and surgeons and, in exceptional cases, as physicians. At the head of the monastery were the prior and the subprior, then almoners played an indispensable role.[80] Particularly gifted brothers from the Bohemian lands were able to receive a university education at medical schools in Vienna or

76 NA, f. APA II, box. 1428.

77 Hlaváčková, Svobodný, *Pražské špitály a nemocnice*, 32.

78 Svobodný, *Pražské špitály a nemocnice*, 32. Bayer, *Beschreibung der öffentlichen Armen-Versorgungsanstalten*, 89.

79 Haas, *Das Krankenmaterial des Spitals*, 11–12. Hlaváčková, Svobodný, *Pražské špitály a nemocnice*, 32.

80 NA, f. KMB Praha, book 115. Inventory of 3.7.1825.

Prague. The main training center for hospital attendants (male nurses) was the hospital in Valtice/Feldsberg in South Moravia, the oldest institution of its kind in the monarchy (*Chirurgie und Krankenpflegeschule*). There were also specialized schools for surgeons (*Wundärzte*) in Prague and Olomouc, but both were soon dissolved as part of the state's efforts to improve surgical care in the mid of nineteenth century.

For both convent hospitals, the range of sources on the therapeutic methods used there is unfortunately rather limited, albeit quite interesting. In 1788 the Brothers' surgeons had at their disposal basic chirurgical instruments. Evidence of the Brothers' advancement, or rather their effort to equip themselves with the most modern therapeutic tools, is the fact that as early as 1794 they used an unspecified electric device to treat Colonel Kopp, who was suffering from mania. In 1825, the hospital disposed of one unspecified electric device with batteries and another electric '*Experimentalaparat mit einem Isoliertentisch und Stühle*', the exact purpose of which is unclear but could be probably related to fashionable practice of mesmerism and electro-magnetic therapy.[81] The Prague civil *Irrenhaus* did not acquire electric devices until much later, with certainty not before 1847.

In the hospital of the Sisters of St. Elisabeth, medical care was provided by a senior physician, who was employed on a fixed salary, an unpaid junior physician, a hospital surgeon, and a head nurse.[82] Medical rounds took place twice a day, at 10 am and 4 pm. If an injury or illness at St. Elisabeth's required a more complicated operation, the patient was transferred to the General Hospital. Sisters worked only as assistants to the physicians, nurses and pharmacists as they were not yet able to study medicine. Nevertheless, they were expected to learn the usual nursing tasks as well as the basic surgery and pharmacy during their novitiate.[83] The sisters looked after the outpatients in the porter's lodge, e.g. pulling teeth or treating less serious injuries, and dispensed medication.[84] Both the brothers and the nurses took care of the patients' hygiene: they took care of the bedding, clothing, food, and chamber pots.[85]

Natural disasters had left their mark and epidemics meant that more and more people needed medical help. The Hospital of the Brothers of Mercy was located on the banks of the Vltava River and its first floor was repeatedly

81 NA, f. KMB Praha, box 156 (year 1794); book 104 (inventory 1788), book 115 (inventory 1825).

82 Postřihač, *Dějiny kláštera a nemocnice*, 23.

83 Weitenweber, *Die medicinischen Anstalten*, 150. Cf. Křečková, Kuchařová, *Dějiny konventu alžbětinek v Praze*, 62.

84 Křečková, Kuchařová, *Dějiny konventu alžbětinek v Praze*, 47.

85 Weitenweber, *Die medicinischen Anstalten*, 150.

flooded in 1784, 1845, and 1891. The floods damaged the first floor of the church and the hospital buildings and affected the gardens.[86] During the Napoleonic Wars, typhus and dysentery were brought into the cities of Prague. Wounded soldiers were treated in both hospitals, and several brothers and four sisters died from these diseases.[87] In 1832, Prague was hit by the Europe-wide cholera epidemic. Both hospitals played an important role in combating this disease, as they did in 1856 when cholera returned.[88] The Brothers of Mercy were also actively involved in prevention, particularly in vaccination with the lymph of smallpox pustules.[89]

Both hospitals encountered and treated practically all diseases known at the time and were able to make a basic medical diagnosis. At the end of the eighteenth and in the first half of the nineteenth century, diagnosis was still mainly based on the observation of symptoms and their typical classification. As in other wards of the hospital, mentally ill patients were diagnosed by the senior surgeon of the hospital of Brothers of Mercy. The diagnoses corresponded to the contemporary but rather older nosological approach and show that the psychiatric science applied by the brothers did not yet take into account the variability of some disorders, in particular the alternation between manic and depressive states in bipolar patients.[90] Nevertheless, it can be assumed that the doctors at the convent hospital gradually absorbed new medical knowledge, as they had an anatomical theatre, practiced autopsies and had been holding clinical classes at the hospital for some time.[91] The gradually growing interest in the internal causes of diseases was reflected in the study of pathological

86 De Deo Sobel, *Geschichte und Festschrift*, 120; Bogar, *Milosrdní bratři*, 202.

87 Bogar, *Milosrdní bratři*, 200, 209. Křečková, Kuchařová, *Dějiny konventu alžbětinek v Praze*, 66.

88 At that time, a record number of 1,134 hospitalized women and another 2,000 female outpatients received care at St Elizabeth's. Křečková, Kuchařová, *Dějiny konventu alžbětinek v Praze*, 66.

89 NA, f. České gubernium, Zemský protomedikát, 1775–1863, book 7 Nemocnice milosrdní bratři a alžbětinky, hlášení 1790–1818; book 17 Zprávy o stavu nemocných – 1820–1830. During a prolonged smallpox epidemic in the city in 1840–1848, the hospital of the Brothers of Mercy admitted a total of 1,267 smallpox patients; see Haas, *Das Krankenmaterial des Spitals*, Tabelle, passim.

90 See Černoušek, 'Nárys historického vývoje psychiatrických klasifikací,' 78. The most frequently listed psychic issues of the religious persons admitted here were 'mania' (51), 'melancholy' (17), and 'amentia' (7), which referred to some form of 'feeble-mindedness'. Relatively common were also post-stroke states ('apoplexy', 12). Much less frequent were cases of states described as *paranoia*, *delirium tremens*, *melancholia religiosa*, *mania religiosa*, or epilepsy (2).

91 Prof. Anton Wenzl Rings, a native of Prague and student of the famous Leiden physician Hermanus Boerhaave, had held private medical course in the hospital of the Brothers of

anatomy, which was possible thanks to the above-mentioned facilities in their hospital.[92]

For the majority of surviving historical records of diseases, it is impossible to make a fully corresponding modern biological-medical diagnosis. The surviving descriptions cannot be mechanically transferred to today's medical systems.[93] Nevertheless, the terminology used in patient registers is a valuable source of information that gives some general idea of the range of diseases prevalent in the period in question. The most common in Prague convent hospitals were various infectious fevers, other unspecified multi-day 'ague' illnesses, and problems with the digestive tract. The next most common group of illnesses were those affecting the respiratory system. Other problems mentioned in the reports included a very wide range of diseases related to internal medicine and obstetrics.[94]

The care of religious persons who were mentally ill resembled the treatment of the physically ill. It was based on the satisfaction of their basic needs, i.e. sufficient sleep and rest, adequate but rather sparing regular food and fresh air. The diet was based on vegetable soups. Most patients received a 'whole diet' (*ganze Diät*) without additional portions of meat, bread, dairy products, beer or wine.[95] Some hospitalized priests complained about the quality and quantity of the food. The aforementioned Josef Kramář stated in October 1809 that: 'On cold nights, I was freezing in my damp cell and the food I received was disgusting and served on a dirty wooden board that may have been unwashed since the days of Jan Žižka.'[96] A few days ago Kramář had a conflict with the prior of the house, Vendelin Sklenczka, because of his excessive drinking. In official correspondence with the consistory, Sklenczka called Kramář as 'a notorious chatterbox' (*geläufige Zunge*).

Mercy in Prague since the mid-1730s. He also later bequeathed his library to the convent; see Kolda, 'Zárodky zdravotnických knihoven.' 219.

92 Grmek, *Histoire de la pensée médicale*, 179–194.

93 Mitchell, 'Retrospective diagnosis,' passim. Karenberg, 'Retrospective Diagnosis,' passim.

94 There were various diseases of the circulatory system, urinary systems, female reproductive organs. Some patients had parasites, external injuries, encephalitis, rheumatism, or gout. Especially the 'coughing up of blood' (tuberculosis), cough, suffocating cough, catarrh of the lungs, pleurisy, and asthma. See NA, f. KMB Praha, a series of books of patients' registers kept almost without interruption from 1620 until 1950, books no. 20 and following. NA, f. AKA Praha 1719–1948(1949), books 20 and following (since 1720). Ebelová, 'Úroveň diagnostiky,' 187–192.

95 NA, f. KMB Praha, box 155.

96 Jan Žižka of Trocnov and Kalich (ca. 1360–1424) was a Bohemian military leader of the Middle Ages. See NA, f. APA II, box 1364.

Mentally ill patients were treated according to the dietary rules of the classical humoral theory, the aim of which was to restore the balance of humors in the patient's body and mind. This was to be achieved primarily through herbs used to make infusions with laxative, detoxifying, anti-inflammatory, and calming effects, such as fermented honey (*oxymelis*). Another group of ingredients were various medicinal salts with similar cleansing or invigorating effects. The Brothers of Mercy also used a so-called 'iron water' (*aqua ferrida*), which was believed in the early modern period to strengthen and invigorate the body and the nerves. The strain on the nerves and all organic tissue in the body was treated by baths, enemas, but above all by rest during hospitalization. Bloodletting was also an important part of the treatment.[97]

Kramář's complaint also reveals that he was asked by the prior of the convent to help fetch wood and serve food at the patients' beds.[98] It is likely that further analysis of the surviving correspondence of the religious patients will reveal similar instances of requests for help in the daily running of the hospital. It is unclear whether the involvement of patients in physical labor was driven by purely pragmatic considerations, was seen as part of therapy through work, or was a combination of disciplinary punishment and healing.

It can be assumed that the treatment of the mentally ill in the Hospital of the Sisters of Mercy did not differ significantly from what was the practice in the ward of the merciful brothers. The Sisters clearly offered their patients temporary refuge from their worries and obligations, regular meals and the necessary rest. The most common diagnoses of the hospitalized patients were female hysteria, melancholia, and epilepsy. However, a partial analysis of sources from the 1810s shows a change in the situation. Whereas in the 1790s the Sisters were still hospitalizing two to three mentally ill women per month, twenty years later there were only three or four per year.[99] This decline can be explained by the changing medical and economic context of the hospital. An "insane asylum" was established in Prague as part of the General Hospital. The care of the mentally ill was made more difficult by a lack of funding, as the hospital was receiving virtually no support for further novices and interest in funding new beds for patients was also declining.[100]

The Hospital of the Brothers of Mercy (as well as the Hospital of the Sisters of St. Elisabeth) was fortunate to have relatively large ornamental gardens and

97 NA, f. KMB Praha, box 155. *Extractus Medicamentorum – Filial-Irrenhaus*, May–June 1815.

98 NA, f. APA II, box 1364.

99 NA, f. AKA Praha, book 26.

100 Schäffner, *Geschichte des Ordens und der Heilanstalt*, 84–86. See also Křečková, Kuchařová, *Dějiny konventu alžbětinek v Praze*, 63.

a recreational area for the sick (*Kranken-Erholungsplatz*), which was used for the therapy of the mentally ill.[101] Peaceful (i.e., not agitated) hospitalized religious were allowed to walk outside the hospital grounds. This was permitted on condition that they returned at a certain hour in the evening and behaved well. With the prior's permission, patients were even allowed to pursue their profession to some extent, i.e. to hold extraordinary masses and preach.[102] This benevolence on the part of the convent administration and the consistory was occasionally abused. A total of 13 (8 priests and 5 secular patients) of the 152 patients' observation in the first half of the nineteenth century had escaped from the ward. In October 1814, for example, a monk from the Prague monastery of the Knights of the Cross with the Red Star, 42-year-old Jacobus Mayer, escaped from the ward after six months. During his escape from the Prague hospital, he stole some kitchen utensils and candles.[103]

Apart from the inventory of the pharmacy at the Brothers of Mercy and a fragmentary list of medicines, research can only deduce medical practice by comparing it with the generally accepted therapy at the time. The patients of the monastery hospital were visited at their bedside at least twice a day. The core of the treatment they received was based on established dietary practice, inherited from antiquity and based on humoral theory. Its cornerstones were adequate nutrition, bed rest and often baths, hot or cold depending on the nature of the illness. Hygiene was of course important, and significant progress was made in this area. The introduction of anaesthesia in the second half of the nineteenth century also brought about some changes.[104]

The best-known physician in the middle of the nineteenth century was Coelestinus Opitz, who was also active as prior. In February 1847, he performed the first amputation of a limb under general anaesthesia with ether in the entire Habsburg Monarchy. For two decades, Opitz performed almost two hundred operations under general anaesthesia, using a simple glass vial with a cloth soaked in ether.[105] Over time, the number of secular doctors in the hospital grew, probably because the brothers had less access to medical training. From 1870s onwards, the friars were no longer able to employ religious physicians in their hospitals but had to hire secular doctors. This decline in the number of physicians from the ranks of religious orders reflected a Europe-wide trend

101 Held, *Kurze Geschichte der Heilanstalt der Barmherzigen Brüder*, 96.
102 Hajdinová, 'Léčba nebo náprava?', passim.
103 NA, f. KMB Praha, book 534.
104 Vlček, 'Nemocnice alžbětinek', 275.
105 Tošovský, *'Neboj se, nic nebude bolet,'* passim. Hlaváčková, 'Nemocnice milosrdných bratří,' passim.

towards the professionalization of medical practice in general hospitals and also manifested itself in the medical institutions administered by ecclesiastical orders in Pest, Vienna, Zagreb and in Prague.[106]

5 Conclusion

The emergence of the 'modern' type of hospital was a Europe-wide phenomenon, even if it naturally established itself in different ways at different time in Würzburg, Pest, Zagreb or Prague. The hospitals in the provincial capitals of the Habsburg Monarchy endeavored to provide the population with high-quality medical care. The state health policy aimed to examine and meticulously register sick inhabitants and then treat them, but also to educate them in better self-control and healthier lifestyles as a basic preventive measure against various diseases. After all, only a healthy population was capable of work and family life – and therefore useful.[107] Compared to the city hospital in Pest and the civil hospital in Zagreb, the convent hospitals in Prague had adequate premises from a very early stage and were able to concentrate entirely on the physical and mental care of their patients. They did not lack premises for clinical treatment and avoided the costly construction or difficult conversion of monastery buildings.

The hospitals of the Brothers and Sisters of Mercy remained indispensable for decades. This was often due to the gradual establishment of new secular healthcare facilities that did not have sufficient capacity. Equally important was the fact that broad societal strata did not immediately accept new type of hospitals. The population trusted the hospitals, which were under the auspices of the church and sought them out not only for the treatment of illness, but also for spiritual care and charity. Pregnant women with less education were more likely to turn to the nuns in convents (although male physicians also worked there, both specialized obstetricians and general *doctores medicinae*) than to the lay physicians and obstetricians in state or municipal hospitals. Patients also appreciated the fact that both the Sisters and the Brothers of Mercy supported them with their prayers.[108]

106 De Deo Sobel, *Geschichte und Festschrift*, 224.

107 Risse, *Mending Bodies, Saving Souls*, 239.

108 Watzka, *Seelenheil und Seelenleid*. It however presents an overview of the negative influence of clergy and Church on the ill with their negative view of the sinful human body being part of the strict Catholic morals. The author focuses on the period 1550-1750.

The hospitals in Pest, Zagreb and Prague, especially those administered by the Brothers of Mercy and the Sisters of St. Elisabeth, were not exempted from the Josephinian reform of institutional provision because of the high standard of medicine they could offer. The emperor's decrees of 1783, which provided the establishment of specialized wards for the treatment of the mentally ill religious, were driven by the court's (and some ecclesiastical authorities') desire to transform church institutions. The new wards were intended to care for a certain privileged group that was now under stricter state supervision because of the reforms. Enlightened priests, monks, friars and nuns were to be faithful servants of the state, and measures were taken to ensure that their moral lapses and mental disorders did not threaten the existing social order.

Thus, the wards for mentally ill religious also served as a place where clerics were interned for disciplinary reasons.[109] The hospitalization of priests who were unable or unwilling to perform their pastoral duties took the form of their long-term isolation, as their presence in public was considered undesirable by both the church and the state. In the first half of the nineteenth century, the convent hospitals continued to have a corrective function. This disciplinary aspect was supplemented by systematic therapy, which was increasingly promoted by the previously small but growing group of medical experts and civil servants who passed on the Josephinian legacy.

Although state authorities in other European cities had created a network of clinical hospitals financed by funds and providing care in close cooperation with the medical schools, the Viennese court was unable and unwilling to fully finance the operation of the convent hospitals. At the beginning of the nineteenth century, they ran into difficulties, as the number of hospitalized persons increased while the convents were chronically underfunded. The Sisters of Mercy found themselves in an even more difficult situation, as they were totally dependent on the charity of the church and the patronage of nobles and burghers.

Without public support, the convent hospitals would hardly have survived the times of economic hardship. The wars against revolutionary France and Napoleon had a negative impact on the material situation of the entire population, including the aristocratic elites, who were the patrons of ecclesiastical institutions. The convent hospitals found themselves in an extremely difficult situation due to inflation, the decline in income, and the rising cost of goods. This went hand in hand with the poor condition of their buildings, which had not been properly maintained for a long time.

109 Hajdinová, 'Léčba nebo náprava?', 14, 29, 40. Hajdinová, 'Péče o choromyslné duchovní v brněnském špitále,' passim.

In the nineteenth century, the convent hospitals in Prague were still perceived as 'places of salvation', providers of charity, consolation and contemplation. Despite this aspect of their functioning, the high level of inpatient and medical care should not be underestimated, as has sometimes been done by anti-religious contemporaries and later by historians who adopted an anti-clerical discourse. The convent hospitals treated various inmates from all walks of life and admitted secular patients if there was sufficient bed capacity. Short stays were the rule, which shows that the hospitals were geared towards specialized treatment and not just a temporary social refuge.

At the same time, clinical teaching and theoretical research into mental illness were no longer carried out in the convent hospitals: This had already been taken over by the doctors of the Prague mental asylum, as it will be presented in the next chapter. The secular doctors employed in the convent hospitals and the physicians who belonged to religious orders however met the standards of a clinical institution. The treatment at the bedside corresponded to the care that patients received in the asylum. The aim was not just to isolate patients, but to provide a wider range of treatment methods. The doctors in the convent hospitals were thus even able to go beyond their original expertise and carry out precise diagnostics. These efforts led to an advance in medical knowledge and a falling mortality rate, which helped them to maintain their position among medical institutions for many more decades than it initially seemed due to the Enlightenment's anti-religious fervor.

Acknowledgement

This study is an output of grant of the Czech Science Foundation (GA CR) no. 2204258S *Anatomy of a Suffering Soul. From the 'passions of the soul' and 'empirical psychology' to a psychiatric hospital in the Czech Lands, 1770–1814*, which has been granted to the Faculty of Arts of the Charles University (Prague).

CHAPTER 5

At the Forefront of Psychiatric Care in the Monarchy: the Prague Mental Asylum as a Model of a 'Protoclinic' in the 19th Century

Daniela Tinková

In the early 1840s, Heinrich Philipp August Damerow, a leading German psychiatrist, critically remarked that there was only one psychiatric hospital in the entire Habsburg Monarchy 'at the level of the new age': the one in Prague.[1] Michael Viszánik, a leading Austrian physician and the inhouse psychiatrist at the Vienna asylum (*Narrenturm*), came to a similar conclusion after critically noting on a research trip through European institutions for the care of the mentally ill in 1843 that there was no psychiatric hospital in the Habsburg Monarchy that met the requirements of the new era. Viszánik was disappointed with the state of psychiatric care and found words of praise for two institutions that cared for the mentally ill: the institute for people with mental disabilities in Hall in Tyrol and the institute in Prague, as the only humane and well-organized ones.[2]

In order to understand the context in which psychiatric institutions developed in Prague, it is important to look at works on the European history of psychiatry in general and in the Habsburg Monarchy in particular.[3] After all, Bohemia had been part of the monarchy for almost four hundred years, and Prague University (along the Viennese University) was one of the most important centers of education within the entire monarchy. A fully fledged psychiatric clinic was only established in Prague only in 1885, but the history of psychiatric institutions in the Bohemian capital began hundred years earlier with a mental asylum (*Tollhaus*), which was founded as part of Joseph II's reforms of welfare provision in the 1780s. And it was this *Tollhaus* that half a century later, in the 1830s and 1840s, thanks to the efforts of Prague psychiatrists, became the best-run institute of its kind in the monarchy and served as a model for similar institutions from the mid-nineteenth century. It also housed

1 Damerow, 'Einleitung,' XXIX.
2 Viszánik, *Leistungen und Statistik*, 25ff.
3 See Watzka, *Vom Hospital zum Krankenhaus*. Lesky, *Die Wiener medizinische Schule*.

 HTTPS://DOI.ORG/10.1163/9789004755062-007

the first ever psychiatric clinic. Its (former) heads and their deputies played an important role in the reform of psychiatric care throughout the monarchy.

The history of psychiatry and psychiatric institutions has a relatively long tradition of research: it is therefore not necessary to repeat it in detail here. It should be briefly noted, however that the optimistic approach of 'Whig' historiography, which interpreted the arrival of enlightened, humanistic psychiatry in the eighteenth and nineteenth centuries in largely a positive terms, was challenged in the last third of the twentieth century by the anti-psychiatric movement, which criticized the internment and abuse of psychiatric 'treatments' and psychopharmaceuticals.[4] Internment of the mentally ill was no longer seen as a largely positive and beneficial measure supported by humane motives. Instead, it was presented as an attempt to get rid of problematic elements in a society that was rapidly industrializing and urbanizing, in which the older forms of social care, especially those of the family or the church, were failing or disintegrating.

In this respect, the psychiatric internment of the eighteenth and nineteenth centuries was not seen as part of the humanistic process initiated by Enlightenment philosophy, but rather as an expression of the dehumanization of the rapidly modernizing capitalist society, as a result of an asymmetry of power between psychiatric patients and their 'doctors'. The same perspective was then applied to the previously celebrated 'discovery' of psychopharmaceuticals, and psychiatric treatment was seen more as a process of enforcing discipline. In the late twentieth and early 21st centuries, social and cultural historians brought a slightly more nuanced and sober perspective to this debate.[5] They sought to distance themselves from the question of the 'right' treatment, stating that it was best left to doctors and psychiatrists to decide. Instead, they focused on the social aspect of internment and modern psychiatry in general, for example by considering the views of the patients' themselves.[6]

Neither the history of the Prague Mental Asylum, nor the history of Prague psychiatric spaces as such has yet been comprehensively studied. Reports on the history of the Prague asylum have so far been presented mainly by Bohemian psychiatrists from the late nineteenth to the second half of the twentieth century. Their aim was to offer a self-reflection of their own field of science

4 See for instance inspiration by the works of Castel, *Le psychanalysme*. Szasz, *Psychiatry*.

5 See Dörner, *Bürger und Irre*. Blasius *Der verwaltete Wahnsinn*. passim Blasius, *Umgang mit Unheilbarem*, passim. Kaufmann, *Aufklärung, bürgerliche Selbsterfahrung und die "Erfindung" der Psychiatrie*, passim.

6 For more on reflecting upon the 'history of madness' in historiography and on the history of psychiatry, see Tinková, "Šílenství" a "psychiatrie" jako předmět kritické historické reflexe, 11–39.

and to define its significance and impact. Their view of the institutionalization of mental health care in the Bohemia tends to reflect the optimistic tone of 'Whig' historiography. Nevertheless, they emphasized the development of biological, pharmacological treatment and laid a solid foundation for future research.[7] Their work was complemented by thorough archive research in several particular areas.[8] The history of the organization and development of psychiatric institutions in Prague was later the subject of rigorous study, while other scholars have placed the development in Prague in a wider context.[9] In recent years, this topic has been explored as part of a joint project.[10]

This chapter deals with the history of the Prague Mental Asylum as an institution that was intended both to care for the mentally ill and to function as a place of scientific research into mental illness. It will describe the Prague Mental Asylum as a model institution for healthcare and propose five main stages that represent the most important steps in the establishment of any psychiatric clinic. These stages can be seen on a more general level as the institutionalization of psychiatry. All these actions subsequently enabled the creation of a fully-fledged 'clinic', i.e. an institution defined by the fusion of the purpose of a hospital with the needs and objectives of a university. In most cases, a clinic is an institution that admits inpatients, participates in both undergraduate and graduate education, is a place of research, and whose expertise and management is provided by university professors in the relevant field of science.

The chapter will focus on the period of about one hundred years in which the Prague Institute functioned as a 'protoclinic', i.e. a place that aimed to combine medical care, scientific knowledge, and the education of medical students and to realize these goals within the limits of its possibilities. It should also be remembered that it was a 'lunatic asylum', administered by the state and later by the provincial authorities – and not a university or private clinic (as was the case in Vienna) – which played a key role in the establishing psychiatry as an independent and eventually academic subject in Prague.

---

7 Heveroch et al., *Zemské ústavy pro choromyslné*. Vencovský, *Psychiatrie dávných věků*. Vencovský, *Čtení o psychiatrii*. Vacek, *O nemocech duše*. Vacek, *Velké psychiatrické případy*. Černoušek, 'Nárys historického vývoje' Černoušek, *Šílenství v zrcadle dějin*. Černoušek, *Studie k dějinám psychiatrického myšlení*. Černoušek, *Studie k dějinám psychiatrického myšlení: určeno pro odborníky*.

8 Hlaváčková, Česká a německá psychiatrická klinika, 133–159.

9 Chaloupková, *Správa a fungování Zemského ústavu pro choromyslné*. Karenberg, Lippert, 'Irrenhäuser in Prag, 331–340.

10 Daniela Tinková's work on the medicalisation of suicide are also relevant to the history of psychiatry; see esp. Tinková, 'Selbstmordstrieb auf den Leib eingeschrieben', 11–33.

As far as sources are concerned, this study is based printed materials, especially dissertations and reports in professional journals published by the heads and deputy heads (*primarii* and *secundarii*) of the Prague psychiatric institute,[11] as well as on written sources that have been virtually unused until now.[12] These include admission records for psychiatric patients, reports with information on their numbers and correspondence between officials of the asylum and the authorities, in particular the Directorate of Medical Institutions and the Provincial Governorate.

To begin with, it is important to say a few words about terminology. In European languages, different terms are used for what are now commonly referred as 'psychiatric hospital' or 'mental health institutes.' When talking about institutions in the eighteenth or nineteenth century, the terms used were pejorative to varying degrees. In English, there are therefore the terms 'madhouse', 'bedlam', 'lunatic' (or better 'mental') asylum. In German there are words such as 'Tollhaus' or 'Irrenhaus' and in Czech, 'blázinec'. In the second half of the nineteenth and in the twentieth century, less derogatory expressions were used, for example 'institute for the mentally ill' and later 'psychiatric sanatorium'.

In this study, the existing terminology was used as follows: To describe institutions that existed during the first phase of the internment of the mentally ill, at the time of the enlightened Josephinist reforms, the term 'madhouse' is used as a direct translation of the contemporary term 'Tollhaus' or the German expression. Typologically or conceptually, it describes this early form of psychiatric institution, which primarily served to discipline and maintain order, as a 'mental asylum'.

In this chapter, the term 'insane asylum' or 'psychiatric institute' is used as a translation of the German term for institution 'Irrenanstalt' that were already distinct, had their own directors, and undertook early attempts at targeted treatment. Conceptually, this corresponds to a 'protoclinic'. It indicates both attempts at targeted treatment methods and the gradual introduction of teaching (and science) into the operation of the institution, which thus gradually took on a distinctly different form. In contrast to the later 'clinics', however, these activities were still improvised, unsystematic, and based mainly on the

11 Especially Riedel, *Prag's Irrenanstalt und Ihre Leistungen*. Nowak, *Notizen über die Prager k. u. k. Irrenanstalt*. Fischel, *Prags k. k. Irrenanstalt*. See Riedel's, Nowak's, Fischel's partial reports in contemporary specialised journals.

12 Especially the following collections of the National Archives, Prague [henceforth NA]: Department I, fond [files, f.] České gubernium – Publicum [Czech Gubernium – Publicum] and NA, Chodovec branch, f. Zemský ústav pro choromyslné Praha [Provincial Mental Asylum].

individual initiative of the individuals involved (physicians who operated the facilities), as opposed to truly institutionalized, systematic, and methodical links between universities and hospitals.

1 From Tollhaus to Irrenanstalt: Institutionalization of the Prague Facility for the Mentally Ill

Until the second half of the eighteenth century, mentally ill patients received no special care. Only then did physicians and philanthropists, influenced by the philosophy of the Enlightenment, begin to demand more humane treatment for the 'insane', in particular their right to appropriate medical care. Leading advocates of this new approach were humanist reformers of psychiatric hospital care such as Vincenzo Chiarugi in Florence, Philippe Pinel in Paris, or William Tuke in York. They began to free mentally ill patients from their shackles and other restrictions and demanded not only a humane approach but also genuine treatment. They were convinced that 'madness' was not a life sentence that could and must be treated. In other words, they believed that mental illness was also a 'disease' that had its causes, whether physical or mental, which could be investigated and therefore it should also be possible to find appropriate treatment. Around 1800 *aliénistique* or 'psychiatry' (a term coined in 1808) started to be considered a branch of medicine in its own right.

Over the course of the eighteenth century, medicine began to diversify. With the growing number of medical professionals, improved diagnostics and the increasing interest of states in the physical fitness of their populations, some medical fields gradually began to crystallize and separate. They then needed their own rooms or even entire hospital buildings. This was particularly true of obstetrics, which was the first to split off from general medicine, but psychiatry (followed by ophthalmology) was also one of the first medical fields to become independent.

As far as mental health care was concerned, the inspiration came mainly from France: the first 'psychiatrists' from (Protestant) German lands usually spent several years in Paris, where they learned about the development of a more humane approach to the custody and care of people with mental disorders. In the 1820s, the first 'reformed' institutions were also established in this region. The Bohemian lands were also influenced by the reforms in nearby Saxony, which became one of the cradles of the new psychiatric care and science in Central Europe. In particular, the Institute for the Mentally Ill established at the Sonnenstein chateau near Pirna, close to the Bohemian border, played a pioneering role, and the first department of psychiatry was founded at Leipzig

University in 1818.[13] Johann Christian Heinroth (1773–1843), a widely respected figure in the German-speaking world who also exerted undeniable influence on the Prague environment, was chosen as its head.[14]

As the example of the hospital in Würzburg shows, the far-reaching changes in institutional provision were heralded by the reforms of enlightened rulers. In Vienna, Prague and later in Pest, Zagreb, and other Central European cities of Habsburg Monarchy, numerous multifunctional church foundations, monasteries and hospitals were dissolved and replaced by a network of new specialized institutions for persons requiring special care. These new institutions were to be controlled by the state, even though the ecclesiastical orders were often allowed to run their own healthcare facilities. Based on the Josephinist so-called 'directive rules' from 1781, persons in need of help were divided into different categories based mainly on their earning capacity (i.e. ability to work). Their needs were then to be met by a network of institutions with a clearly defined purpose in the provincial capitals of the Habsburg Monarchy.[15]

The mentally ill were to be given their own institution, a *Tollhaus*. This was also the original purpose of the very first separate building intended for the internment of the mentally ill, the infamous panoptical *Narrenturm*, the 'Tower of the Mad' in Vienna. However, one could not speak of treatment or 'humane conditions' here: the asylum was more reminiscent of a prison. As late as 1839, the completely shocked Michael Viszánik, whose words were quoted at the beginning, dragged several tones of chains away from there, determined to improve the degrading conditions of the mentally ill. But it was a longer process. In Prague, then the capital of the Habsburg province of Bohemia, the situation was similar.[16]

The Prague *Tollhaus* was closely linked to the general hospital and its administration and was run by its management. It also shared its medical staff: it did not have a doctor appointed specifically for the madhouse and only the orderlies were its own. Until 1828, the *Tollhaus* was managed by the senior physician (*primarius*) of the Department of Internal Medicine of the General Hospital,

13 Bach, *Die "Heil- und Pflegeanstalt Sonnenstein,"* 288–290.

14 See Steinberg, '*Die Errichtung des ersten psychiatrischen Lehrstuhls*', 303–307. Steinberg, 'Johann Christian August Heinroth'.

15 See Hlaváčková, Svobodný, *Všeobecná nemocnice*. Hlaváčková, Svobodný, *Pražské špitály a nemocnice*.

16 Nevertheless, one should bear in mind that there also existed municipal hospitals which, too, provided an asylum to the mentally ill. As an exceptional case, however, one should mention the southern Moravian town of Znojmo, which had a hospital dedicated to the mentally ill since the 15th century.

who from 1811 was usually also a professor of internal medicine at the university. One of these department heads was also the physician Jan Theobald Held, on whose initiative the name of the institute slowly changed from the pejorative *Tollhaus* to the more neutral *Irrenhaus* between 1806 and 1811. A busy schedule made it impossible for the head of the department to concentrate systematically on the care of mentally ill patients, so the *Tollhaus* was probably run by its deputy, the *secundarius*.

The first important stage in the institutionalization of psychiatric care was the gradual separation of a dedicated department from other institutions of broad-based social care and the recruitment of the hospital's own medical staff. The separation from the general hospital, probably on the initiative of the Directorate of Medical Institutes in collaboration with the Provincial Governorate, led to the establishment of the position of its own medical management in the form of a senior and junior physician (*primarius* and *secundarius*) and own nursing personnel, who could thus focus solely on the mentally ill patients. In 1829, the *Irrenhaus* was given its own management in the form of a senior and junior physician (*primarius* and *secundarius*).

The first person to be appointed head of the institute was the long-serving *secundarius* Josef Pelikán, but his tenure was short-lived. He was soon followed by Karl Damian Schroff, who began a relatively long line of notable personalities who headed the institute until the end of the nineteenth century. Both positions, that of senior physician (*primarius*) and junior physician (*secundarius*), were held by prominent figures who advocated reform and a humanistic approach to psychiatry. Their work was influenced by the reform efforts of Pinel, Tuke, or Conolly.

However, both Schroff and his successor Wenzel Friedrich Rilke did not remain in psychiatry: Schroff became professor of pharmacology in Olomouc and then in Vienna; Rilke and his *secundarius*, Nowak, decided to devote themselves to pathology. The management of the institute was thus opened up to a young doctor who had started there as Schroff's *secundarius*, and who continued their reform work: Josef Gottfried Riedel (1803–1870). During Riedel's tenure as head of the *Irrenhaus*, the Prague psychiatric institute became completely independent of the general hospital. In the mid-nineteenth century, it was placed under the director administrative control of the provincial government, and its name was changed to the Provincial Institute for the Mentally Ill (*Landesirrenanstalt*). As the Prague institute gained a significant reputation under Riedel's management, Riedel was called to Vienna in 1851 to build a completely new institute for the mentally ill in Brünnlfeld, a Viennese suburb surrounded by gardens and fields.

2 Expansion of Capacities and Acquisition of Further Buildings

As part of the implementation of the Josephinian directive to establish public hospitals, a relatively large hospital complex was built in the late 1780s in the Karlov district of Prague's New Town. It was created by adapting earlier facilities run by foundations and a monastery. Like the municipal hospital in Pest and the civil hospital in Zagreb, which were founded somewhat earlier, but whose construction was delayed due to financial obstacles, the new hospital complex in Prague included a general hospital, a maternity hospital with a foundling ward, a hospital for the disabled people (*Siechenhaus*), and a madhouse (*Tollhaus*), which was an integral part of the Josephinian compound.

The *Tollhaus* received its own new building in 1790. This three-story, rectangular site was located in the immediate vicinity of the General Hospital and was surrounded by a wall. It was the work of the outstanding engineer Franz Herget, who equipped it with a system of sewage disposal, heating- and air circulation that was unusually sophisticated for the time.[17] The facility with a capacity of 54 beds was completed in the fall of 1790 and admitted its first patients in December of the same year.[18]

The second important step in the internal organization of the institute was to expand its capacity by acquiring additional buildings in response to growing demand, which allowed for a better functional division of space, including a rational distribution of patients, whose numbers were growing rapidly. In early 1820s, the institute succeeded in acquiring the nearby abolished St. Catherine' Convent, surrounded by gardens. This made it possible to separate the less severe and treatable cases, which could (and did) receive more targeted treatment. Thus, the curable female patients were transferred from the Herget's *Irrenhaus* built in 17903 to the smaller of the two buildings, while the men were moved to the main convent building. From then on, the original *Irrenhaus* was reserved for patients who were considered untreatable, unclean, or agitated ('rabid'). Later, the adjacent St. Catherine's Church, which had been specially converted for their needs, was also available to the patients.

17 Above the entrance stands the inscription CUSTODIAE MENTE CAPTORUM. IOSEPHUS II. LEOPOLDUS II. MDCCXC. (For supervision of the mentally ill built by Emperors Joseph II and Leopold II, 1790).

18 Hlaváčková, Svobodný, *Všeobecná nemocnice*, 243–259. Hlaváčková, Svobodný, *Pražské špitály a nemocnice*, 48–62. See also Bayer, *Beschreibung der öffentlichen Armen-Versorgungsanstalten*, 48–52.

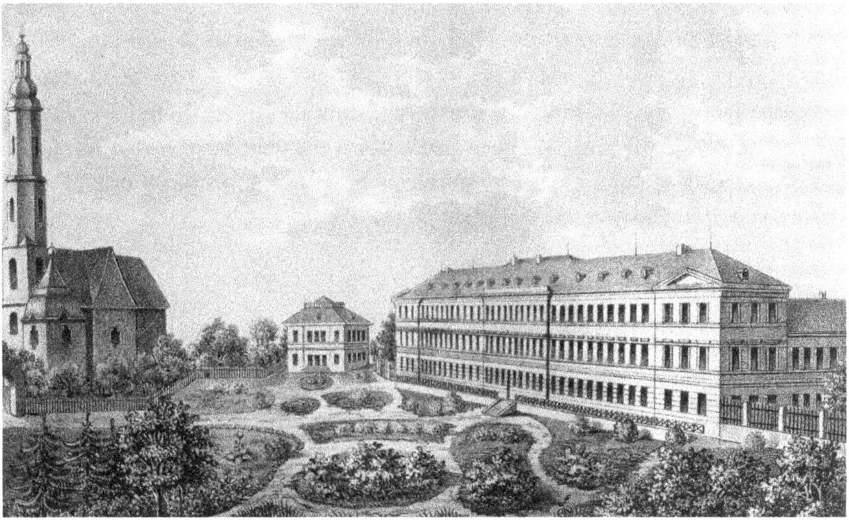

FIGURE 5.1 View of the Prague *Irrenanstalt* around 1850. In Jakob Fischel, *Prag's K. K. Irrenanstalt und ihr Wirken seit Ihren Enstehen bis incl. 1850*, Erlangen, Ferdinand Enke, 1853

In the 1830s, the capacity of the expanded institute was no longer sufficient, and negotiations began on the construction of a completely new building. Josef G. Riedel, the head of the institute, acquired both the necessary permits and the funds to erect a new, spacious building in the garden of the former monastery. It was completed in 1846, and Riedel not only proposed the design but also worked closely with the builders. All the buildings were surrounded by extensive gardens and fields, which were used by the patients for occupational and work therapy (see picture). The complex was the largest of its kind in the Habsburg Monarchy. This 'New House' (*Neubau*), as it was later called, was intended exclusively for patients capable of undergoing treatment. The building could accommodate 170 male and 75 female patients. The incurable patients were now all housed in the building of the former St. Catherine's Convent. In total, the institute was now able to treat over 500 mentally ill as inpatients, which corresponded to one-eighth of all psychiatric beds in the monarchy.[19]

After Riedel's departure, a young Austrian, Franz Köstl (1811–1882), was appointed as the new head of the Prague Irrenanstalt. He and his successor

19 See esp. Fischel, *Prags k. k. Irrenanstalt*, passim.

Jakob Fischel responded to the rapid increase in patients' number by further expanding the Prague institute. They established new branches in Prague and helped to create new institutions for the mentally ill in southern (Opařany), western (Dobřany u Plzně), and northern Bohemia (Horní Beřkovice, on the ground of the castle). All of these institutes were to receive for some of the patients that the Prague institute was struggling to care for, and they still fulfill their original purpose today.[20]

3 Division and Classification of Patients

From 1811, Jakob Fischel, the institute's assistant physician, compiled lists of patients.[21] Fischel's information shows that the number of psychiatric patients in the Prague institute increased dramatically in the first half of the nineteenth century and amounted to 4646 persons. The asylum's catchment area was mainly Prague and Bohemia in general, but patients from other parts of the monarchy were also found here, albeit rarely and in small numbers. However, there were also persons from neighboring countries and other parts of Germany. During the Napoleonic Wars, the institute even treated several Russian soldiers.

Given the majority religion in Bohemia, most of patients were Catholics. There were also a relatively small number of Jewish patients, while Protestants were rare, and most of them were foreigners, especially German speaking persons from the German lands. Even rarer were patients of Orthodox Christian denomination, namely Greek Catholics from Russia.[22]

In terms of occupation, craftsmen and tradesman made up the largest group, which is not surprising given their percentage of the population. This corresponds to the fact that most patients belonged to the third income class, followed by the category of people with no regular income. Wealthier people from the first- and second-income classes were less numerous. It can therefore be assumed that mentally ill persons from the wealthier and better educated strata of society could count more on the help of their families, who could afford a more individual form of isolation. They did not need to send their relatives to an institution, which – like the general hospital – was supposed to serve as a safety net for the poor and helpless.

20 Heveroch, *Zemské ústavy pro choromyslné*, passim.

21 Based on Fischel, *Prags k. k. Irrenanstalt*, passim.

22 NA, Zemský ústav pro choromyslné Praha (Mental Asylum Prague), ZÚs-CH Praha, kniha 10 (*Irrenhausstandesprotocoll* anfangend vom Jahre 1790), No. 1–91.

Most patients stayed in the institution for three to six months, but some stayed for many years. The mortality rate was relatively high, partly because the people who came here were old, neglected or in poor health to begin with. Most of the patients were between 30 to 40 years old. The number of men was a third higher than that of women. This is perhaps because mentally ill women generally did not pose such a threat to their environment as mentally ill men and are therefore more often cared for by their family.

For reasons of better organization and capacity of the institution, the patients were divided into several categories. On the instructions of the senior physician, the *Irrenanstalt* only admitted patients who were classified as a danger to themselves or others. This was intended to reduce the growing number of potential inpatients by limiting them to the most severe cases. However, the result was that many mentally ill patients remained at home, in the care of their families, and there is no information about them. The actual distribution of patients within the institute was mainly determined by gender and income class, which determined the standard of material care. Other important criteria were the patients' expected response to treatment and the degree of disruption they were likely to cause. It should be noted that the classification was not dictated by the patients' diagnosis, which was ultimately problematic and elusive.

After admission, the patients were divided into men and women: To maintain 'morale', each gender was assigned to a separate part of the building. The nursing staff were also separated by gender. In Herget's original building, each gender had its own floor, in St. Catherine's separate building, and in the New House a wing of this large building. The division of patients into curable and incurable patients was of central importance. On the basis, patients either received only 'care' (and were disciplined) or 'treatment', which could therefore be maximally effective. The incurable patients initially remained in Herget's building. After the construction of the New House, they were mainly in St. Catherine's, while the New House was reserved for patients who could hope for a cure or at least a significant improvement. The division of patients into *'rabid'* and *'placid', 'clean'* and *'unclean'* was supposed to ensure the isolation of 'dangerous' and aggressive patients and the special care of those who needed a special hygiene cure.[23]

As in the municipal hospital in Pest and the civil hospital in Zagreb, patients in the Prague institute were also classified according to their socio-economic status. The 'rich' and 'poor' categories determined the level of comfort, privacy,

23 Fischel, *Prags k. k. Irrenanstalt*, passim.

and quality of food. Patients in the first three classes paid for hospitalization, while patients in the fourth class did not pay on the basis of a poverty certificate. The first two classes naturally received more comfortable accommodation, more privacy and better food. The patients in the third class, which was the most numerous, usually had to make do with modest comfort, roughly equivalent to that of the patients in the fourth class.

The distinction between the educated and the uneducated sometimes coincided with economic criteria but not necessarily. This classification was decisive for the allocation of the main activity: while the members of the educated classes could mainly pursue intellectual or artistic activities and therefore had a library, art equipment, musical instruments, but also billiards, for example, at their disposal, the less educated patients were mainly occupied with manual labor, handicrafts, agriculture, gardening, etc. The 'uneducated' women worked mainly in the kitchen, in the laundry, or were engaged in handicrafts, especially in the processing of textiles. The products of their work supplemented the furnishings of institute (furniture, clothing, linen, and other items produced by the patients) or helped with the running of the institute (work in the institute's kitchen and various maintenance tasks). This work was not unpaid: the patients were paid for their work and could take their earnings with them when they were released.[24]

Since the end of the eighteenth century, European psychiatrists have attempted to classify psychiatric disorders, the best-known being French classifications systems. Unfortunately, these systems were not necessarily suitable for use in institutions dealing with actual patients. For a long time, there was no clear definition of a 'mental' disorder, not even a clear distinction between a 'physical' and 'mental' illness. Doctors asked whether a 'mental' illness was one that resulted from an injury to the brain, i.e. whether it was an organic disorder, such as epilepsy or syphilis. It clearly has physical causes, but it also affects mental health. They wondered what the connection was between a 'mania' and 'melancholia' as you often find both in the same patient: they didn´t know whether it was one illness or two.

In the first decades of existence of the Prague Institute's existence, the admission records did not in fact contain any information on the diagnosis: the illness ('Krankheit') section remained empty. This may be because the *Tollhaus* was seen as an institution whose purpose was to maintain order and provide social care. In other words, it was not necessarily seen as a medical

24 Fischel, *Prags k. k. Irrenanstalt*, Viszánik, *Leistungen und Statistik*, 15.

institution: Neither treatment nor diagnosis were as important as welfare and safety for patients and the public.

It was not until the second half of the 1820s that diagnoses began to be recorded more systematically. Based on reports from local physicians who recommended hospitalization, as well as on his own observation, the head of the institute, Josef Pelikán attempted to divide the patients into certain classification categories. In most cases, however, the 'diagnosis' was not determined immediately upon admission: the doctors were aware that different psychiatric illnesses could merge or influence each other, possibly just coexist, and, besides, the taxonomy was at that time still quite rudimentary at that time. The junior physicians tended to focus their dissertation on identifying different factors or triggering mechanisms without aiming for any kind of monocausal explanation, and their ambitions in terms of establishing of diagnosis were rather modest.

In contrast to Riedel's comprehensive classification, which ranged from feeblemindedness over general 'insanity' with fixed ideas and was based on the textbook by the influential Leipzig psychiatrist Heinroth,[25] the Institute's regular reports only distinguished between 'idiocy' (*anoia*) and various types of mania, melancholia, and epilepsy, which were easy to differentiate.[26] The Prague doctors were well aware of the possible connection between mania and melancholia and knew that the two conditions could manifest themselves as two poles of a disorder (today bipolar disorder).

The doctors at the Prague Institute were not interested in the diagnosis as such, but in circumstances and factors that could have contributed to the development of the mental illness. To this purpose, they prepared a very detailed manual for the local medical professionals, whose opinion was to supplement the application for admission of a particular person to the Prague institute, for the preparation of a thorough anamnesis of potential patients. If provincial authorities – members of the police, the estate administration (reeve or magistrate), and the medical experts – came to the conclusion that a person was mentally ill and should be interned in the Prague institute, they had to attach six basic documents to their application.

---

25 Heinroth, *Lehrbuch der Störungen des Seelenlebens*, 153, § 194.

26 Josef Riedel in his 1830 study presents information covering the past three years (1827–1829), when he worked in the Prague institute. In tables for 1826, he thus based on older records uses the following classification: *Blödsinn* (feeble-mindedness/idiocy; 43 persons), *Fallsucht mit Geisteszerrüttung* (epilepsy with a confusion of mind; 22 persons), *Manie* (mania/rage; 67 persons), *Melancholie* (45 persons), *Allgemeiner Wahnsinn* (general madness/hallucinations; 10 persons), *Fixer Wahnsinn* (madness with fixed ideas, etc.; 12 persons). See Riedel, *Prag's Irrenanstalt und ihre Leistungen*, 42.

Four of these documents concerned the patient's material care (residence, financial situation): Based on this information, the patient was placed in a certain class and a fee was set or it was decided that the person was poor and not have to pay. Two further documents were then issued by medical professionals: the first by the family doctor or surgeon who was familiar with the sick person's condition, the other by an 'official' (regional or municipal) doctor who would attach an 'official' report justifying why this person should be admitted to the psychiatric institution. From the very first trip to the psychiatric institution, future patients were therefore accompanied by an anamnesis, which in the words of the junior physician Jakob Fischel, formed – a 'double image' (*doppeltes Bild*). The first part contained the patient's medical history, the other a description of the patient's current condition. The doctors and physicians who prepared such reports were, as mentioned above, provided with clear instructions for their preparation.[27]

In addition to the basic information about the date and place of birth, the medical history should also contain details about the mental state and temperament of grandparents, parents and siblings. Of particular importance, of course, was any occurrence of mental illness in the family, its nature and duration, as well as information about suicides, including probable causes or triggers. More detailed information about the parents was also considered relevant, such as their age and health at the time of the patient's conception, the influence of 'passions', lifestyle, various injuries or happy and unhappy events in the expectant mother's life at the time of conception. Other questions investigated the patient's birth history, the number of children in the family and their physical state or cause of death.

The physicians were even interested in nutrition in early life and childhood diseases, including those that could damage the nervous system. Childhood and adolescence were examined with different questions.[28] The following section focused on the circumstances of marriage, whether it was for mutual sympathy and inclination (*Neigung*) or other reasons, what the relationships were like between the couple and between the couple and their children, what the course was (for women) of their pregnancies, births, deliveries, and weaning.

---

27 See Fischel, *Prags k. k. Irrenanstalt*, 89–91. Similarly, also Riedel, *Prag's Irrenanstalt und Ihre Leistungen*, 113–119.

28 As: formation of reason, phantasy, religiosity, education, clothing, treatment of the child by its parents, the onset of puberty, menstruation, its disorders, and possible nervous conditions linked to them, satisfaction of the sexual drive with special focus on masturbation, its duration, and intensity, extramarital children and other excesses, the influence of reading materials, bad company, or bad examples, but also for instance the effect of seclusion in a convent or monastery.

There were also sections on 'passions', 'household circumstances' and 'various happy circumstances.' Other questions related to the potential patients' material provision and their occupation or sources of income.

This was followed by the 'second image' in the form of a description of the manifestations of the current illness, the forms of contact with the patient and medical care provided in the past and its outcome.[29] This protocol included a physical description of the patient, in particular elements that may indicate illness, such as the color of the cheeks, the shine of the eyes, the state of the pupils and function of the sensory organs. The prevailing mood, inclinations, affects, passions and personal characteristics were also relevant. The doctors even measured the temperature of various parts of the patient's head (!).[30]

In stark contrast to these maximalist claims formulated by the Institute's physicians, the actual reports submitted by rural healthcare professionals were much shorter and less detailed. They were usually based on the author's knowledge of a particular patient and their family, although most patients spoke to the doctor in person and often had no problem describing their past lives in detail. The doctor then sometimes confronted their statements with those of family members, the local priest or other local authorities.

The records of the *Irrenanstalt* show above all what behavior tended to be perceived as 'madness'. Due to the limited capacity of the institute, its management emphasized that admission was only intended for people who had become dangerous to themselves or others – and only if their condition promised prospects of improvement. An analysis of some of the admission records from the 1830s does indeed show that a large proportion, perhaps even the majority, of patients drew attention to themselves through aggression towards others or suicide attempts. In such cases, the authorities were usually called in, who then also contacted a doctor or a surgeon. In cases of attempted suicide or injury to another person, it was usually the surgeon who had been called in to treat injured person who subsequently suspected a psychiatric disorder. Another group of patients those who were already 'visible' to an authority, usually either in prison or in the army. These people had not a family network to back them up, so the path to institutional care was usually shorter.

Then there were also patients who had obvious health problems, even physical ones, for which either they themselves or their relatives went to see a local medical professional, usually a surgeon. So relatively common were

29 Fischel, *Prags k. k. Irrenanstalt*, 91–92.
30 Fischel, *Prags k. k. Irrenanstalt*, 90–92.

cases where someone had suffered an injury – usually to the head[31] – and their behavior and way of thinking changed as a result. The doctor usually took note of this, and if the thinking and behavior did not return to normal, he considered hospitalization. Similarly, in cases of chronic or acute illness or pain, which led the patient to see a doctor, the physician could then monitor any changes in the patient's behavior.

Interesting in this context is the case of Franz Rustler from Milíkov (Miltigau) near Cheb (Eger), in Western Bohemia, who went to the care of the local estate doctor after suffering a spinal injury in a fall from the attic. The surgeon gradually began to unravel the story of his life, which was unproblematic until his dismissal from service as a farm laborer. It was at this point that he allegedly began to show a 'propensity for theft'. His thefts seemed particularly odd because Rustler made no attempt to hide the stolen items and was not at all concerned about whether he might be observed. Furthermore, he did not even attempt to use the stolen property, such as a pipe filled with tobacco. In this case, no one would probably consider committing him to a mental institution if the surgeon had not taken the initiative.[32]

This touches on another group of persons whose behavior or thinking did not conform to existing norms and who not infrequently pushed the boundaries of what was acceptable in daily life. Then there was a wide range of different manifestations of madness and confusion that the family (or the community, if the person had no relatives) could not cope with. In such cases, the request for hospitalization was usually made by the local authorities in collaboration with the local doctor or surgeon, who then turned to the regional (municipal) physician for an opinion.

When a local doctor or surgeon began to investigate such behavior, the initiative for internment usually came from him. The Suchards from Rumburk (Rumburg, Romjbor) in Northern Bohemia, for example, complained in September 1837 about their own adult son who was apparently mistreating them. Their complaint was eventually supported by medical experts.[33] In the summer of the same year, Josef Hübner, a carpenter, complained about the 'dangerous madness' of his wife Veronika, who apparently destroyed the household furnishing and even made noise in the street. Josef Grosse, a doctor from Frýdlant

31 Riedel, *Prag's Irrenanstalt und Ihre Leistungen*, 73ff. In the year 1829, Riedel described the case of a laborer B. M. who suffered an injury to the head when carrying a heavy log. Since that time, he had a constant urge to destroy things. In the institute, he had apparently recovered.

32 NA, f. Provincial Mental Asylum, carton [box] 8, not foliated, 1836, Franz Rustler.

33 NA, f. Provincial Mental Asylum, box 8, not foliated, report from September 1837 and following, Josef Sucharda.

(Friedland), wrote a report, in which he concluded that the woman in question was 'indeed mad (*wahnsinnig*) and harmful (*schädlich*) and dangerous (*gefährlich*)', to her surroundings, which was the criteria for hospitalization.[34]

Another theme that emerges from the admission records is the suspected causes or rather factors and circumstances that led to the mental illness. In some cases, the life or future patient was influenced by negative personal events or circumstances. In the case of several women, it was an unhappy marriage,[35] abuse by the husband or the death of a child.[36] Long-term stress, deprivation, or sudden tragic events led these women and mothers either to deep melancholy, bordering on complete apathy, or in 'madness with delusions.' These 'delusions' could manifest themselves, for example, through excessive religiosity, conversations with the deceased persons, or feelings of guilt, sometimes linked to the conviction of possession by the devil or despair over eternal damnation.[37]

In their reports for Prague, Austrian and German (Berlin-based) medical or psychiatric journals, the Prague physicians attempted to describe in detail the characteristic features and symptoms of certain diseases in detail using specific cases, but their efforts did not end there. They investigated various pathogenic factors that could have triggered the disease or at least facilitated its progression. They were aware that some of these factors could be purely physical (e.g. in diseases caused by brain dysfunction or injury) but also purely psychological. Prolonged financial problems or trauma related to a sudden emotional shock from the death of a loved one or unhappy love could therefore be as important as the brain damage related to 'idiocy' or epilepsy. Various hypotheses were then either confirmed or refuted by the autopsy if the patient died while still in the hospital. The Prague *Irrenanstalt* thus became a genuine

---

34 NA, f. Provincial Mental Asylum, box 8, not foliated, report from August 1837, Veronika Hübner/ová.

35 See Riedel, *Prag's Irrenanstalt und Ihre Leistungen*, 50–59. Riedel describes the case of a woman, 24 years old, admitted to the institute in December 1829. After her stay in the hospital, where she was treated for gloom and melancholy persisting for six years (the entire time of her marriage), she apparently returned home 'cured'. It should be noted, however, that shortly afterwards she got divorced. Also see Riedel, *Prag's Irrenanstalt und Ihre Leistungen*, 80–86. In the year 1828, Riedel outlined the case of a 24-years-old W.B. who became melancholy in marriage with a brutal drinker. See also Riedel, *Prag's Irrenanstalt und Ihre Leistungen*, 88–96. Riedel mentioned a case of 'utter loss of will' in F. K., a female servant who had been seduced and then abandoned.

36 Riedel, *Prag's Irrenanstalt und Ihre Leistungen*, 77ff. In the year 1828, Riedel described the case K.R., eventually qualified as a case of 'religiöse Melancholie'.

37 Riedel, *Prag's Irrenanstalt und Ihre Leistungen*, 105ff.

'research laboratory' that produced enough 'empirical material' to be able to make comparisons and generalizations.

4 Disciplining and Healing

There was a gradual change from an institution whose purpose was to protect 'public order' to a fully-fledged 'hospital'. Originally disciplinary measures and the emphasis on maintaining order changed to attempts to find treatment norms based on non-violent methods without the use of restraints. This was related to the introduction of new treatment methods. For most of the time, one cannot really speak of 'treatment' in the sense of therapy. What existed were merely different ways of dealing with patients. Moreover, there was no direct link between the way patients were treated and their diagnosis. The main objectives of such treatment were, essentially disciplinary in nature. There focus was on calming the agitated or 'rabid' patients and stimulating the apathetic, e.g. the melancholics. To this purpose, European institutions for the mentally ill around 1800 used various old and completely new means and methods. In addition, all 'insane asylums' had various restraining devices such as belts to strap patients down (usually to their beds) and straitjackets.

For the first decade of the Prague asylum, there is no detailed information about the methods used. It is known that 'raving' patients could be immobilized by handcuffs attached to the bed. Around 1830, there was a special room for the spinning chair, a device invented around 1810 by the English physician Joseph Mason Cox. Its purpose was generally to 'expel' harmful thoughts and induce vomiting, thus also cleansing the body. For the Prague Institute, such a swivel chair was apparently based on the model of the German psychiatrist Christian A. F. Hayner.

The Institute also had special leather gloves for onanists who were to be under special supervision. They wore a straitjacket at the same time – including women[38] who showed 'tendency to onanism'.[39] Such patients were even accompanied to the toilet by nurses and had to sleep in leather gloves. Various 'aberrations' of sexual life – which Riedel and Nowak usually referred to as erotomania, nymphomania or 'excessus systematis sexualis' – were also treated by daily cold baths and cold showers, particularly directed at the crotch. A gifted and educated 23-years-old student, in whose case the doctors (the report was

38 See Nowak, *Notizen über die Prager k. u. k. Irrenanstalt*, 50–59.

39 On this more generally Riedel, *Prag's Irrenanstalt und Ihre Leistungen*, 24.

written by Nowak) came to the conclusion that the main cause of his nervous breakdown, apart from a melancholic and contemplative nature, was the above-mentioned onanism, thus had to sleep with leather gloves on his hands in addition to the above-mentioned straitjacket.[40] After six months of this treatment he was apparently cured.

At this time, various strange procedures were carried out with the aid of 'pain-inducing apparatus' (*schmerzregende Apparat*). The aim was apparently to deliberately inflict pain in order to awaken the patient (especially a melancholic one) from a state of 'self-absorption' (*Insichversunkenheit*).[41] For example, Riedel repeatedly mentioned the pulling of their hair cord (*Ziehen des Haarschnur*), referring to an operation in which a cord was threated under the skin at the back of the patient's neck: It was used, for example in the treatment of epilepsy patients.[42] The so-called 'Autenrieth balm', an irritant concoction based on potassium tartar, had a similar effect: it was applied to the shaved skin on the head or neck, where it caused painful irritation by inducing inflammation and necrosis with swelling. In principle, it could have been aimed at 'Brownian' stimulation of apathetic (asthenic) patients.

Riedel's dissertation also repeatedly mentions of classical the 'antiphlogistic' treatment, which included bloodletting, the use of leeches, but above all the prescription of various types of purgatives (laxatives or emetics used for *Eckelkur*, i.e. induction of vomiting) for the purpose of 'cleansing' the patient's body. These were used in combination with a relatively strict diet.

After the 1830s, both the senior and junior doctors proudly claimed that no (literally) 'torturing' instruments were used in the institute and that of the restraining instruments, only straps and straitjackets were in use for raging patients. They introduced a system that became known as the 'non-restraint system.' Various hot and cold-water application had been available for physical stimulation since the 1820s. For this purpose, the institute had converted several rooms on the first floor of the former convent of St. Catherine and later in the New House. From 1847, the institute also had an electromagnetic device for stimulating the neuromuscular apparatus by galvanic (direct) current.

A far more important group of 'treatments' was based on dietary change and discipline, i.e. a strict daily regimen and work. The treatment focused on three aspects: Firstly, isolation, i.e. removal from the previous environment, which was seen a crucial 'pathogenic' factor that had contributed to the development of the illness. It was believed that continued residence in such an environment

40 Nowak, *Notizen über die Prager k. u. k. Irrenanstalt*, 50–69.

41 Riedel, *Prag's Irrenanstalt und Ihre Leistungen*, 96–102.

42 See for instance, Haarseil, https://de.wikipedia.org/wiki/Haarseil (accessed 19 May 2018).

would only exacerbate the sufferer's condition. Secondly, there were coercive measures aimed at preventing undesirable behavior (outbursts of rage, vandalism, screaming, onanism). To this end, patients were tied up in straitjackets or strapped to beds. Thirdly, the way of life and the daily rhythm were changed, with strict regularity being observed. This aspect of the treatment was based on the principles of classical (ancient) dietetics, i.e. the regulation of the 'six things not inborn'.

Instead of locking patients to their room, emphasis was placed on them spending time in fresh air. For this purpose, the patients had several gardens and even a field at their disposal. As far as nutrition was concerned, the patients were served moderate portions at regular intervals. The main staple foods were thin soups and vegetables: dairy products and meat were only served to supplement the diet. Patients were also sedated with various medications and emetics and laxatives were still used to 'cleanse' the organism. Since the 1840s, there have also appeared records of regular drinking of mineral water from various parts of Bohemia.[43] Exercise was provided by regular work, which was seen as a central aspect of the treatment regime. Work therapy formed the core of the Prague Institute's therapeutical approach.

The emphasis on activity has been found in various European psychiatric institutions since the late seventeenth century and it is also known as 'occupational therapy', 'treatment through work' or 'ergotherapy'. In Prague, patients were kept busy with agricultural activities that took place in the Institute's gardens. This approach was based on the belief that patients' minds and bodies should be kept busy. The doctors emphasized that a body tired from work can rest better and achieve a better sleep, which has a positive effect on the healing of the soul and prevents any fights. Rest and sleep were precisely defined and took place at regular times. Craftsmen had various tools at their disposal, while women were usually offered work in the kitchen, maintaining the house, or light manual labor, especially with textiles.

By working in the garden, helping in the kitchen, making furniture or sewing clothes and bed linen, the patients personally contributed to the furnishings of the Institute. They were also paid for this work, so that most patients received at least a small amount of money that they had saved up when they were discharged. Members of the educated classes could use a 'carefully furnished' library with literature on geography, natural sciences, and other subjects (although religious literature was deliberately not available). The Institute also had musical instruments: aside from string instruments, in addition to string

---

43 Viszánik, *Leistungen und Statistik*, 28. Riedel, *Erfahrungen über die Wirksamkeit*, passim.

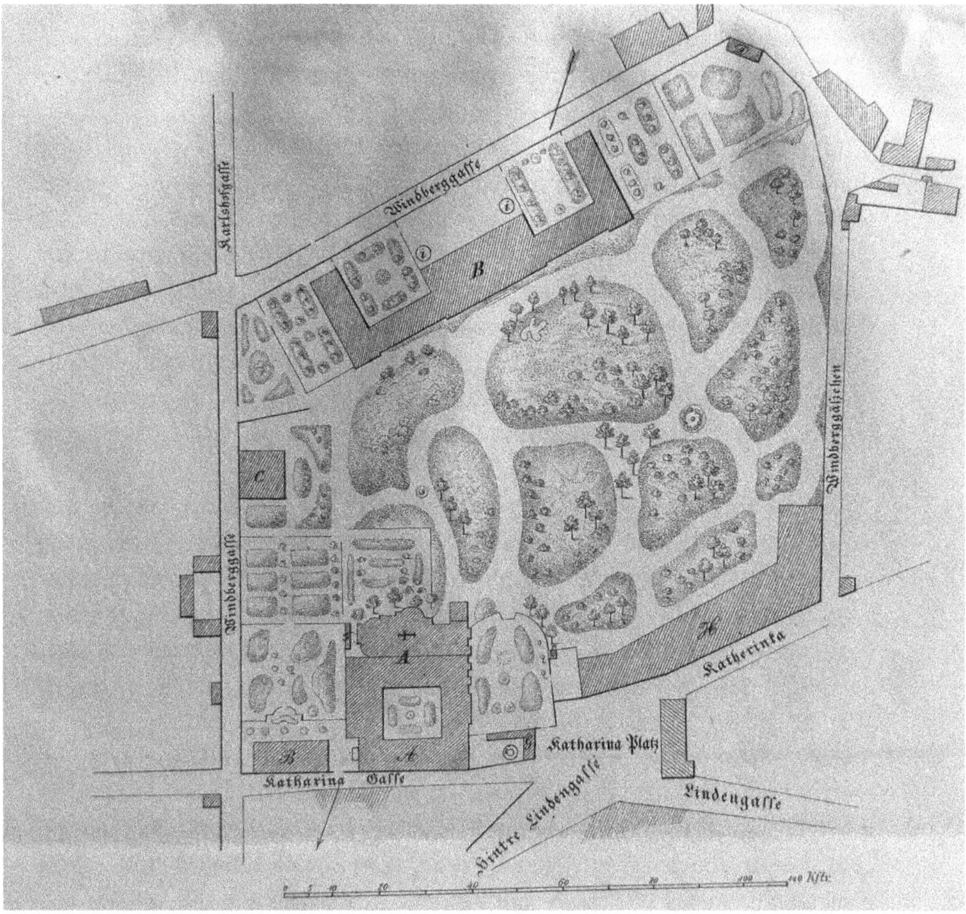

MAP 5.1 Situation plan of the Prague *Irrenanstalt* around 1850. In Jakob Fischel, *Prag's K. K. Irrenanstalt und Ihr Wirken Seit Ihren Enstehen Bis Incl.* 1850, Erlangen, Ferdinand Enke, 1853

instruments, three pianos were mentioned in its inventory. Patient concerts were apparently a regular part of life in the Institute.[44]

Excretions were carefully tracked and recorded. Their regularity or absence was clearly connected associated with a mental disorder (e.g. menstruation in women), while a return to regularity was seen as a prerequisite for the healing of the soul. The elimination of all elements that could cause 'passions of the soul', i.e. strong emotions, was also considered important. It seems that this was also the reason why some 'acute' patients were initially confined to

44 Nowak, *Notizen über die Prager k. u. k. Irrenanstalt*, 24.

darkened isolation room and on admission and only transferred to 'friendlier' (*freundlich*) room once they had shown some improvement. This regular cure was intended to free the patients from their previous condition, in which they had succumbed to various 'passions and excesses.'

In general, strict discipline was expected throughout the premises and there was a clear emphasis on regular structuring of space and time. A detailed schedule was drawn up for each day and each category of person had their clearly defined role. Finally, this also applied after to the nursing personnel, who had to meet high moral and disciplinary standards. It is no coincidence that Riedel was tried to give preference to hiring former soldiers: they were used to discipline and often also had the necessary physical strength. In short, order and regularity, work and light exercise were viewed as the prerequisites for regaining the lost harmony of the mind, which was closely linked to restoring balance to the body.

During the period under study, one can trace the transformation from an institution based mainly on disciplinary measures and methods of subjugating patients to one that sought to improve the mental state of hospitalized persons. At the same time, a clear difference becomes apparent between the 'care' of incurable patients and the 'treatment' that developed through the introduction of new treatment methods for patients who were considered curable. The 'treatment' consisted of a combination of strict disciplinary measures (isolation, reassurance, pacification) and classical dietary rules that were not specific to mental disorders but were considered the backbone of any treatment. These included various methods that today are more commonly referred to as 'leisure activities' or 'wellness.' Other methods were based more on the Brownian concepts of sthenia and asthenia, where the aim was to stimulate the apathetic and calm the restless or angry. This was achieved using some pharmaceuticals but also through baths, showers and electrotherapy.

5 Institutionalization of Psychiatric Training

The hospitals in Pest and Zagreb presented so far have drawn attention to the emphasis that the enlightened reformers placed on clinical teaching. This legacy of the Enlightenment was also found in facilities for the mentally ill. From 1821, various 'Habsburg' medical schools started to introduce lectures in psychiatry given by professors of internal medicine. In Prague, such lectures were probably organized at irregular intervals in the *Irrenhaus*, which the professors of internal medicine visited regularly. Unfortunately, the content, frequency or academic level of these lectures remains unknown. Twenty years later, Josef

Gottfried Riedel, the senior physician of the *Irenhaus*, successfully applied for permission to offer optional lectures in psychiatry. Riedel was appointed a public lecturer – the first (private) associate professor (‘*Dozent*’) of psychiatry in the monarchy.[45]

Riedel’s lectures took place twice a week in the *Irrenhaus*. Their attendance is only documented by fragmentary lists of students who attended compulsory and elective lectures in 1842, 1843, and 1844.[46] The lectures were probably intended for graduates of medical and surgical studies, whose education they were intended to expand. Younger students, medics, rarely attended. Most of the participants were aged 26- and 30-year-old, with the youngest being just 21 and the oldest 40. In 1842, the first year these lectures were announced, a record number of 19 students had enrolled, but only nine attended regularly (five physicians, two medical graduates without an academic title and only two physicians).

It was a ‘department without a chair’ and Riedel taught for free of charge. Later, such voluntary courses were organized by Riedel’s successors. In 1864, Franz Köstl succeeded in obtaining an extraordinary professorship for psychiatry – at a time when a similar, partially ‘systematized’ department was being set up in Vienna by Professor Maximilian Leidesdorf. The full professorship followed in 1873/4 and the person who received it was Jakob Fischel (who was appointed practically parallel to the better-known Theodor Meynert in Vienna).[47]

It was not until 1885 that first fully-fledged university psychiatric hospital (clinic) was established in Prague. This was fifteen years after Vienna, the capital of the monarchy, where a psychiatric university hospital had been transformed under the direction of Theodor Meynert from the Provincial Institute for the Mentally Ill (*Landesirrenanstalt*) in Brünnlfeld in 1870. The original founder of the Institute, Josef G. Riedel had died that year.

Unsurprisingly, the Prague psychiatric clinic was established in the building of the New House of the Prague *Landesirrenanstalt*. It consisted of two clinics, because in 1882 the Prague University split into a Czech and a German part, and the analogous ‘dualism’ was then applied to all its parts. The German psychiatric clinic was headed by Arnold Pick (1851–1924), a prominent Prague psychiatrist of international renown, while the Czech clinic was headed by Benjamin

45 Second was the physician and poet Ernst von Feuchtersleben, who was appointed Dozent of psychiatry at the University of Vienna in 1843.

46 Archiv Univerzity Karlovy [Archive of the Charles University, AUK], f. *Verzeichnis der ordentlichen und aussenordentlichen Vorlesungen, welche an der Universität zu Prag gehalten werden*, box 89, 90.

47 See Hlade, *Theodor Meynerts (1833–1892) Physikalisierung des Ich*, passim.

Čumpelík, the founder and leading figure of Czech psychiatry. Seventeen years later, in 1903, psychiatry became a mandatory subject for all medical students: the lectures were held five times a week during the summer semester. In short, this time witnessed the birth of a 'clinic' which, like its Viennese counterpart, could build on a century-long gradual formation of psychiatry. It took place primarily in this 'protoclinical asylum' and not at a university.

6 Conclusion

This chapter traced the changes that this 'protoclinic' underwent over the course of a century, from 1790 to 1885, before it became a fully-fledged 'clinic', i.e. a university hospital. During this period, the Prague *Irrenanstalt* was transformed from a disciplinary institute focused on social welfare and charity into a place of treatment, but in a certain sense also into a research institution. This process was followed in five stages of development, focusing on innovations that took place mainly in the first half of the nineteenth century.

First, between 1790 and 1850, the Prague Institute for the Mentally Ill gradually gained full independence from the Prague General Hospital and other institutions of social and medical care. It was placed directly under the provincial government and was given its own medical staff in the form of a senior and junior physician (*primarius* and *secundarius*) as well as nursing staff, who were thus able to concentrate fully on the mentally ill patients.

Secondly, towards the middle of the nineteenth century, the Prague Institute had several buildings at its disposal, which enabled a functional organization of the premises and the distribution of patients: The Herget's building from 1790, which housed incurable and problematic patients but was gradually abandoned, modified facilities of the former convent of St. Catherine, which were used for incurable patients; and finally a new building, the so-called New House, which had been erected in the gardens of the former monastery and was intended for patients receiving more 'targeted' treatment. In the mid-nineteenth century, the Institute expanded into further premises and acquired branches outside Prague. This expansion of the Institute's capacity was a response to growing spatial and medical requirements.

As already mentioned, the smooth operation of the Institute was supported by the organization and classification of patients. The distribution of patients within the Institute's premises was based primarily on their gender and income class (wealth), which determined the quality of the material care they received. Other important criteria were the curability of the patients' affliction and whether the patient in question was disruptive (by being 'unclean', 'noisy' or 'agitated'). At this stage of the Institute's development, diagnoses played a subordinate role, were formulated rather cautiously and generally. The doctors of the *Irrenanstalt* were primarily interested in the circumstances and factors that could have contributed to the occurrence of the patient's mental disorder.

The Prague *Irrenanstalt* was gradually developed from a 'disciplinary' institution into a 'hospital' where efforts were made to provide appropriate treatment. From the initial disciplinary and restrictive measures through some topical and more brutal 'reform' efforts, by the 1830s and 1840s at the latest, the doctors working in hospital arrived at a combination of disciplinary and dietary measures, the use of an electromagnetic machine, but above all occupational therapy and psychological methods. The 'treatment' was mainly based on strict discipline and diet with an emphasis on activity and work, which were further combined with various other therapeutic methods such as baths, showers or electro shocks, but also drugs and mineral water. Nevertheless, there were already indications to relatively drastic restraining or stimulating (irritating and generally quite painful) measures in the 1830s. No general conclusions about the possible use of psychological methods can be drawn from the surviving sources – therefore it is not yet possible to speak of specific 'psychiatric care'.

The Prague *Irrenanstalt* played a key role in the establishment of psychiatry as an academic discipline. The first lectures on psychiatry were held here in the 1820s and private lessons were given here from 1841 at the direct request of J. R. Riedel, i.e. since Riedel became the first lecturer (*'Docent'*) in psychiatry in the Habsburg Monarchy. In the 1860s and 1870s, the senior physicians of this institute, Franz Köstl and Jakob Fischel, were appointed extraordinary and later ordinary professors of psychiatry, and after 1885 two psychiatric university clinics were established in Prague. It should also be mentioned that it was an (initially state, later provincial) 'madhouse', an institution intended to help the poor who could not afford their treatment, and not a university or some private sanatorium, which played a completely irreplaceable role in the establishing psychiatry as an independent and ultimately academic discipline in Prague. In the second half of the nineteenth century, this institution served as a model for other provinces of the monarchy and other institutes were modelled on it: in various parts of Hungary, but also in Vienna, thanks mainly to Josef G. Riedel, who was appointed to the imperial capital for this purpose. Other institutes were then founded by his students or former assistants such as Josef Čermák, who transferred the Prague experience to other places and situations.

The Prague Institute accepted patients based on an expert opinion drawn up by the relevant local health officials. Potential patients had to fulfil several key criteria: They had to be a danger to themselves or others and there had to be some hope of recovery. From the chief physicians' reports and other records, it appears that most patients came from the lower social strata. This is indicated by the fact that most patients belonged to the income third- and fourth-income classes, i.e. the groups of patients who paid little or nothing for their treatment. It can be assumed that wealthier and better educated patients preferred private treatment to public facilities.

The senior and junior doctors at this Institute tried to gather as much information as possible about their patients as possible and to systematize what they had learned about mental illness and ways of treating. Even if they did not produce large scientific volumes or groundbreaking studies, and even if they did not become university professors and their lectures were not part of the compulsory program for medical students, their meticulously recorded empirical observations and protocols, as well as the reports published in professional journals, had undoubtedly contributed to the development of a new science: psychiatry.

The heads of the Prague Institute regularly published their reports in medical journals in Vienna and Prague, but also in the first German journal devoted exclusively to psychiatry. In this way, they naturally wanted to draw attention to the strengths of the Prague Institute they were establishing, but also to contribute to the knowledge about mental illnesses and their optimal treatment. From the very beginning of their reform efforts, they were therefore actively involved in the formation of a new, mainly German-speaking community of doctors – psychiatrists. Not surprisingly, the Prague Institute was frequently visited by mainly German psychiatrists.

One should also take note of the effect that the publications of the doctors who worked at the Prague *Irrenanstalt* had on the general awareness of mental disorders. By publishing different texts about the mental asylum, they contributed to the destigmatisation of mental illnesses, pointed out the possibility of treatment and recovery and fought against the widespread prejudices about 'madness.' Finally, they also took note of the 'moral' but above all the social and economic roots and causes of mental disorders.

The establishment of a 'mental asylum' in the Bohemian capital had an impact on the perception of mental disorders and mentally ill persons outside Prague. The process of admission to the Prague Institute placed fewer demands on doctors practicing in smaller towns and rural areas: they were asked to take notice persons whose behavior indicated mental disorder and, if these persons posed a danger to themselves or others, they were to cooperate in their admission. They were also asked to take their medical history, which in practice meant talking to them to reconstruct their personal history, the story of their body and mind. Then they could perhaps try to classify their unwanted behavior to fit into one of the categories of 'madness' defined by contemporary doctors. In this way, the concept of 'insanity' – or rather mental illness – began to enter the general discourse and consciousness of even the rural population.

Acknowledgement

This study is an output of grant of the Czech Science Foundation (GA ČR) no. 2204258S *Anatomy of a Suffering Soul. From the 'passions of the soul' and 'empirical psychology' to a psychiatric hospital in the Czech Lands, 1770–1814*, which has been granted to the Faculty of Arts of the Charles University (Prague).

CHAPTER 6

The Persistence of Provincial Autonomy: Habsburg Governance and Institutional Care of the Mentally Ill in Brno/Brünn, 1785–1864

Zdeněk Nebřenský and Pavlína Pončíková

In July 1864, the Moravian Provincial Committee, in consultation with the chairman of the Provincial Diet, set up a commission to ensure that the newly opened Provincial Institute for Mentally ill in Černovice/Czernowitz near Brno/Brünn would fulfil its purpose in the best possible way. The commission consisted of committed citizens, politicians and doctors who discussed conceptual and operational issues relating to the Institute at their meetings. One of them dealt with the question of whether the Institute should specialize exclusively in the treatment of mentally ill people or whether it could have a broader care giving focus of care and accept incurable patients as well. The recently elected mayor of the provincial capital, Alfred Skene, said:

> We have a hospital for the mentally disordered people and not a nursing home … I am not a doctor, but it's basically proven that patients who are not cured within six or eight years are incurable and belong in a detention facility.[1]

Mayor Skene pointed out the pressing issue that divided members of the commission, whether they came from political, civic or medical circles. The fundamental difference in the care of physically and mentally ill patients was seen in the duration and therefore the cost of treatment. For "the mentally disordered people", the shortest standard length of stay in hospital was six to eight weeks, after which they could be discharged if they responded well. Patients who did not recover within two months, had to leave the hospital. If they could not be cared for in their home community, they were transferred to a facility for the terminally ill at the municipal expense, which multiplied the number of chronically incurable inmates. As a result, hospital treatment for people with mental disabilities took much longer than treatment for other illnesses or injuries.

1 Moravský zemský archiv [Moravian Provincial Archive, henceforth MZA], files [f.], A8 Zemská registratura, karton [box, ka.] 154, Signature [Sign.] A45/5, Folio [fol.] 811.

 | HTTPS://DOI.ORG/10.1163/9789004755062-008

However, the nature of the health facility and the extent to which it should care for incurable patients was not officially determined, and there were long disputes about it. Some members, such as the director of the St. Anna's General Hospital, Ignaz Mayer, pointed out that the capacity of the Institute in Černovice was sufficient to take in incurable long-term patients as well as "the mentally disordered people". According to him, it was still too early to decide what the actual focus of the Institute would ultimately be. He explained that this would change over time and would only become clear in a few years' time. The director of the Institute, Joseph Czermak, on the other hand, argued that there had already been care facilities in Brno for several decades. The newly opened Institute was therefore built according to the principles of psychiatry. These included that it should meet the needs of humanity, and particularly the requirements of science.[2]

Committed citizens and politicians were generally concerned about the running costs of Institute, which some believed would rise for the incurable patients. Other members of the commissions claimed that savings could be made because terminally ill persons did not need a doctor or a guardian and did not need such good food.[3] From 1864, all welfare and health facilities throughout the Habsburg Monarchy were transferred from the state to the provincial administration. Hospitals, orphanages and asylums became the property of the individual provinces, and the operation of health facilities was financed from the provincial budget, which had an impact on more than just the institutional care of "mentally disordered people".[4]

The construction and opening of the Institute marked the end of a period in the eighty–year history of institutional care for the mentally ill in Moravia. This started with Emperor Joseph II's decision to build according to the model of the Vienna General Hospital, the United Poor Relief House (*Vereignites Armenversorgungs-Haus*) in Brno/Brünn, from which later the St. Anna's General Hospital and Ward for Mentally Disabled persons gradually separated.[5] In 1785, the House initially served to care for the sick, mothers, foundlings, orphans and people with mental disabilities under one roof. It consisted of hospital (*Krankenhaus*), house for mothers and foundlings (*Gebähr- und Findelhaus*), house for orphans (*Waissenhaus*) and house for mentally disabled persons (*Tollhaus*). As the number of ill persons increased and treatment became more specialized, the care of individual patient groups reached the organizational

2 MZA, f. A8 Zemská registratura, ka. 154, Sign. A45/5, fol. 815.
3 MZA, f. A8 Zemská registratura, ka. 154, Sign. A45/5, fols. 816–817.
4 Topp, *Freedom and the Cage*, 39–40.
5 Vitecek, *Der Wiener Narrenturm*, 36–38.

and spatial limits of the old monastery grounds. The heads of the various medical wards, which had become increasingly independent, were confronted with temporary operating conditions that were not suitable for a modern healthcare facility. Citizens and politicians alike realized that additional, if not new, buildings would be needed to improve the quality of medical care.

Historians have already studied the reforms of public asylums, which repeatedly changed medical conditions and provided spatial solutions to "insanity". These studies have clearly shown how facilities for people with mental disabilities were built by all institutional and non-institutional actors.[6] The buildings often structured the care of people with mental disabilities and influenced this care in very ambiguous ways. The spatial division of the asylum into equal halves for men and women, the offices for the administration and the layout of the rooms within each building were defined in detail.[7] To prevent infection and contain the outbreak of disease, the doctors ordered architectural changes and sanitary revisions to the building. Planners began to dream of a hospital as a collection of small buildings, each filled with narrow, rectilinear rooms, separated from other spaces and surrounded by open air.[8] Not only were the physical aspects of the asylum studied, dividing patients into wards according to the severity of their illness, but also the humane treatment of patients in the gardens.[9] Similarly, historians have paid attention to how patients perceived the places in which they were housed and how the day-to-day running of hospitals could be gendered without regard to patients' needs.[10] However, despite the wealth of advanced medical knowledge and practices, the design of healthcare facilities has yet to be definitively clarified.[11]

Following this basic history of hospital spaces in the late nineteenth century, this chapter examines the extent to which the establishment of hospitals in general, and the design of asylums in particular, depended on the state and the public authorities who decided on the institutional care of mentally ill. It looks at the history of hospital care for the mentally ill in Brno from its beginnings in the late 1780s to the founding of the psychiatric institute in the 1860s. Although Joseph Czermak, the head of the "insane asylum" in Brno and later the first director of the Institute, had a wealth of experience in hospital administration and familiarized himself thoroughly with the treatment in

6 Moran. Topp, Introduction, 2–6.
7 Topp, *Freedom and the Cage*, 116.
8 Kisacky, *Rise of the Modern Hospital*, 14–15.
9 Collins, *The Architecture and Landscape of Health*, 100–118.
10 Ankele, *Alltag und Aneignung*, 130–149.
11 Pawlowsky, *Mutter ledig – Vater Staat*, 257–262.

German mental asylums on his study trips, this may not have been sufficient for the long-term operation of a modern psychiatric facility. The development of a hospital institution could be reversed. Its professional orientation had to be constantly defended vis-á-vis the political authorities.

The chapter is based on the analysis of archival sources that emerged from official communication, i.e. reports issued by the House's administration for meetings of the Moravian Provincial Committee. Some parts of the reports dealt with both important organizational changes and the daily work of the House. In view of this fact, it is impossible to decide whether the Committee's inundation with trivialities, reflected a relationship of subordination between the intendant of House (later the director of Institute) and the members of the Committee, or whether it was a strategy of the intendant to distract the Committee from larger decisions, such those concerning the handling of funds, which were made by the intendant behind the Committee's back. For the initial period in which the House was constituted, the court decrees are taken into account, which primarily confirmed the annual allocations of imperial and provincial funds.

The first part of the chapter presents the state-building efforts of the Habsburg rulers and their advisors during the Enlightenment, when the institutional framework for the modern hospital care of people with mental disabilities was created. The second part of the chapter examines how the administration of the hospitals changed in the wake of the Napoleonic Wars and declining revenues, which led to financial support and intervention by the court authorities. Later, the hospital administration was separated from the provincial health administration and the individual hospital wards were given more autonomy. In the third part, the chapter focuses on the activities of Joseph Czermak, who was appointed head of the mental asylum. He immediately built on the efforts of his predecessors and was able to push through the construction of the new institution for the mentally ill on a greenfield site.

1 Enlightenment Transformation

The wars over the Austrian succession threated to destroy the Habsburg Monarchy. Military campaigns decimated the health of the population and famines undermined the conscription of men into the army. This and other factors spurred Empress Maria Theresa to introduce reforms. The changes introduced in the state administration were of fundamental importance for the development of care institutions, which were to operate on a uniform basis throughout the monarchy. This purpose was served by the General

Medical Regulations (*General-Medicinal Ordnungen*), which were gradually issued for the individual provinces and were based on some older domestic models as well as on the current medical edicts from the German lands. The Medical Regulations for Moravia, which came into force on December 15, 1752, was no different from the regulations issued in other hereditary lands: it weakened the power of the manorial authorities and mentioned, for example, procedures for regulating the public space against the spread of epidemic diseases. No less important were the conditions for the various categories of medical personnel and the instructions for their work in the healthcare facilities, which were aimed, among other things, at combating "sleazy and treacherous medicine".[12]

On the basis of the new medical regulations, the former health administration was separated from the other official agendas and placed in the hands of the supreme health authority, the so-called Medical Court Deputation (*Sanitäts-Hofdeputation*). This consisted of doctors with the rank of health advisors who supervised the provincial health commissions that already existed in the various lands of the monarchy. The Moravian Health Commission in Brno was also headed by a provincial health advisor who supervised the regional doctors and surgeons (*Kreisphysikate*). These looked after the health of the population in each of the six Moravian administrative regions. In agreement with the regional physicians, the health advisor could commission municipal, manorial and private physicians to carry out tasks on behalf of public health, including health care in the convent hospitals. Thanks to the generosity of noble men and women who followed the empress's example and invited the Brothers and Sisters of Mercy to the provincial towns and parishes, the convent hospitals were built on the sites of former farmhouses and inns. Later, hop fields or meadows near the riverbank were added to the original property, the hospital grounds were extended, and the patients stay in the hospital garden could become part of their convalescence.[13]

---

12 Comlos, *Nutrition and Economic Development*, 119–120, 125–127. Voth, Height, Nutrition, and Labor, 627–636, here 630. Godsey, *The Sinews of Habsburg Power*, 235. Sinkulová, *Lékaři, stát a zdraví lidu*, 30–31. Tinková, *Tělo, věda, stát*, 291–293. Hlaváčková, Veřejné zdravotnictví, in *Velké dějiny zemí koruny české*, 213.

13 *Kurzgefasste Geschichte der Versorgungs- und Kranken-Anstalten der Hauptstadt Linz, verfasst von Kaspar Aufschmid, Protomedikus und Direktor der Versorgungsanstalten*, Oesterreichische Staatsarchiv, HHStA, Haus A, Hofreisen, Sign. 44-1-103, fols. 126, 130–133. Bernt, *Systematisches Handbuch des Medicinal-Wesens*, 17. Kopetz, *Österreichische politische Gesetzkunde*, 258–259, 271. Kretschmayr, *Die österreichische Zentralverwaltung*, 377–381. Lesky, *Österreichisches Gesundheitswesen*, 11, 19–24, 67. Bernard, The Limits of Absolutism, 205. Tinková, *Tělo, věda, stát*, 294. See also Knörlein, *Kurzgefasste Geschichte*, 14–16.

The Provincial authorities and the magistrates of the towns donated the materials for the construction of healthcare facilities and supported the establishment of foundations to cover the costs of running the hospital beds. Convent hospitals were part of the monastery buildings. One could gain access through a gatehouse with decorative portals. The first floor of the wing facing the street usually housed pharmacies that were open to the public. The interiors were dominated by long, wide halls with high ceilings, containing several dozen beds and an altar, which was still indispensable at the time. A few isolated rooms were reserved for the mentally ill. Hospital care by religious doctors, pharmacists and nurses of both sexes was intended for old, sick and poor men, regardless of their religion, language, or status, as theoretically envisaged by the content principles. The female patients, including some pregnant, prostituted and women with mental disabilities, were then treated in the hospitals of the Sisters of Mercy, who had no medical training, but in more complicated cases sought the help of the medical staff of the merciful brothers or the municipal doctors.[14]

In 1770, the Viennese authorities issued the Comprehensive Medical Normative (*Generale normativum in re sanitatis*), which standardized the health care regulation of the individual lands. It also deepened the earlier regulations of the medical professions and their obligation to improve the health of the population. In the context of the establishment of the civil hospital in Zagreb, it has already been explained in detail how the Normative contributed to the formation of a sanitary cordon in the south-eastern provinces of the monarchy and to protection against the spread of the plague, which from then on was dealt with directly by the War Council in Vienna. In Brno, the former authorities responsible for combating the plague were merged with Provincial Health Commissions under the direction of the chief provincial physician (*Protomedicus*). Until then, the Protomedicus had formally supervised the regional doctors, but now he now began to direct them. With the help of the Normative, the empress and her advisors created a centralized health administration that extended from the court through the provinces to the regional level. They attempted to subject former estate bodies such as the regional physicians to court power and turn them into state authorities.[15]

---

14 *Kurzgefasste Geschichte*, fol. 127–128, 133. Kopetz, *Österreichische politische Gesetzkunde*, 271. Horáčková, Menšíková, Vargová, *Zdravotní péče*, 7–8, 15. See also d'Elvert, *Geschichte der Heil- und Humanitats-Anstalten*, 216, 220–221.

15 Lesky, *Österreichisches Gesundheitswesen*, 68–69. Sinkulová, *Lékaři, stát a zdraví lidu*, 36–37. Tinková, *Tělo, věda, stát*, 293–294.

The separate administration of health matters lasted until 1776, when the Court Health Deputation was dissolved, and its powers were transferred to the court offices responsible for the affairs of the individual provinces. It cannot be said that the empress abandoned the earlier reform efforts in return for maintenance of political stability, as her decisions are sometimes interpreted. The *Protomedicus* continued to influence the operation of caregiving facilities, including hospitals, foundlings wards and maternity houses. He was responsible for the foundation and construction of a new type of hospital (*Krankenhaus*). The division of the medical professions according to their field of activity also remained unchanged. Sonnefels's population principle that the state's interest lay in further increasing fertility and preserving the lives of infants met with broad approval in the growing ranks of physicians and led to experiments with the establishment of the first maternity wards, as exemplified in hospitals in Pest, Zagreb and Prague. With the decline of the plague epidemics, the pesthouses were considered superfluous, which was a welcome reason to redirect their funding to hospitals dedicated to the treatment of the sick.[16]

A similar approach was taken in the decentralization of poor relief and the removal of the homeless persons, but not actually sick, from hospitals into the care of local parishes. The orphans were given to people of good repute in return for a daily allowance for education and care. The benefactors received a certain amount of pocket money, and the sick were cared for in other ways. The savings made in the poor relief were intended to free up additional funds for healthcare facilities. By taking away part of the income of the caregiving institutions, there was theoretically the possibility of making a new type of hospital materially independent.[17]

The court advisors found themselves at a crossroads and had to decide which path to take. Should places scattered in many different facilities be converted into beds in new-type hospitals or should these several hundred patients be concentrated in one institution? The court physicians argued in favor of the first, more medical approach. But, Emperor Joseph II, impressed by a visit to the Hôtel-Dieu in Paris, ultimately opted for the second, economical approach. In Pest, Zagreb and Prague, the provincial authorities, often after personal consultation with the emperor, began to search for suitable former

16 Bernt, *Systematisches Handbuch*, 343–345. Bernard, The Limits of Absolutism, 205–207. Hochedlinger, Die Sanitätshofdeputation, 606–609.

17 Vitecek, *Der Wiener Narrenturm*, 26–27, 34–36. See also *Kurzgefasste Geschichte der Versorgungs- und Kranken-Anstalten*, fol. 127.

almshouses in which the largest number of patients could be accommodated after the necessary structural alteration.[18]

Parallel to the changing clientele of the individual hospitals, their funding was also adjusted. Ever since the Theresian reforms of health administration were pushed forward, court officials kept a watchful eye on the charitable foundations and assets supporting the running of the caregiving institutions. In the 1780s, many of them were abolished as dispensable and their funds were used to build new health facilities for the medical care of the urban population. Although the first steps had been taken to control church property, especially the monasteries, this did not mean that a new type of hospital immediately emerged. The diversity of health facilities prevented effective control, and even the Directive rules (*Direktivregeln*) issued by Emperor Joseph II. In April 1781 did little to change this. The emperor attempted to divide the facilities according to the target groups for which they were intended. In provincial capitals of the Habsburg Monarchy, this was not always possible for organizational and spatial reasons, so that these institutions often remained part of the general caregiving facilities and the sick, mothers, orphans and people with mental disabilities could be housed under one roof.[19]

In Pest, Zagreb or Prague, the municipal, civil or convent health institutions continued to have their diverse "early modern" focus and were guided by the principle of Christian love for one's neighbor. However, the Josephinist regulations were of decisive importance, as they created a political framework for the establishment of new hospitals in provincial towns based on the Viennese model.[20] In Staré Brno/Altbrünn, for example, the emperor ordered the Dominican monastery of St. Anne to be dissolved and new public hospital to be built in its place. On December 1, 1785, the new facility was opened under the name 'United Poor Relief House' (*Vereignites Armenversorgungs-Haus*). Mothers, foundlings, the sick and mentally ill found refuge here thanks to the emperor's donation from the Main Poor Relief Fund (*Hauptarmenfond*) which received a financial share of the assets sold after the abolition of the

18 Risse, *Mending Bodies, Saving Souls*, 266. Bernard, The Limits of Absolutism, 209–210. Grois, *Das Allgemeine Krankenhaus*, 27, 33, 38–39. Knörlein, *Kurzgefasste Geschichte*, 19. Vitecek, *Der Wiener Narrenturm*, 33–35.

19 Kopetz, *Österreichische politische Gesetzkunde*, 258–259. Knörlein, *Kurzgefasste Geschichte*, 19. Grois, *Das Allgemeine Krankenhaus*, 27–31. *Quellen zur europäischen Spitalgeschichte*, 303. Scheutz, Weiß, Spital als Lebensform, 186. Vitecek, *Der Wiener Narrenturm*, 33–34, 39–41.

20 *Kurzgefasste Geschichte der Versorgungs- und Kranken-Anstalten*, fols. 127, 132.

ecclesiastical brotherhoods. It seems that the House opened at the right time, as the doctors and staff treated more than 700 patients in the first year alone.[21]

The medical part of House – the hospital consisted of two large rooms with 80 beds, one of which was occupied by sick men and the other by women. The hospital had two departments – one for internal diseases (mainly fever and joints) and one for external diseases (especially skin diseases, but also all diseases requiring surgical intervention). The original plan of the House did not provide for the establishment of a separate ward for infectious diseases, so a temporary solution in the form of two wooden houses in the garden had to be chosen. One was used for the isolation of smallpox patients and the other for patients with rabies. The special ward for patients with venereal diseases, which was an important institution on the way to the development of modern hospitals in Pest, Zagreb and Prague, was not initially mentioned in connection with St. Anne's House.[22]

As early as the late eighteenth century, court decrees defined the categories of hospital professions that ensured the smooth running of healthcare facilities. Important decisions about treatment were of course made by the head physician and surgeons. The nursing staff then followed the treatment procedures and progress of individual patients. Most of the nurses in the House were not staff in the medical sense, but wardens (*Wärter, Wärterinnen*) who were to assign patients to rooms according to gender and illness. They cleaned the instruments, performed night duty and took care of bedding and clothing. They monitored compliance with visiting times. The wardens were supposed to be kind to friendly to patients and were expressly forbidden to demand additional payment form patients for their services. If patients expressed special wishes, they reported them to the head physician, who decided whether they were justified.[23]

In the Poor Relief House of St. Anne, the Emperor's Privy Councilor Thomas Pötzl was entrusted with official control and a leading provincial physician Franz Michael Valenzi with medical supervision. And as Valenzi with his successors were not always able to fully perform their administrative duties, they brought in two officials from the Prague Provincial Governate to assist them.[24]

21 Kopetz, *Österreichische politische Gesetzkunde*, 259. Czermak, *Die Mährische Landes-Irrenanstalt bei Brünn*, 1–2. Horáčková, Zdravotní péče, 19. Weiß, *Geschichte der öffentlichen Anstalten*, CXXXIV–CXXXV. See also d'Elvert, *Geschichte der Heil- und Humanitats-Anstalten*, 216–221.

22 Horáčková, Zdravotní péče, 19–20. Czermak, *Die Mährische Landes-Irrenanstalt*, 1–2. See also d'Elvert, *Geschichte der Heil- und Humanitats-Anstalten*, 194.

23 MZA, f. A8 Zemská registratura, ka. 148, Sign. A45-3, fol. 22.

24 MZA, f. A8 Zemská registratura, ka. 148, Sign. A45/2, fol. 51.

The patients were treated by the hospital doctor who was assisted by a surgeon. The staff took care of daily routines such as providing food, laundry and washing clothes, including equipping the room with a small cupboard for medicines and personal belongings.[25] The patients were cared for by more than two dozen wardens who made sure that the minimum air volume for each bed was not exceeded. The midwife and her assistant took care of the mothers in the 20-bed maternity ward. If a mother was unable to care for her child, lit was left in the 20-bed facility for foundlings. The children in the 20-bed orphanage were supervised by caregivers and breastfed by wet nurses.[26]

The authorities issued special regulations for the treatment and admission of the mentally ill, who were segregated and could only be visited from with permission from outside. Officially, various facilities consisting of reinforced walls and raised windows with bars were permitted for acute and "disturbed" patients. They were guarded by wardens who lived in their immediate vicinity. Although additional restraining devices were introduced, patient who were diagnosed as "less dangerous" were allowed to be in the garden or yard as part of their therapy.[27] The "insane asylum" was set up in a closed off part of the House with five chambers for the internment of people with mental disabilities. These were closed with an iron door and received light through a small, well-barred opening. The inside of the chamber consisted of a layer of straw and a chain attached to the wall. In the first year of operation, 15 mentally ill patients were housed here one after the other.[28]

2 Revolutionizing Hospital Administration

Like the General Hospital in Vienna, the administrative and medical management of the provincial hospitals were separated after the death of Joseph II. While the court officials attempted to alleviate the financial deficits of the General Hospital, the provincial authorities in Brno had a say in the management and profitability of St. Anne's House. However, their control, could often only be formal, as they were preoccupied with many other issues. In particular, the *Protomedicus*, who was supposed to oversee most of the facilities, very rarely

25 MZA, f. A8 Zemská registratura, ka. 148, Sign. A45/2, fols. 76, 81, 86.

26 MZA, f. A8 Zemská registratura, ka. 148, Sign. A45/2, fol. 4. Czermak, *Die Mährische Landes-Irrenanstalt*, 1–2. See also d'Elvert, *Geschichte der Heil- und Humanitats-Anstalten*, 194.

27 The first court decrees for "insane asylums" in Prague and Graz were issued in November 1790 and January 1796 respectively. See Kopetz, *Österreichische politische Gesetzkunde*, 264. See also *Kurzgefasste Geschichte der Versorgungs- und Kranken-Anstalten*, fol. 135.

28 Horáčková, Zdravotní péče, 19–20.

appeared in the individual hospitals, as he was responsible for health care in the entire province. Thus, executive power in the House was assumed by the intendant, who, together with the controller was responsible for personnel, financial and administrative matters relating to admission and discharge of patients. The importance of the intendant grew with the increasing number of employees, whose control became crucial to the operation of the hospital. For example, the intendant coordinated the chambermaids who were responsible for preparing the beds, minor repairs and keeping the hospital rooms clean. He also arranged for the proper installation of corridor heating outside the rooms, which was the latest technical innovation.[29]

The hospitals in Pest, Zagreb and Prague, including the foundling wards, orphanages and asylums, were financed by charity, legacies and endowments. As the number of patients grew, they struggled to maintain a balanced budget. The cost per bed increased, while the contributions from the funds remained stable for several years. Everyday items, such as straw mattresses, bed linen and bedding could only be replaced once the patient was cured, which took many months for the long-term and mentally ill patients. Health and hygiene were much more important to the medical staff than financial issues. For example, the Provincial Accounting Office, which administered the financial records of St. Anne's House, complained in the summer of 1795 when irregularities were discovered in the handling of the *Krönungsfond*. As a result, a lengthy investigation was launched, and a new calculation was made to ensure that no more money was missing.[30]

According to the court's calculations, the combined funds used to finance hospital operations showed a slight surplus for several years. However, the sharp increase in state expenditure in connection with the military campaigns shook this balance considerably. The income from the poor relief and savings funds, which covered hospital operations, fell rapidly.[31] In order to pay off the hospitals' debts, Emperor Franz issued several court decrees, which were also extended to health facilities in the provinces. They permitted the collection of fees from wood, charcoal and inheritances for the benefit of the hospital funds. The fees for hospital admission and care were also increased.[32]

29 Czermak, *Die Mährische Landes-Irrenanstalt*, 1–2.

30 MZA, f. A8 Zemská registratura, A45/2, ka. 148, Sign. A45/2, fols. 76–78.

31 *Kurzgefasste Geschichte der Versorgungs- und Kranken-Anstalten*, fol. 128. Grois, *Das Allgemeine Krankenhaus*, 77, 83–84. Knörlein, *Kurzgefasste Geschichte*, 21–23.

32 *Kurzgefasste Geschichte der Versorgungs- und Kranken-Anstalten*, fols. 128–129. Nachricht des mährisch-schlesischen Landesgubernium aufgrund des Hofdekretes vom 23. Mai 1804 betreffend die Erhöhung der Aufnahms- und Verpflegstaxen des brünner Kranken-,

It soon became clear that the hospital's budget was insufficient to cover most living costs, especially during the harsh winter of 1805, when the administration of St. Anne's House had to cut food rations for the inmates. Due to the general rise in prices, more and more people fell into poverty and illness. Patients were no longer able to pay for medical treatment and the hospital's income continued to fall.[33] The administration of the House flooded the Moravian Estates and the emperor with requests for annual contributions from the domestical and coronation fund, the release of which had to be negotiated at length.[34] The court authorities supported the demands, including the increase in the annual contribution, but the Estates, from whose funds additional amounts were to be paid, did not agree to the court decisions on the grounds of insufficient finances, with the result that the contribution was not increased for several years.[35]

In March 1811, because of the state bankruptcy, the well-known financial patent was published, which, among other things, divided up the *Stiftungsfond* and *Versorgungsfond*. In order to prevent both funds from being quickly exhausted at the same time, the municipalities were obliged to pay hospital fees for their inhabitants who were admitted to health facilities.[36] This applied in particular to inmates of the poorhouse and the mental asylum, whose treatment was more costly. A persistent and unsatisfactorily resolved problem that the heads of the House struggled with for more than two decades was the charges for military patients, which were lower than for civilian patients. In peacetime, this problem was not as pressing as in times of war.[37] The worsening financial difficulties prompted the heads of the hospitals to turn to the judicial authorities to obtain an increase in the daily rate they received from the respective funds for the treatment of patients.

Some of these requests were granted, depending on how well connected the heads of the hospitals were with the relevant court dignitaries. A few institutions were declared state-owned, while others continued to be administered by the provincial authorities. The state and provincial administration of health facilities began to separate arbitrarily in the individual provinces.[38] As the

---

Siechen-, Toll- und Gebär- und Findelhaus und des olmützer Versorgungshaus, in ÖStA, FHKA SUS Patente, Sign. 456.3, fols. 353–354.

33 MZA, f. A8 Zemská registratura, ka. 157, Sign. A45/6, fols. 945–946.

34 MZA, f. A8 Zemská registratura, ka. 157, Sign. A45/6, fols. 951–953.

35 MZA, f. A8 Zemská registratura, ka. 157, Sign. A45/6, fols. 963–964.

36 Grois, *Das Allgemeine Krankenhaus*, 85–86. Knörlein, *Kurzgefasste Geschichte*, 24.

37 MZA, f. A8 Zemská registratura, ka. 148, Sign. A45/2, fol. 49.

38 *Kurzgefasste Geschichte der Versorgungs- und Kranken-Anstalten*, fol. 130. Knörlein, *Kurzgefasste Geschichte*, 26–27. Knörlein, *Die Irren-Angelegenheiten*, 14.

number of people treated increased, the expenses of the Brno House rose to such an extent, that the Poor Relief Fund could no longer meet the demands placed on it. In the almost three decades of its existence between 1786 and 1814, the asylum alone treated 500 mentally ill patients, an average of 19–20 persons per year, although it had ten beds.[39] The state subsidies in the form of tax surcharges on firewood, wine and levies from estates could not cover the running costs. In order to cover the costs of the House and to counter the constant financial difficulties, a court ruling ordered that the part of the requirements could be paid from the state coffers.[40]

The adjustment of funding and the interference of state officials in the institutional affairs were not reflected in the administration of the House, which was formally held by the head provincial physician, but executive power was given to the intendant. This only changed after almost half a century in November 1830, when a prominent Moravian physician, governor's councilor and protomedicus Joseph Steiner Edler von Pfungen resigned as director of the House at his own request.[41] The office of director of the House was separated from the office of Protomedicus, and the Moravian Provincial Governate was given the power to appoint a new director with medical training. So that the director could devote his time to curing patients, three scribes assisted him in his official duties. A second doctor, Paul Olexik, worked with the director in the treatment of prominent patients and became a key figure in the medical diagnosis of the House. A surgeon and an assistant in the operating theatre dealt with emergencies.[42]

Due to the increasing number of patients, three separate wards were set up. The maternity and the foundling wards were moved out of the House, giving the asylum additional space in a separate courtyard and gradually increasing its capacity to 120 beds. As a result, the asylum became more autonomous and was able to employ two specialists for the treatment of the mentally ill. They generally acted as deputies for first doctor and were in frequent contact with most of the patients. The second doctor looked after the running of the hospital in terms of order and cleanliness, prescribed medication and controlled the work of the nurses. He supervised the good manners and behavior of the hospital staff and patients. He also initiated the introduction of more humane

39 *Kurzgefasste Geschichte der Versorgungs- und Kranken-Anstalten*, fol. 136. Kopetz, *Österreichische politische Gesetzkunde*, 259. Czermak, *Die Mährische Landes-Irrenanstalt*, 2. See also d'Elvert, *Geschichte der Heil- und Humanitats-Anstalten*, 194.

40 Czermak, *Die Mährische Landes-Irrenanstalt*, 2.

41 MZA, f. A8 Zemská registratura, A45-2, ka. 148, Sign. A45/2, fols. 25–27.

42 Kopetz, *Österreichische politische Gesetzkunde*, 265.

treatment: the shackles for the mentally ill were abolished and the chambers were equipped with better furniture. The patients were clothed and given the same standard diet as the patient in the other wards.[43]

In the 1850s, tensions between the central and provincial authorities increased. Initially, the government in Vienna maintained its power, infiltrating offices at all levels, operating in the provinces and asserting court authority over provincial institutions.[44] This policy, the most fundamental of the last half century, was far from enabling a restructuring of the "insane asylum", which was set up according to the cell system and still functioned more as a detention than as a health facility. The administrative conditions of the combined caregiving facility prevented its development. Progressive medical practices were undermined by the spatial limitations of the premises. The asylum's leading doctors repeatedly tried to persuade provincial governate officials to expand the premises. One of them was Joseph Czermak, who had a wealth of experience as second physician at the Prague *Irrenanstalt* and was appointed as a senior doctor of the asylum in 1855. Czermak's aim in Brno was to reform the care of the mentally ill. After taking up his post, he undertook a study trip to selected institutions in German countries and began planning the reorganization of the asylum.

The first task was to justify the fact that any changes, including the construction of a new building at were necessary at all. With the help of the gendarmerie, Czermak commissioned a survey to find out how many mentally ill were living in Moravia, as there was no proper official registration of these people. The results of this survey showed a considerable territorial disparity; on average, two to three times fewer mentally ill people were recorded in Moravia than in the other provinces of the monarchy. Nevertheless, the number of mentally ill was high and it was clear that the facilities available for their treatment were inadequate. The old building of the former Dominican monastery did not allow for any major structural changes, and it was not structurally feasible to adapt it to modern facilities. Czermak suggested demolishing it and replacing it completely with new premises.[45]

It should be remembered, however, that the asylum was under the direction of the Poor Relief House, which in turn was controlled by the provincial committee and the governate. Czermak's actions were bound by official procedures, and any initiative, no matter how small, that deviated from the official routine had to be approved by the central authorities. The Ministry of

43 Czermak, *Die Mährische Landes-Irrenanstalt*, 2–3.
44 Deak, *Forging a multinational state*, 107–112, 130–134.
45 Matoušek, Vzrůst počtu choromyslných na Moravě, 131–134.

the Interior Alexander Bach initially rejected Czermak's proposal and the Provincial Governate recommended that the project be revised in more detail. Czermak proposed to build a facility with a "pavilion" system, but the construction was technically and financially demanding. He was forced to change his proposal and work out a simpler, less expensive project with a "corridor system," which was positively evaluated by the consultants on site through the committee.[46]

In the end, the Ministry of the Interior and the Provincial Governor concluded that the submitted project was sufficiently modified to proceed with the construction of a completely new institute. The subsequent success of the Czermak's proposal was mainly due to the fact that influential persons promoted it. The high provincial engineer Joseph Seyfert drew up the architectural design of the building and the health officer of the provincial committee, Alexander Engel, helped to push through a building project in the Provincial Governate on the grounds that Moravia needed an institute of this kind. The location was chosen near the village Černovice/Czernowitz, which was on the edge of the historic suburbs, a quarter of an hour from Brno. It was accessible from the city, but isolated from the urban "unhealthy" environment. The seclusion of the facility was intended to limit external influences, which was one of the treatment methods.[47]

The design of the institute's complex, which Czermak drew up together with the architect Seyfert, envisaged a dividing the complex into individual pavilions, which were to provide the mentally ill with more comfortable medical care (see Figure 6.1).

However, this concept was somewhat ahead of its time and was rejected by the authorities, who stuck to the existing "corridor" arrangement, that had been common practice since the middle of the nineteenth century and was supported by most doctors.[48] The Ministry of the Interior, together with the Provincial Governate recommended the "corridor" arrangement as it allowed that more patients could be accommodated. The administration building was connected to the men's and women's wings under one roof (see Figure 6.2).

In the original project, the layout of the day lounge was wider, so that the interior of the hall offered a more generous view, a larger space for setting up the tables and benches. Following the example of the Vienna *Irrenanstalt*, the Ministry of the Interior proposed replacing the lounge with paved corridors and transforming large room into a dining room for all patients, who were

46 MZA, f. A8 Zemská registratura, ka. 152, Sign. A45/5, unpaginated.

47 Czermak, *Die Mährische Landes-Irrenanstalt*, 3–4. See also Moravský zemský ústav, 311–312.

48 Topp, *Freedom and the Cage*, 29–33.

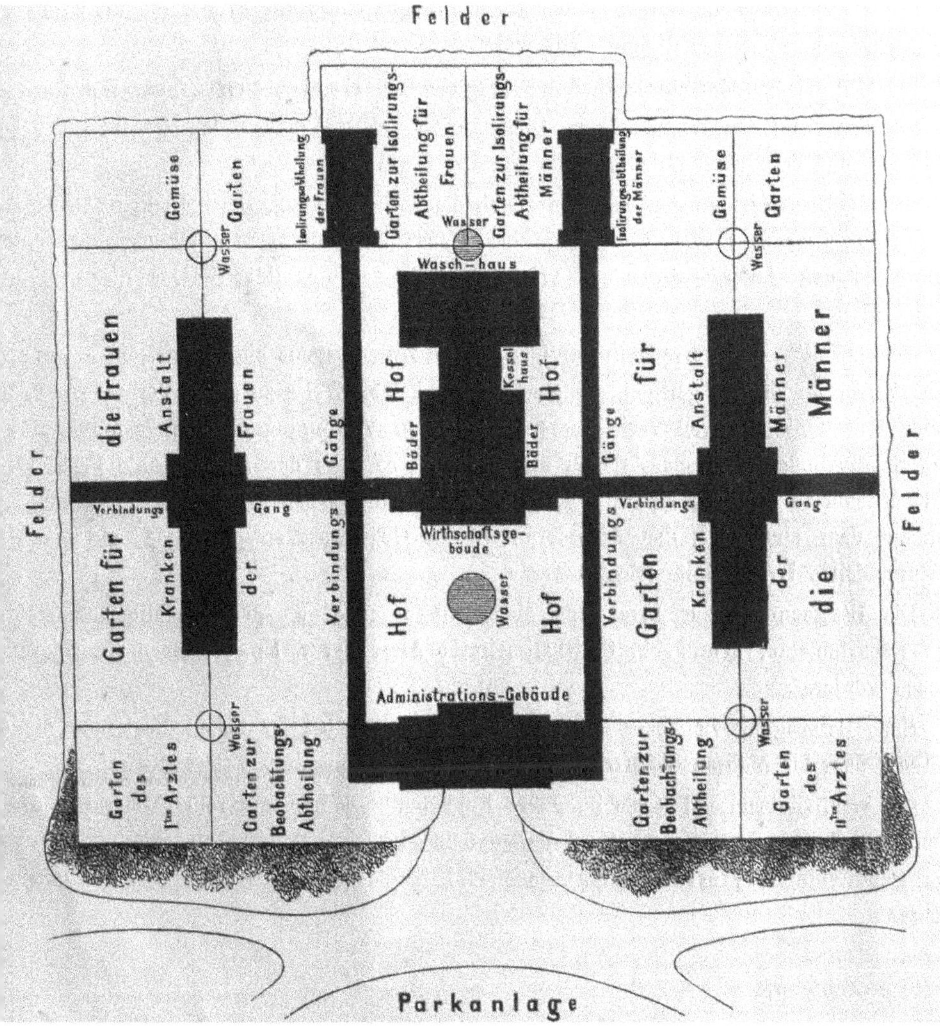

FIGURE 6.1 Original plan for the Institute of Mentally Disordered Persons in Černovice/Czernowitz. In Josef Czermak, *Die mährische Landes-Irrenanstalt bei Brünn, ihre bauliche Einrichtung, Administration, ärztliche Gebahrung und Statistik*, Wien: K. Czermak, 1866

to meet there in the morning, at lunchtime and in the evening. During the day, they were to stay in their rooms or be able to spend time in the corridor. Director Czermak and architect Seyfert rejected the ministerial amendment and insisted that the corridors should remain part of the lounge. The corridors were nevertheless roofed over, heated and fitted with double windows. The proposed large dining hall was not built, as suggested by the Ministry. The bedrooms were closed during the day and the inmates could move freely in the day

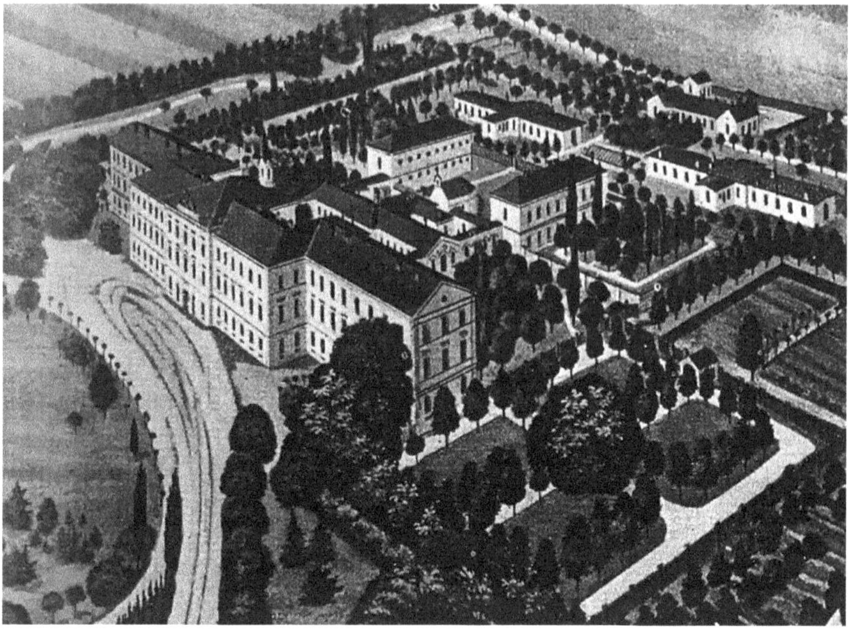

FIGURE 6.2 The Moravian Provincial Institute for the Mentally Ill in Černovice/Czernowitz. Moravské zemské muzeum. Oddělení pro historii biologických věd, fond Zapletal inv. no. 4812.

room. They were easy to supervise and ate there so that they did not have to be carried around when the food was served.[49]

In order to obtain a solid building at the lowest possible cost, the Ministry of the Interior published the tender in the newspaper. The Provincial Governate collected all bids for the construction and the selection committee appointed by the governorate assessed their suitability.[50] No wonder it took another three years before the authorities completed all the formalities and the project could start. By decree dated May 4, 1860, the Ministry of the Interior approved the construction of a new mental hospital and ordered the purchase of a 25-acres square plot of land from provincial funds. Due to further adjustments in the implementation of the building plan, the foundation stone was not laid until a few months later. The construction works was mainly carried out by small firms from Brno and Vienna under the supervision of the provincial building officer in collaboration with Joseph Czermak.[51]

49 Czermak, *Die Mährische Landes-Irrenanstalt*, 10.
50 MZA, f. A8 Zemská registratura, ka. 152, Sign. A45/5, unpaginated.
51 MZA, f. A8 Zemská registratura, ka. 152, Sign. A45/5, unpaginated.

3 Arrangement of the New Institute

In October 1863, the Moravian Provincial Institute for the Mentally Ill was officially opened. The newly appointed director Czermak immediately began to organize the transfer of patients from St Anne's Hospital. The capacity of the psychiatric ward was greatly reduced, as the old hospital building was extensively remodeled. After its completion, an observation and diagnostic department was available there only for mental patients from Brno. The existence of two departments for the care of the mentally ill led to some tensions, as the quote at the beginning of the chapter suggests. The St. Anne's Hospital took advantage of closer links with other health facilities and provided help in acute cases. However, it was not specifically equipped for long-term psychiatric treatment and terminally ill patients were sent to Černovice/Czernowitz, to which Czermak and his colleagues objected, pointing out that the new Institute was not a warehouse.[52]

A total of nine buildings and smaller structures were erected on the grounds of the Institute during this construction phase. The three-story main building had two wings, the right wing for male patients and the left wing for female patients. In addition to the operating theatres, the main building also housed offices, lounge areas and hospital administration departments. In the middle of the connecting corridor on the first floor there were rails on which wagons with firewood and coal were transported from the cellars by trained dogs.[53] The Institute's chapel was built behind the main administration building, near the rooms for the "educated" patients. It was connected to the institute's kitchen and baths and had a room for hydrotherapy.[54] The 100-metre-long main part of the building was entered through a representative gatehouse. Its front part was laid out according to the design of the Brno city gardener Anton Schebanek, while the rear part consisted only of ornamental beds at the time. The entire area was surrounded by a wall.[55]

The main building and several surrounding buildings provided 300 beds, which were initially occupied by 114 men and 94 women brought from St. Anne's Hospital. Within a few weeks, 7 more patients were admitted. From January 1864, Czermak negotiated with the director (and his former boss) Riedel for the admission of 12 women and 19 men from the Vienna Irrenanstalt, which was run by the state and was therefore obliged to admit patients regardless of

52 Hádlík, Poznámky k vývoji péče o duševně nemocné, 32.
53 Czermak, *Die Mährische Landes-Irrenanstalt*, 8–9. Hádlík, Poznámky k vývoji, 35.
54 Czermak, *Die Mährische Landes-Irrenanstalt*, 14–15.
55 MZA, f. A8 Zemská registratura, ka. 154, Sign. A 45/5, unpaginated.

their residency status. As these people were originally from Moravia, it was decided under pressure from the authorities that they should be transferred to the Institute in Černovice. This decision immediately triggered fears among provincial representatives that the Institute would be overcrowded, would not be able to accept patients from Moravia and would therefore no longer fulfil its medical mission, as it would turn into a "confinement" facility.[56]

Even before the patients were accommodated, Joseph Czermak, together with the second physician Franz Langer and the surgical assistant Friedrich Palliardi, whose position was being questioned for economic reasons, divided the hospital inmates into groups according to their ailments.[57] The state of health of some people was complicated, and if the doctors did not want to jeopardize the therapeutic purpose, safety and order, the patients had to be assigned to the appropriate departments. Outside the main building, two pavilions with their own fenced gardens planted with hawthorn were set up for "disturbed" patients. There, the more dangerous patients were isolated in a separate room. The allocation had to be approved by the Provincial Committee, as two of the Institute's wards were not yet in operation and the doctors requested access to them.[58]

Compared to other hospitals, the Institute had the smallest possible number of wards, whose furnishings and equipment were reduced to a minimum for reasons of economy. The necessary number of beds in the individual wards was adjusted and staffed with wardens, as medical conditions often changed suddenly, and patients could be transferred from one ward to another. The variety of symptoms required the greatest possible utilization of all wards. The originally intended temporary closure and reservation of two wards proved to be irresponsible, as this could have disrupted the healing process.[59] Czermak's concept of the psychiatric institute did not assume that one ward after another would be occupied, depending on how many patients of all kinds arrived and where a bed was available. The Institute's wards were constantly staffed by trained personnel, so that any patient could be accommodated at any time, even just one for whose diagnosis the equipment on that ward was intended. Medical judgment alone determined the staffing of wards, the suitability of the patients and their allocation to various groups, regardless of the administrative difficulties.[60]

56 MZA, f. A8 Zemská registratura, ka. 154, Sign. A45/5, fols. 818–821.
57 MZA, f. A8 Zemská registratura, ka. 154, Sign. A45/5, fols. 840–841.
58 MZA, f. A8 Zemská registratura, ka. 152, Sign. A45/5, unpaginated.
59 MZA, f. A8 Zemská registratura, ka. 156, Sign. A 45/5-3, fols. 91–93.
60 MZA, f. A8 Zemská registratura, ka. 156, Sign. A 45/5-3, fols. 93–94.

Czermak laid down the rules of the Institute, which in principle did not differ from those he had learned in detail at the Prague *Irrenanstalt*. There were two known versions of these rules. In the latter, adjustments were necessary mainly regarding the changes brought about by the provincial laws on the operation of health care facilities. Czermak emphasized that the Institute in Černovice/Czernowitz was a charitable institution for the treatment of curable patients and the guarding of incurable and dangerous patients.[61] Only patients who were recognized as mentally ill, had legal residence status and a person who was guaranteed to pay for their hospital stay could be admitted.[62] Patients had to undergo an initial examination in the treatment room, during which their current physical and mental condition, in particular their symptoms and the stage of their illness, were assessed. The initial examination also included the preparation of a proposal for treatment at the Institute.[63]

Similar rules were adopted by the healthcare facilities in various provinces of the monarchy, although there may have been some exceptions. According to the Institute's rules, each patient had to be examined twice a day by a doctor who made rounds, and an appropriate protocol had to be drawn up to assess the patient's current state of health. Great emphasis was placed on humane treatment and friendliness. The guards had precise instructions on how to treat the patients. They were not allowed to decide on the use of coercive measures themselves. Insults and swearing were forbidden. Relatives could be admitted but always had to obtain the director's consent. Visits without a close relationship to a particular patient were only possible in exceptional cases, mostly for professional and scientific purposes. The general public had no access to the Institute's premises. Correspondence and the receipt of parcels from the family were possible but were usually controlled by the wardens.[64]

Although Czermak did not like to do so, he sometimes abandoned these demands because he had to remember to be as economical as possible. If he did not think enough about economy, the administrator of the Institute was there to remind him. The administrator took care of the economic operation of the institute, kept the books and dealt with official matters. His salary, which corresponded to that a second physician, showed the importance of his position. Jakob Drapal, a former accountant at St. Anne's Hospital, was appointed the first administrator of the Institute. His duties included officially receiving patients, processing payments for their stay and keeping their medical records.

61 Czermak, *Die Mährische Landes-Irrenanstalt*, 28.

62 Schelleová, Schelle. *Civilní kodexy*, 44.

63 Czermak, *Die Mährische Landes-Irrenanstalt*, 115.

64 Czermak, *Die Mährische Landes-Irrenanstalt*, 50, 82.

Drapal had assistants who could take over some of his duties, especially the preparation of protocols and the handling of official correspondence. These assistants were not employees of the Institute, but were sent by the provincial committee, to whose control the Institute remained subject.[65]

The mentally ill were looked after day and night by wardens who received monthly salary, meals and clothing. They lived in the Institute and shared rooms near the patients' bedrooms. At this time, there were no other nursing staff in the Institute.[66] In addition to caring for the patients, the wardens had to have a training certificate to supervise the workshops where the patients worked as part of their therapy. Originally, there was supposed be one warden for every six patients, which seemed excessive to the committee, as the Institute's rules stipulated a ratio of one warden for every seven patients. Czermak tried to explain that the number of mentally ill patients was increasing and that it was necessary to have trained staff on the hand, to which the committee members had reservations for financial reasons.[67]

Since the founding of the General Hospital in Vienna, four types of payment for patients' stays in the hospital had been introduced in its statutes. This was adopted by hospitals in Pest, Zagreb and Prague, only the amount of the fees and the services provided changed over the decades.[68] The statute stipulated that all patients could be admitted to public hospitals without distinction of class, gender or religion. Only those suffering from protracted and incurable diseases were not admitted. The guilds had the option of paying annual lump sums to the hospitals for their journeymen, apprentices and laborers, who could then be admitted to the hospital free of charge in the event of illness. Like in Pest, Zagreb and Prague, people from different regional and social backgrounds, including servants who had no fixed abode, could be admitted on the recommendation of the parish priest and the district doctor. In some cases, patients could also be treated at the request of homeowners who wanted to take the sick person out of the house.[69]

Similar to the procedures for admission to the Prague mental asylum, the district physician examined the patients and determined whether hospitalization was necessary or whether the patients could be treated at home under medical supervision. Based on the results of the examination, the parish priest decided to release an amount from the poor relief fund to cover the hospitalization

65 Czermak, *Die Mährische Landes-Irrenanstalt*, 6.

66 Czermak, *Die Mährische Landes-Irrenanstalt*, 33.

67 MZA, f. A8 Zemská registratura, ka. 154, Sign. A45/5, fols. 859–860.

68 Watzka, Psychiatrische Anstalten in Österreich, 364.

69 Kopetz, *Österreichische politische Gesetzkunde*, 261.

costs. Hospitalization for poor patients with residency status was paid for by the home municipality (village community). Severe cases where "insanity" was obvious did not require confirmation from the district doctor and the formalities completed later. As the psychiatric hospitals were not only intended for poor patients, who were treated free of charge, but also for patients from the "middle class" who could not be cared for at home due to their personal circumstances, admission was paid for.[70]

At the Institute, patients were divided into three classes of paid and one free class according to their means. Payments had to be made one month in advance. The patients themselves were forbidden to handle the money, so the payer had to be a person outside the hospital, usually a relative or guardian. If the stay was not paid for on time, the patient was officially assigned to another class.[71] The 215 patients who passed through the gates, 5 male and 5 female patients, formed the first and second class. They paid 1–2 gulden per day for a two- to four-bed room, which was supervised by a warden. They could have their own clothes and linen, the meals served were of the best quality and consisted of a meat, vegetables and drinks. From a medical point of view, they all belonged to Ward A, where "calm" and "clean" patients were accommodated. They could visit the library and the music room, for which a range of board games and instruments had been purchased.[72]

While the highest-class patients received more comfortable accommodation and better care, the third patients were housed en masse and received fewer hearty meals. There was also a difference in care, as one guard was responsible for several patients. In the Ward B, third-class patients paid 60 kreutzer per day for a ten–bedroom with hospital clothing and linen, and nutritious food consisted of less expensive ingredients.[73] More than a third of the patients did perform domestic work outside of their detention. Occupational therapy was provided in the workshops, the laundry and the washroom, which were located in the southern part of the grounds. On their own initiative, some of them were able to earn some extra money by gardening as part of their treatment. The senior doctors and the janitor had their own gardens in the immediate vicinity of the main building. Some greenhouses and steam bath with kitchen gardens were used to supply the Institute's kitchen.[74] Many different flowers also grew in the greenhouses, and since the corridors lacked the decorative flowers that

70 Kopetz, *Österreichische politische Gesetzkunde*, 260.
71 Czermak, *Die Mährische Landes-Irrenanstalt*, 30–31.
72 MZA, f. A8 Zemská registratura, ka. 156, Sign. A 45/5-3, fol. 93.
73 MZA, f. A8 Zemská registratura, ka. 156, Sign. A 45/5-3, fol. 93.
74 Czermak, *Die Mährische Landes-Irrenanstalt*, 163.

were considered a suitable distraction for the resting patients, Czermak asked the provincial committee if the gardener Schebanek could arrange the flowers in the interior rooms of Institute.[75]

Although the Institute began its work, the authorization session was delayed and the provincial authorities did not complete the review and correction of all accounts for another five months.[76] Since the handover of the Institute, minor construction work continued to be carried out, including by the five male patients as part of their occupational therapy.[77] They contributed from their earnings for room and board. When one of them died, income was transferred to the provincial treasury for the "Insane Fund" (*Irrenfond*), which partly covered the treatment of "disturbing", "unclean" and physically weak patients who could become very dangerous and required constant supervision. These were free class patients who were housed in the two pavilions outside the main building (referred to as wards F and G).[78]

Most patients were accommodated in wards C and D, where the number of patients increased every year. They were still the third class, and the level of care and food was the same as for patients in Ward B. However, most of patients were physically frail and bedridden and required nursing care. Ward D patients were "less clean", sometimes had seizures and became dangerous.[79] There were some third-class educated patients on ward E who were classed as convalescents and needed special attention and care. Two male patients helped in the office.[80] Czermak wanted to enrich the treatment and ordered the production of gymnastic equipment after the provincial committee had agreed to pay the salary of the gymnastics master of the Provincial Academy, Herzel, who came to the Institute two or three times a week to train with the patients.[81]

In the hospitals, the spiritual needs of the sick were respected and cared for by competent people, often priests from the local (Catholic) parishes. Larger healthcare facilities could afford to employ their own clergy. In theory, the hospitals also accepted patients from other confessions, mostly Christian denominations. Chaplain Jakob Zažímal from the Komárov/Kumrowitz parish served in the hospital together with a Protestant priest and a rabbi on a "part-time"

75 MZA, f. A8 Zemská registratura, ka. 156, Sign. A 45/5-3, fols. 63–64.
76 MZA, f. A8 Zemská registratura, ka. 154, Sign. A 45/5, fol. 734.
77 MZA, f. A8 Zemská registratura, ka. 154, Sign. A 45/5, fol. 798. See also Czermak, *Die Mährische Landes-Irrenanstalt*, 163.
78 Czermak, *Die Mährische Landes-Irrenanstalt*, 30–42.
79 MZA, f. A8 Zemská registratura, ka. 156, Sign. A 45/5-3, fol. 93.
80 Czermak, *Die Mährische Landes-Irrenanstalt*, 163.
81 MZA, f. A8 Zemská registratura, ka. 156, Sign. A 45/5-3, fols. 99–100.

basis. Together they administered the sacraments to the sick and dying. Those who died in the hospital were taken to the autopsy room and the mortuary, which were set up in the north-eastern part of the hospital grounds. The hospital was also able to bury them in the Institute's cemetery at the family's expense, depending on the class of paying patients.[82] Most of patients admitted were Catholic, followed at a great distance by Jews and least of all Protestants. The few Jewish patients admitted to the Institute were female manual laborers. Within a few years, the number of Jewish and Protest patients fell slightly.[83] Citizens who professed the Israeli religion preferred to be treated in the Jewish hospitals, which were rapidly built in the second half of the nineteenth century.[84]

The Institute in Černovice/Czernowitz mainly admitted residents from Moravia. That did not mean that patients without Moravian residency status could not be admitted to the Institute. However, a respected "Moravian" had to guarantee and pay for the treatment of patients with "non-Moravian" residence status. Furthermore, only patients who belonged to one of the three paying classes without residency status could be treated at the Institute. Due to the geographical proximity to Silesia, where there was no mental asylum, most patients without residency status came from there. In 1864, several patients from Bohemia, Galicia and Hungary were also admitted to the Institute. Only two mentally ill patients came from the Austrian lands. Individual female patients from Prussia, England and Italy who were treated in the Institute were a rare exception. Not much changed in the first decade.[85]

The Institute had an equal number of places for men and women, but male patients slightly outnumbered females.[86] The most strongly represented age group was persons between the ages of thirty and forty. They made up a fifth of all patients.[87] The Institute also admitted children, as there was no formal school or other educational facility, they were taught by a chaplain. Most of the patients worked as day laborers and workers before being admitted to the Institute, the second largest group being former craftsmen. Only a few individuals came from the ranks of merchants, employees and teachers.[88] There were three main diagnoses of mental illness. The patients were most frequently

82 Czermak, *Die Mährische Landes-Irrenanstalt*, 6, 46, 83.

83 Regarding the religion, there were 91% Catholics, 6.2% Jews and 2.8% Protestants in 1870. See MZA, f. A9 Zemský výbor, ka. 6873, sign. P 7/1-2, fol. 1206.

84 Wölfler, *Das alte und neue Wiener Israeliten-Spital.*

85 MZA, f. A9 Zemský výbor, ka. 6873, sign. P 7/1-2, fol. 1198.

86 MZA, f. A9 Zemský výbor, ka. 6873, sign. P 7/1-2, fol. 1206.

87 Czermak, *Die Mährische Landes-Irrenanstalt*, 126–127.

88 Czermak, *Die Mährische Landes-Irrenanstalt*, 126–127.

treated with mania, followed by melancholia and anoia. Melancholia was associated with depression, anxiety and sadness. Mania was characterized by excessive energy, agitation, and general restlessness. Anoia was an all-encompassing term for mental weakness. Several patients with temporary types and subtypes of mental illness were also recorded such as epilepsia cum psychosis or anoia cum paralysis.[89]

After the departure of Czermak to Graz and the appointment of Franz Langer as the new director in 1869, the number of patients at the Institute increased. In 1872 there were only just over 400 beds in the Institute, four years later there were already over 500 inmates hospitalized. One reason for the deteriorating capacity was certainly the amendment of the in 1874, when a decree of the Ministry of the Interior came into force and general practitioners were obliged to register the mentally ill in their district, even those who were not in institutional care.[90] The doctors had to ensure that the mentally ill were cared for in such a way that they were not harmed in any way and lived in appropriate conditions. If the practitioners found that the "home care" of the mentally ill was not in order, they were to arrange for them to be admitted to a psychiatric institution.[91]

The area surrounding the Černovice Institute could provide building plots for the construction of new pavilions, but the Provincial Diet did not allow any new buildings on the site. It argued that construction costs would increase and agricultural land on site would be significantly reduced, which would jeopardize the Institute's self-sufficiency in food production.[92] The director of the Institute had to obtain official approval from the provincial committee approval for any expenditure. The daily problems with laundry, heating and food supply worsened the hygiene and undermined the treatment.[93] Due to shrinking capacity, permanently incurable and dormant patients were discharged home for treatment. Beds were placed in rooms with fewer patients and rooms that were not intended for patients were converted for medical purposes. The director also acquired additional beds by gradually transferring chronically ill men to the new branch, which was set up in the premises of the Convent Hospital of the Brothers of Mercy in Staré Brno/Altbrünn.[94]

89 Czermak, *Die Mährische Landes-Irrenanstalt*, 139.
90 Matoušek, Vzrůst počtu choromyslných, passim.
91 Preininger, *Sbírka zákonů a nařízení o zdravotnictví*, 373.
92 Hádlík, Poznámky k vývoji, 36.
93 MZA, f. A8 Zemská registratura, ka. 156, sign. A45/5-3, fols. 42–43.
94 MZA, f. E45 Milosrdní bratři Brno, ka. 86, sign. 344/1891, fol. 8.

4 Conclusion

Since the Enlightenment reforms, transformation of caregiving institutions in the early 1780s had been dedicated to "the mentally disordered people". Developments in Brno did not differ significantly from those in Pest, Zagreb and Prague. Initially, wards for people with mental disabilities were reserved within hospitals. The mental asylum was integrated into the United Poor Relief House founded by Emperor Joseph II in 1785. The sick, mothers, foundlings, orphans and people with mental disabilities came together under one roof. The House thus followed the institutional and administrative model of the General Hospital in Vienna. Just as in the *Narrenturm*, the care of the mentally ill in the asylum could hardly be described as medical treatment. The patients were severely restricted in their freedom of movement, lived in inadequate sanitary conditions and had reduced food rations, which were considered a panacea.

The House initially combined a kind of poorhouse and hospital care. The beds for terminally ill patients took up a considerable part of its capacity, which brought it close to early modern infirmaries. Despite the numerous administrative staff, the management of the House was in the hands of the chief provincial physician, who supervised most of the health facilities in Moravia and could not take their special features into account. The Moravian Estates represented in the provincial diet and its committee carefully monitored the expenses of the House and moderately compensated for the intervention of the court authorities in Vienna. However, the increasing obligations to the poor of the province during the Napoleonic Wars limited the support of Estates. The House lacked the funds for its daily operations and became dependent on subsidies from Vienna.

An ambiguous situation, in which the House was able to survive thanks to state funding without the provincial committee having to relinquish its influence, led to further changes in the hospital administration. The authority of the intendent was strengthened, who, together with the office assistants, took care of the day-to-day running of the House and ensured a balanced budget, sometimes even at the expense of medical care. Preparations for the advancing cholera epidemic presented the provincial head medical officer with additional organizational tasks. In the House, this was underlined by the separation of the post of director from that of provincial head physician in 1830, when the provincial authorities were given the power to appoint a new director with medical training. Second physicians and additional medical staff were recruited and special hospital departments, including the ward for people with mental disabilities, could be established within the House (later called St. Anne's Hospital).

At the same time, the development of medicine and the spread of diseases in the industrial suburbs of Brno placed increased demands on the hospital doctors, whose insight could no longer be ignored. The Provincial Committee was interested in improving medical care, including the treatment of the mentally ill. It requested reports from hospital directors in other provinces of the monarchy on how they were tackling the problem of care and capacity. The Committee's representatives responsible for health care, sought out trained physicians who brought a wealth of experience, not only in medical care, but also in hospital management. In 1855, the Provincial Committee recruited Joseph Czermak from the Prague Irrenanstalt, which enjoyed a very good reputation at the time. The committee appointed Czermak as the first doctor of the mental asylum at the St. Anne's Hospital in order to make changes in line with the latest medical practices.

From the early 1850s, the leading Habsburg physicians undertook study trips to psychiatric institutions in German lands and elsewhere with the support of the provincial authorities. On their return, Czermak and his colleagues attempted to apply the knowledge, they had acquired, in their local hospitals. Although the doctors moved from one institution to another and spread their experiences throughout the monarchy, the operation of the "insane asylums" changed only slowly. The rooms overcrowded with patients could hardly provide an appropriate environment for care. The Moravian provincial committee partially complied with the doctors' demands and rented additional buildings to house separate medical departments. The stubborn problem, however, remained the layout of the St. Anne's Hospital, which was difficult to convert into a modern facility. The large monastery buildings, with their similarly designed corridors, were more suited to the work of the wardens than to the treatment of patients.

The important prerequisite for the transformation of the St. Anne's Hospital was the administrative reforms in the late 1850s. The city administration of Brno annexed larger suburban districts and some of the obstacles arising from the spatial limitations of local municipalities were removed. The provincial committee was considering an area-intensive reconstruction of the hospital and its wards. However, there was a difference between the proposals of the medical circles, mainly represented by the heads of the medical wards and those of the authorities. Joseph Czermak, for example did not consider a mere increase in capacity to be a systematic solution. In his opinion, it would have been much more effective to establish specialized institutes and concentrate on care in the so-called pavilions. With the later pavilion-type facilities, it was much easier to add smaller buildings or place them on the site. This type of facility could also be built and commissioned more flexibly to respond to current medical trends.

However, the political authorities rejected the pavilion-type hospital due to the financial and structural requirements. The original project had to be abandoned, and a proposal was drawn up that mixed element of both building types and united the hospital wings and individual wards under one roof. If one compares this unrealized plan for the hospital grounds with the system of villas ("pavilion") that prevailed in the monarchy in the 1890s, clear differences become apparent. It cannot be said that they were the same type of complex. The inpatient wards were to be close to the main administrative building and connected to it by a covered corridor on the first floor. The same applies to the hydrotherapy building and the baths. There should be one pavilion for men and one for women, each with five wards.[95]

The Ministry of the Interior together with the Moravian Provincial Committee approved the modified design for the construction of new institution and appointed Czermak as the first institution's director. The administration and rules for the treatment of patients, which were based on legal norms, represented the changes that institutional care had undergone since the middle of the nineteenth century. Patients who were diagnosed with mental illness and who had the means to pay for their hospital stay were admitted to one of five specialized wards. Diagnosis was tailored to this, dividing patients into three basic forms of illness, but with a range of transient symptoms and characteristics in individual patients.

The opening of the Institute coincided with the imminent handover of the health care facilities to the provincial administration, which the central authorities agreed to after several years of negotiations. However, this decision, ultimately restricted the further development of institutional care for the mentally ill. The Provincial Committee responsible for the healthcare facilities came under pressure from persons in political and medical circles who tried to expand the focus of the Černovice Institute and to place terminally ill patients there. This plan did not work out, but the number of patients grew rapidly. Subsequently, a tension developed between the specialized medical care of mentally challenged patients as highlighted by psychiatrists and the institutionalized confinement of allegedly dangerous persons as emphasized by politicians and doctors from general hospital.

Acknowledgement

This study is an output of grant of the Czech Science Foundation (GA CR) no. 2204258S *Anatomy of a Suffering Soul. From the 'passions of the soul' and 'empirical psychology' to a psychiatric hospital in the Czech Lands, 1770–1814*, which has been granted to the Faculty of Arts of the Charles University (Prague).

95 See Topp, *Freedom and the Cage*, 29–35.

CHAPTER 7

With the Emperor's Support: Plans and Obstacles of Psychiatric Institutionalization in Hungary between the 1840s and 1860s

Janka Kovács

The late eighteenth century and the early decades of the nineteenth century saw the rise of the custodial mental asylum in several countries of Europe, among them some regions of the Habsburg Monarchy, especially the Austrian and Bohemian territories. In Hungary, however, the first private and subsequently state-funded asylums were established well into the nineteenth century.[1] Until then, the place of the mentally ill within the gradually evolving system of social and health care was subject to debate in the country,[2] and even though a small group of health care and social reformers were actively seeking a solution to the so-called "mad-problem" and the first plans to establish a mental asylum for the Kingdom of Hungary were devised as early as the 1790s, the early history of the institutionalization and professionalization of Hungarian psychiatry is characterized by unrealized plans. These, however unsuccessful they might have been, are worthy of closer inquiry, as they reveal how official and expert attitudes towards the mentally ill evolved and transformed throughout the decades characterized by the struggle to establish a mental asylum for Hungary.

The period of institutionalization – spanning roughly between the late eighteenth century and the late nineteenth century – shifted into the focus of social historical inquiries mainly from the late 1970s until the early 2000s. In these decades, inspired largely by the critical attitudes expressed in antipsychiatry and the seminal works of Michel Foucault, Erving Goffman, R. D. Laing, or

1 The first state-run asylum was opened in Nagyszeben (Sibiu, today in Romania) in 1863. Transylvania, however, did not belong to Hungary administratively until 1867, and the Royal National Asylum in Nagyszeben remained a provincial institution even after the Austro–Hungarian Compromise. Until the turn of the century, three major public asylums were opened in Hungary: The Royal National Asylum in Lipótmező in 1868, the Angyalföld Mental Asylum in 1884, and the Nagykálló Asylum in 1896.

2 See for example: Daday, Adatok a magyarországi, 449–451. Horánszky, A Magyar elmegyógyászat, 37–53. Pándy, *Gondoskodás az elmebetegekről*. Vikár, Az elmeápolás kezdetei, 37–53. Zsakó, Az egykori országos, 84–107.

 | HTTPS://DOI.ORG/10.1163/9789004755062-009

Thomas Szasz reinforcing different agendas and approaches toward contemporary psychiatry from the early 1960s onwards, the first "national histories" of institutionalization and more general accounts on the first formative decades of psychiatry have been written, especially in Western European contexts.[3] Early works inspiring further inquiry reflected on the abuses and insufficiency of institutional psychiatry in the mid-twentieth century and the differing perceptions of the concept of "madness" even going to the extremes of delegitimizing psychiatry as a medical enterprise and a "unique policing profession".[4] Later inquiries attempted to map the social history of institutions and institutionalization tended to accept the medical framework and the medicalized interpretations of "madness", working in this vein to reconstruct the respective national histories of psychiatry.[5]

Despite significant international examples, in Hungarian medical historiography, so far, no attempts have been made to delve into the earliest plans – enjoying both professional and political support – for an asylum in Hungary and consider them as "building blocks" in the conflict-ridden and difficult process that led to the opening of the Royal National Asylum in Lipótmező in 1868. Most historical accounts, both older literature produced by psychiatrists and newer, more professional works on the history of mental health care in Hungary[6] refrained from an in-depth investigation of archival documents and an analysis of questions based on primary materials that did not explicitly concern the attempts aimed at establishing an asylum. Nevertheless, this scholarship allowed for the issue of institutionalization to shift into the focus of medical and social discourses. This resulted in a narrative which characterizes the long process of institutionalization as a series of "failed projects", which eventually bore fruit in the late 1860s. While this is by and large true, earlier research did not take into account that preparing the ground for opening a public asylum in 1868 was a complex process, lasting between roughly the 1790s and the 1860s. The way the members of the Hungarian medical community fostered discussions on the issue from the late eighteenth century onward and the way they came to terms with their own possibilities and limitations in the first half of the nineteenth century, yields a more thorough and multifaceted analysis.

3 See for example: Engstrom, *Clinical Psychiatry*. Goldstein, *Console and Classify*. Shorter, *A History of Psychiatry*. Scull, *The Most Solitary of Affictions*. Porter, *Mind Forg'd Manacles*. Kaufmann, *Aufklärung*. Castel, *L'Ordre psychiatrique*. Dörner, *Bürger und Irre*.

4 Though this concept has been present in his work earlier, Szasz reflected most comprehensively on this notion in one of his later books, cf. Szasz, *Coercion as Cure*.

5 See a critical reflection on the approaches to the histories of madness and mental history in Kirk et al. *Mad Science*.

6 Lafferton, *Hungarian Psychiatry*.

This entails the concurrent study of questions, such as the limits of medical education, the lack of professional psychiatric knowledge and thus the lack of advocates within the medical circles for an asylum project as obstacles and the evolution of "alternative spaces" (e.g., wards in general hospitals or hospitals run by religious orders) and the first individual and collective initiatives to create a functioning hospital space for the mentally ill as the building blocks of the institutionalization process.

This study discusses the first findings based on archival research as a survey chapter written within the framework of a postdoctoral project, the aim of which is to make a first attempt to uncover the fundamental documents related to and discourses revolving around the early phase of the institutionalization of psychiatry in Hungary. For the sake of clarity, the article follows the thread of plans and considers the main obstacles to reveal the main currents of the discourse around mental asylums in the period leading up to the opening of the Royal National Asylum. After a short discussion of the first (unrealistic) initiatives and the main obstacles to the institutionalization project, the article zooms in on the first two serious plans conceived in the 1840s and the planning process of the Royal National Asylum that was directed from Vienna in the second half of the 1850s and the 1860s – considering not only the plans, but also the actors, theories, and possible models involved in this decades-long project.

1 The Idea of an Asylum Is Born: Motivations and Obstacles

Although the problem of the place and care of the "mad" within the evolving system of social and healthcare had gained traction already in the earlier decades of the eighteenth century[7] – especially in the medical discourse intensifying from the 1770s , the first proposals to establish a mental asylum in Hungary were not discussed until the Diet of 1790–1791, held shortly after the opening of the asylum known as the "Narrenturm" as part of the General Hospital in Vienna in 1784 and the Prague asylum in 1790. At this early instance, no particular medical ideas were involved in the discussions (even though the most modern ideas had already circulated in Hungary at the time[8]), rather,

7 See more on the discourses of state medicine and the possibilities of institutional care for the mentally ill: Kovács, "Finding a Place for the Most Unfortunate?".

8 It is evidenced, for example, by Mihály Haffner's proposal in 1793 to open a hospital for the city of Pest following the model of the Viennese General Hospital. In his detailed plan, he discussed the placement and isolation of mentally ill patients and the organization of their ward and rooms, reflecting the – by contemporary means – most modern ideas, such as humane treatment or meaningful activities. Cf. Haffner, *Versuch eines Vorschlages.* and Kovács, 1798: Megnyílik a Rókus kórház.

their nature was partly philanthropic and practical, and partly financial. At the Diet, the Hungarian estates urged the collection of funds for the establishment of an asylum and the reassignment of a part of the funds of the monasteries and contemplative orders that were dissolved by Joseph II from 1782 onwards. As a result, 122,032 gulden were assigned to the national asylum fund which – in the later decades – was further expanded via donations and bequests.[9]

The practical reason and urgency of this step was that in the other parts of the Habsburg Monarchy – following the foundations in Vienna and Prague – the establishment of further smaller (custodial) asylums ensued at the turn of the eighteenth and nineteenth centuries, in, for example, Graz, Linz, or Brno. Consequently, isolation and a type of rudimentary care had already been accessible to a limited number of patients[10] in the Austrian, Bohemian, and Moravian parts of the Monarchy, while no similar institution was available for Hungarian patients. In theory, they were eligible for care in asylums anywhere within the Monarchy (in practice, this primarily meant Vienna, being the closest to Hungary), however, this violated the rule of reciprocity, which meant that individuals could only be admitted to different health care institutions if they could offer the same to individuals from the other parts of the Monarchy.[11]

9 In 1869, an audit commissioned by the Ministry of the Interior to compile a report inquiring into the circumstances and mistakes of the building of the Royal National Asylum in Hungary. This report contains a substantial historical part, which details the earliest attempts with references to the most important documents and regulations related to the planning and building process from the Diet of 1791 until the opening of the asylum. This bulky, almost 300-pages long report serves as a good point of orientation for the discussion of the earliest plans and also for later archival research. Cf. Magyar Nemzeti Levéltár Országos Levéltára [National Archives of Hungary, Central Archives, hereinafter referred to as MNL OL] K 150 Box 559. 3258/76. Jegyzőkönyv a lipótmezei magyar orszg. tébolyda intézet felülvizsgálatáról [Report on the audit commissioned to inspect the Royal National Asylum in Lipótmező]. See the order to reassign a part of the funds and create a national asylum fund for Hungary: Concl. Cons. No. 15711. die 26. Aug. 1791. Regni Gyrgathum instaurandum. In: Linzbauer, *Codex Sanitario-Medicinalis Hungariae* 3/1, 665–666.

10 On the operation, statistics, and therapeutic practices of the Viennese and Prague asylums in the first half of the nineteenth century see the reports published by their primary and secondary physicians: Fischel, *Prags k. k. Irrenanstalt*. Riedel, *Prag's Irrenanstalt*. Riedel, *Ärztliche Berichte*. Viszánik, *Leistungen und Statistik*.

11 Until 1814, the principle of reciprocity did not even prevail in cases when similar institutions (i.e., general hospitals) were accessible, and payments had to be settled by the respective authorities (the localities the patient originated from, or via the poor fund created from the funds of the dissolved religious orders further supplemented by donations and bequests in later decades). This was subject to change after 1814 with the order of the United Court Chancellery (Vereinigte Hofkanzlei) stating that Hungarian patients – except for the mentally ill – have to be treated free of charge in Viennese hospitals and the other way around. Cf. Concl. Cons. No. 23756. Gratuita reciproca intertentio in Nosocomiis

Since Hungary had no mental asylum, this quickly resulted in conflicts mainly with the Viennese authorities. Hungarian patients, who could finance their stay in the asylums in any way – through their families or local authorities – could in theory be admitted to asylums anywhere in the Monarchy, but in several instances, the institutions refused to accept them. And although by 1829 this question was officially settled[12] and the agreement was annulled only after 1852,[13] the questions of admittance and financing continued to cause problems as testified by a number of requests handled either by the Staatsrat or the different departments of the Locumtenential Council[14] until 1848 and between 1861–1867, pointing at the urgency of setting up an asylum for Hungary and this issue serving as a main driving force behind the institutionalization project.[15]

Although the collection of funds had almost been continuous from the late eighteenth century onwards, the Napoleonic Wars significantly slowed down the process, and the issue of establishing a mental asylum came to the fore again only in 1808–1809, when the Locumtenential Council set up a committee led by the *protomedicus* (chief physician) of Hungary, Endre Pfisterer to make plans for a national asylum and find a location that would be sufficient for the purposes of isolation and healing. Pfisterer's plan, which was completed by

---

Hungariae et Viennae, die 13. Sept. 1814. In: Linzbauer, *Codex Sanitario-Medicinalis Hungariae* III/2, 445. See the outline of the evolution of reciprocal care and the history of its frequent setbacks in: Linzbauer, *A magyar korona országainak*, 33–40.

12 The Viennese asylum was ordered to admit Hungarian patients if they were able to finance their stay in the hospital. Cf. Concl. Cons. No. 7849. Numerus Maniacorum hungaricorum et extraneorum in Regno gratis intertentorum; – Principium Reciprocitatis hoc quoque in puncto qum Provinciis germanicis et Gyrgato Viennensi introductum, die 31. Martii 1829. In: Linzbauer, *Codex Sanitario-Medicinalis Hungariae* III/3, 356–358.

13 Linzbauer, *A magyar korona országainak*, 40.

14 The Locumtenential Council (also known as the Vice-Regal Council) was the most important internal governmental organ of the Kingdom of Hungary, which operated under the Hungarian Court Chancery and was supervised by the palatine. It was set up in 1723 and operated until 1848. It also operated for a short while between 1861 and 1867; thereafter its functions were taken over by different ministries. See more on the Hungarian government bodies between 1526 and 1918 and the availability of their resources in: Ress–Niessen, Hungary, 43–81.

15 See for example some cases centered around the questions of admittance and financing: Österreichisches Staatsarchiv, Haus-, Hof- und Staatsarchiv, Kabinettsarchiv, Staatsrat 1835/1008; 1841/251; 1842/1008; 1846/6628. The requests were sent in the greatest numbers to the Department of Secular Foundations of the Locumtenential Council (cf. MNL OL C 80) until 1848 and the Department of Public Health between 1861 and 1867 (cf. MNL OL D 210 XX. Magyar Királyi Helytartótanács Közegészségügyi Osztály [Locumtenential Council, Department of Public Health]; MNL OL D 217 IV. Egészségügyi kútfő [Medical records]). A thorough analysis of these sources will be the task of future research.

1809, described a small asylum for altogether 70 patients (20 paying and 50 non-paying), where they would have been separated according to their behavior and cleanliness ("calm and clean" and "furious and unclean"). Furthermore, Pfisterer proposed the employment of a director who would also be the primary physician of the asylum, as well as other medical staff, among them an assistant physician, an assistant surgeon, and six nurses and non-medical staff, such as a caretaker, a priest, a cook, and two servants.

In the plan, several potential locations were identified primarily in Buda and Pest – as it was generally agreed on that a central location within Hungary would be of paramount importance.[16] As none of the chosen locations seemed sufficient or affordable enough, the search continued throughout the 1810s. After Buda and Pest, other, non-central locations were also considered in the process, such as various monasteries in different parts of the country.[17] After careful inspection, none of the empty areas were deemed sufficient for establishing an asylum and reconstructing existing buildings except for the Kiscell and Pécs monasteries – was also not considered a viable option. What is more, in the meantime, the latter two ecclesiastical buildings were utilized for other purposes – as a military depot and military hospital and an orphanage.[18]

The establishment of an asylum in the first decades of the nineteenth century was hindered not only by financial reasons and the lack of a suitable place, where it could be built. Discussions on psychiatric institutionalization were limited to a very narrow circle involving largely those medical officers who held positions within the Hungarian Locumtenential Council such as chief physicians Mihály Lenhossék or Ignác Stáhly. The medical community as a whole was essentially left out of the discussions and most doctors were either unaware of or uninterested in the urgency of the problem. This was largely due to the structure and content of medical education and the role and place of psychological and psychiatric knowledge within the curricula of the University of Pest. While the content of education was fundamentally similar at the universities within the Monarchy – due to the uniformizing initiatives of the University of Vienna from the late eighteenth century onwards, which were only partly successful –, and psychological and psychiatric knowledge gradually

---

16 Pfisterer proposed the following locations: the ground near the so-called Újépület/Neugebäude (in the 5th district of today's Budapest), Káposztásmegyer (in today's 4th district), the vicinity of the Botanical Garden (in today's 8th district), Vérmező (in today's 1st district), and the location of the old military cemetery in Buda (in today's 1st district). Cf. MNL OL K 150 Box 559. 3258/76, fol. 2.

17 Fekete, Intézetünk megalapítása.

18 MNL OL K 150 Box 559. 3258/76, fol. 3.

began to appear within medical education from the turn of the eighteenth and nineteenth centuries, medical psychology and/or psychiatry was not taught as a separate subject until the 1840s in the region.[19]

Nevertheless, from the early nineteenth century, the traditional Hippocratic–Galenic approach to medicine was gradually replaced in subjects which contributed largely to the development of the, to use a modern term, psy-sciences. In textbooks on physiology, pathology, therapy, medical semiotics, and state medicine (*medizinische Polizey* and forensic medicine) the approaches of neurophysiology and neuropathology were introduced, having a "particularist" approach to both physiological and psychological phenomena instead of a holistic view. At the same time, at the two-semester courses on state medicine, a "social view" was introduced into medical education, viewing madness and its consequences from a broader social perspective, offering possible – institutional and extra-institutional – solutions to the problem.[20] The dissertations compiled and written by medical students show how students appropriated psychological knowledge, while the case histories from the University of Pest demonstrate how this type of bookish knowledge on mental illnesses was converted into practice – even though in a very marginal and limited way.[21]

What is more, while in Vienna and Prague there were institutions that could eventually serve as spaces for clinical instruction, the lack of such an asylum or at least a clinical ward impacted the development of Hungarian psychiatry, the motivations of individual physicians, and the possibility of fostering a meaningful discourse on its social role in a negative way. In both Prague and Vienna, there had already been initiatives in the first half of the 1840s to establish a chair for psychiatry. The University of Pest,[22] due to the lack of expert lobbyists

---

19 The introduction of psychological and psychiatric knowledge in medical education in the nineteenth century has only been superficially dealt with in secondary literature, even in otherwise well-researched areas, such as Great Britain, where research has only begun recently. Cf. Merkulova, *Pedagogy and the Building of British Psychiatry*. On the University of Vienna, see: Lesky, *Die Wiener medizinische Schule*, 175–191.

20 On this issue with particular focus on Hungary within the context of the Habsburg Monarchy see: Kovács, The darkest field of medicine, 17–46.

21 More on how mental illnesses were represented in dissertations and clinical case histories in late eighteenth- and early nineteenth-century Hungary see: Kovács, "Érzelmi nyavalyák", 67–84. Kovács, *A lélek tudománya*.

22 The first plans for clinical instruction were sent to the Court Commission of Studies (Studienhofkommission) by Josef Gottfried Riedel from Prague and Michael Viszánik from Vienna in 1841 and 1844 respectively. Eventually, Riedel became the first professor in the Monarchy to hold clinical lectures in the Prague asylum, while theoretical lectures on medical psychology were held by Ernst von Feuchtersleben and clinical lectures by

and an asylum where clinical lectures could be held, had lagged behind until the 1860s.[23] Therefore, in the 1830s and 1840s, even though establishing a mental asylum for Hungary was on the agenda of the official authorities and the highest-ranking members of the medical community (such as the chief physicians and councilors), most members, especially those studying at the medical faculty of the University of Pest in increasing numbers from the early nineteenth century,[24] could not receive training either in theoretical or clinical psychiatry. And although it was an option to receive practical training in the Viennese asylum (which still operated as part of the Allgemeines Krankenhaus in the so-called "Narrenturm"), it did not attract Hungarian-born physicians in large numbers. Nevertheless, both Ferenc Schwartzer, the founder of the first private asylum in Hungary in 1850 and the "father of Hungarian psychiatry" whose pupils would later lead the first broader discourses on mental health reform from the 1860s and 1870s onwards, as well as Emil Schnirch, the first director of the Royal National Asylum in Nagyszeben/Hermannstadt (Sibiu, today in Romania) in Transylvania opened in 1863 and Lipótmező opened in 1868 completed their practical years there as secondary physicians next to Michael Viszánik.

The Hungarian medical community, beginning to define itself as a professional group with physicians organizing themselves into associations and

---

Viszánik from the mid-1840s in Vienna. See their petitions in ÖStA AVA Unterricht StHK Akten Teil 2 315 5Prag Med 2988/385, Psychiatrie, Allerunterthänigster Vortrag der treugehorsamsten Studien-Hofkommission über das Gesuch der Primarärztes des Irrenanstalt zu Prag, Doktor Riedl um Bewilligung daselbst unentgeltliche außerordentlich Lehrvorträge halten zu dürfen, 15 Mai 1841; ÖStA AVA Unterricht StHK Akten Teil 2 243 4Med 825/924, Psychiatrische Krankheiten, A. o. Vorlesungen über Psychiatrie, 16 November 1844, fols. 1–66.

23 In 1847/48, Szilárd Pomutz (also known as Konstantin Pomutz) held lectures on psychiatry. (Cf. Hőgyes, *Emlékkönyv*. Rigó [ed.], *A Budapesti Orvostudományi Egyetem*, 21.) However, from 1847/48 until the early 1860s, it becomes difficult to reconstruct the structure of lectures and those responsible for teaching a given subject (especially in the case of minor subjects, such as psychiatry), as the curricula were discontinued after the Revolution and War of Independence in Hungary in 1848–1849. In the 1860s, theoretical lectures were introduced, and clinical lectures were held by Ferenc Schwartzer in his private asylum opened in 1850 located in Buda in Kék Golyó utca (in today's twelfth district in Budapest, where the National Institute of Oncology operates). Clinical instruction eventually began at the psychiatric ward of Saint Roch's Hospital as well, led by the most eminent pupil of Schwartzer, Károly Bolyó. Cf. A Királyi Magyar Tudományegyetem Tanrendje, 1860/1861–1867/1868. https://adt.arcanum.com/en/collection/ELTE_EgyetemiTanrendek/?decade=1860#collection-contents (last accessed: February 2, 2024).

24 Cf. Lafferton, *Hungarian Psychiatry*, 49.

launching their first journal[25] *Orvosi Tár* (Medical Collection) in the vernacular, created its first forums for (public) discussion from the 1830s onwards. Yet, the shortcomings in medical education concerning mental pathologies visibly surfaced in their professional activities. While individual mental illnesses were increasingly dealt with in a variety of medical books published either in Latin, German, or the vernacular Hungarian[26] from the last third of eighteenth century, the question of institutionalization rarely came up either individually or as part of the discussions on organizing public health more effectively, and – as compared to the urgency and significance of the issue – the question was seldom featured in *Orvosi Tár*.[27] If so, it rarely reflected "original" ideas or plans, rather, they reproduced foreign knowledge.[28]

Apart from public forums, such as books and journals, the issue of institutionalization rarely came up at the more enclosed professional forums of the medical community, such as the Royal Budapest Society of Physicians (Budapesti Királyi Orvosegyesület) established in 1837 or the Society of Hungarian Physicians and Naturalists (Magyar Orvosok és Természetvizsgálók Egyesülete) established in 1841.[29] At their monthly and annual meetings, which served as opportunities to discuss individual cases and the burning issues of public health, mostly those areas came forward that dealt with averting more immediate dangers to society (such as epidemiology) or were more established and institutionalized fields, having a broader impact on wider layers of society (such as obstetrics or surgery).

Even in the late 1840s, when the first serious plans of settling the situation of the mentally ill were conceived (to be discussed below), these forums

25 On the significance of scientific journals in organizing professional communities see: Dawson–Lightman–Shuttleworth–Topham, eds., 2020.

26 On the emergence of the discourse of psychology and psychiatry see: Kovács, *A lélek tudománya*. 19–94.

27 See for example the following short articles: Bugát, Őrjintézet Pesten. N. N. Viszánik külföldön. Stadler, A pesti polgári kórház. Esze, Az elmekórházakról.

28 See the comprehensive discussions of mental health care and penal institutions based on foreign examples by Szaniszló Töltényi, surgeon and professor at the Josephinian Military Academy of Surgery in Vienna: Töltényi, Közlemények, 337–345. Töltényi, Közlemények, 354–362. Töltényi, Közlemények, 2–8. Töltényi, Közlemények, 17–26. Töltényi, Közlemények, 226–233. Töltényi, Közlemények, 242–248. Töltényi, Közlemények, 370–377.

29 On the history of the two societies see: Chyzer, *A Magyar Orvosok*. Simon, A Budapesti Királyi. Salacz (ed.), *A Budapesti Királyi*. Stráner, Város és tudomány.

largely ignored the question of psychiatric institutionalization.[30] This is well exemplified by the competition announced by the Society of Hungarian Physicians and Naturalists in 1847, asking the competitors to devise a complex plan for the reform of public health in Hungary. While several plans were sent to the Society, and some of them, such as the works of Imre Bittner, József Csorba, or Sebestény Endre Kovács, the formative physicians of the age, also appeared in print, none of them included in their proposals a serious plan for settling the situation of the mentally ill, and some, like Bittner, failed even to mention the issue.[31] Thus, while a scattered and unorganized discourse unfolded on the problem and urgency of institutionalization, the ideas and plans to settle the situation of the mentally ill in Hungary remained largely behind "closed doors" as a problem dealt with mainly by official authorities and a few chosen representatives of the medical community.

---

30 During the Reform Era in Hungary, the only longer and thorough lecture at the itinerary congresses of the Society of Hungarian Physicians and Naturalists was held by Ferenc Bene in 1847, however, the proceedings of the congress – due to the events of 1848–1848 and the following retaliation – were only published and could reach a larger audience in 1863. Cf. Bene, A lélekgyógytan, 79–85. At the congresses, besides the plenary lectures, smaller group meetings were also held, where individual cases were discussed. At the 1844 congress in Kolozsvár (Cluj-Napoca, today in Romania), the issues of mania and alcoholism were discussed. Cf. Semmelweis Orvostörténeti Múzeum, Könyvtár és Levéltár [Semmelweis Medical History Museum, Library, and Archives, hereinafter referred to as SOMKL] I. Magyar Orvosok és Természetvizsgálók Vándorgyűlései [Congresses of the Society of Hungarian Physicians and Naturalists], Box 1. A' Magyar Orvosok és Természet Vizsgálók 1844dik évi öszelö 2–6. napjaiban Kolosvárt tartott gyülekezete Orvos-Sebészeti szakosztályának jegyzőkönyve [The Minutes of the Congress held at Kolozsvár on September 2–6, 1844 of the Society of Hungarian Physicians and Naturalists, Department of Physicians and Surgeons], fols. 6r–v. At the 1847 congress, besides Bene's lecture, Pál Almási Balogh discussed the relationship of psychiatry and criminal law. Cf. SOMKL I. Magyar Orvosok és Természetvizsgálók Vándorgyűlései [Congresses of the Society of Hungarian Physicians and Naturalists], Box 1. A Magyar Orvosok és Természetvizsgálók VIIIik nagygyülése Sopronban Augustus 11-kétöl 17-ig bezárolag 1847. Második közülés augustus 15kén Kismartonban [VIIIth Congress of the Society of Hungarian Physicians and Naturalists in Sopron between August 11–17, 1847. Second public meeting on August 15 in Kismarton (Eisenstadt, today in Austria)]. At the monthly meetings of the Royal Budapest Society of Physicians, mental illnesses and individual cases were often discussed, however, no comprehensive plans for mental health reform were devised by the Society during the 1830s and 1840s. Cf. SOMKL I. Budapesti Királyi Orvosegyesület [Royal Budapest Society of Physicians], Boxes 1–2. (1837–1848).

31 Cf. Bittner, *Eszmék a közorvostan.* Csorba, *Észrevételek az álladalmi.* Kovács, *Javaslat az álladalmi közegészség.*

2 Searching for Models: the First Realistic Plans?

To establish a well-functioning, curative asylum – the idea of which had already been circulating in Europe by the 1830s –, it was imperative to find a location that would support this function. On the long run, creating a space for medical education was also a necessity to train mad-doctors, or, to use a contemporary term, "alienists", and since the Medical Faculty was located at Pest, either Pest, Buda, or Óbuda would have served as suitable locations. In 1824, plans were made to set up an asylum near the former military hospital in Pest (in today's 5th district), however, according to contemporary calculations, it would have cost 314,430 gulden, which far exceeded the amount available in the national asylum fund at the time. To help supplement the fund, in the late 1820s, the Locumtenential Council began collecting money from individuals, the clergy, and municipalities. In 1829, the town of Buda offered 1000 gulden supplemented with a further 1000 if the asylum were to be built in Buda, a plot where the building and its gardens could be located, along with building materials, such as rubble-stone and limestone.[32]

The first realistic plan to establish an asylum, however, is linked to a smaller municipality north of today's Budapest and a bishop's see, Vác, where the building of the Theresianum, a former boarding school following the Viennese model,[33] was found appropriate for the purpose. In 1832, when the issue was raised at the Diet held in Pozsony (Bratislava, today in Slovakia), the building stood empty. Although it was supposed to be repurposed before, as in 1808, the Ludovica Military Academy was established here (hence the later name of the building, Ludoviceum, which also appears in the sources), the plans fell through. In 1832, Archduke Joseph of Austria, Palatine of Hungary had already sent a committee to assess the state of the building and decide whether it was suitable for the purpose of an asylum. According to the final report of the committee, the building – while in theory it could cater to patients –, cannot be purchased, as the price and the costs of rebuilding would have exhausted the national asylum fund completely.[34] Therefore, the building of the former Theresianum stood empty until 1834, when the Bishop of Vác, Ferenc Nádasdy purchased it and donated it for the purposes of an asylum.

---

32 MNL OL K 150 Box 559. 3258/76. fol. 4.

33 The boarding school operated between 1767 and 1784, therefore, by this time, it had been out of use for decades, which left its mark on the state of the building causing further problems and making its potential reconstruction a financially more challenging project.

34 MNL OL K 150 Box 559. 3258/76. fols. 5–6.

In 1836, the Locumtenential Council set up another committee to assess the condition of the building and calculate the price of the reconstruction, while Mihály Lenhossék, the chief physician of the country was sent to Germany on a so-called "technological journey"[35] to study the construction and management of its most modern asylums and apply the knowledge thus gathered in Hungary. At the same time, another campaign was launched to collect funds, petitioning the monarch to reassign part of the income of some of the bishoprics for the purpose.[36] While the documentation of Lenhossék's journey has not been uncovered so far, and thus it is not known, which asylums in Germany he visited, his plan for an asylum is included in the historical part of the 1869 report compiled by the committee that was ordered by the Ministry of the Interior to inquire into the building process of the Royal National Asylum. According to this plan, Lenhossék proposed an asylum for 400 patients, where the general division of patients would have been applied: besides separation by gender, he would have separated them along curability and behavior. He would have also introduced three payment categories and 180 places for non-paying patients. According to Lenhossék's plans, completed by 1839, the staff would have counted 148 individuals, a significant number as compared to the available beds in the institution.[37]

However, in their original form, these plans were never to be realized, as the final calculations amounted to twice the funds available in the national asylum fund.[38] Therefore, the plans were recalibrated for 117 patients and the Royal National Asylum in Vác was intended to serve as a temporary solution until a suitable and more favorable option would come up in Pest; thereafter, the building in Vác was to house incurable patients. The amount allocated for this project – 148,682 gulden – would have covered the reconstruction of the building.[39] Concurrently, the plans were re-examined and since they were found inadequate professionally and financially, construction work was halted in 1841. Three years later, Ferdinand V ordered the preparation of new, more cost-effective plans and an account of the available amount in the national asylum fund. The new plans were prepared by the then chief physician of Hungary, Ignác Stáhly for 196 patients, which were recalibrated by the Court

35 On medical travel and its sources see: Müller, 2004. On technological journeys in the Hungarian context more recently: Kurucz, 2022a; Kurucz, 2022b.

36 MNL OL K 150 Box 559. 3258/76. fol. 6.

37 MNL OL K 150 Box 559. 3258/76. fols. 7–8.

38 The available amount was altogether 340,561 gulden, while repurposing the building would have cost 681,498 gulden.

39 It was supposed to be completed by the contractor Mátyás Zitterbarth, and in 1840 an initial amount of 14,000 gulden was paid to him to start the construction works.

Building Commission (Hofbaukommission) for 180, while by a court decision in 1846 the final number of patients to be taken care of in the Vác asylum was limited to 90 (80 paying and 10 non-paying patients).[40]

In 1847, Stáhly also elaborated a plan for the number of individuals to be employed in the asylum, their payment, and accommodation. According to this, the future chief physician (*primarius*) of the asylum, who would have also served as the director of the institution was to make 800 gulden per year (and an extra 100 if he were to take up directorship); the two secondary physicians were to make 300 gulden per year, while the caretaker was to be employed for 600 gulden a year. The details of payment are not included in the case of the scribe, the portier, the 16 nurses (eight male and eight female nurses), and a servant who would also have been employed in the Vác asylum. Servants and nurses were to be accommodated in separate houses owned by the town of Vác, as constructing new buildings in a temporary asylum for the staff were to be – according to Stáhly – unnecessarily costly. Stáhly, however, was hesitant about accommodating the chief physician of the asylum in a separate building. His presence at the institution was imperative in many cases – but providing the suitable rooms for him (and potentially his family) would have necessitated reconsidering the plans already accepted by the Court Building Commission. Stáhly was also preoccupied with the person of the chief physician (and director) of the future asylum, as there had already been three applicants for the post, Ferenc Schwartzer, the then secondary physician of the Viennese asylum, Konstantin Pomutz, secondary physician of the Viennese general hospital, and Edward Herdegen, professor of chemistry at the Josephinian Military Academy of Surgery in Vienna.[41] Out of the three, Stáhly found Ferenc Schwartzer to be the strongest contender, and he advised that he be sent to on a European study tour to examine the most up-to-date technologies of asylum management and techniques.[42] Even though the plans of the Vác asylum had fallen through in 1847, this journey had eventually taken place and was financed by the national asylum found.

In July of the same year, Archduke Stephen of Austria, Palatine of Hungary halted the process of rebuilding the Ludoviceum in Vác by ordering a committee to examine whether the plans of the Court Building Commission and the Hungarian Royal Building Committee (Königliche Landes-Bau-Oberdirection)

40 MNL OL K 150 Box 559. 3258/76. fols. 9–10.

41 See their applications from 1846 in MNL OL C 66 Dossier 479. 1847 F 31. 4104/504/1846 and 8150/1030/1846 respectively.

42 MNL OL C 66 Dossier 479. 1847 F 31. No. 20/401/847, May 9, 1847.

fulfilled the modern requirements of building therapeutic asylums.[43] The main question of the committee was whether Vác as a location would be profitable on the long run, as the building – due to its bad condition – would require thorough reparations that would cost more than building a new one and would be too far from the University of Pest posing difficulties for clinical instruction. Apart from these, other serious shortcomings of the plan were uncovered, such as the impossibility of separating patients due to the lack of space and creating solitary cells for paying patients. It was also due to the lack of space that certain – required – rooms could not be created, such as the laundry, kitchenettes, or a room for the chief physician/director of the institution, the centrality of which within the building would have been imperative for the uninterrupted operation of the hospital.

Furthermore, the crumbling building was not only small, but also damp, lacking light, air and an appropriate view to the surrounding area.[44] According to the report, the conclusions of which were supported by the Locumtenential Council's later petition to the monarch signed also by Ignác Stáhly as councilor,[45] the plans of the Prague asylum,[46] a modern, contemporary institution befitting the needs of moral therapy,[47] should serve as a model for a new and purpose-built Hungarian national asylum at a central location. Thus, instead of adhering to the current plans, the councilors proposed to sell the building of the Ludoviceum,[48] find a suitable location in Pest, and – echoing and earlier idea – send the future chief physician abroad to learn about the new techniques of asylum management and therapy.[49]

The two physicians, who were eventually sent abroad were Ferenc Schwartzer and Konstantin Pomutz, who in August 1847 petitioned Archduke Stephen to send them on a European journey, arguing that all "civilized countries" in Europe have institutions dedicated to the mentally ill – the Habsburg Monarchy included, with the notable examples of Hall in Tyrol, Prague, Graz or Linz – and that it would be urgent to establish an institution for Hungary that is very similar in its structure and operation to these. The doctors also argue that it would be vital to provide theoretical, as well as practical training

---

43 MNL OL C 66 Dossier 479. 1847 F 31. No. 31.357/847, July 10, 1847. fols. 91r–93v.

44 Ibid.

45 MNL OL C 66 Dossier 479. 1847 F 31. No. 14056/1847. July 20, 1847.

46 MNL OL C 66 Dossier 479. 1847 F 31. No. 31.357/847, July 10, 1847. fol. 93r.

47 On moral therapy and its application see: Digby, 1985. 22–87.

48 According to the 1869 report, the main problem with the project was that the plans relied solely on the national asylum fund that was entirely unsuited to support such an ambitious undertaking. Cf. MNL OL K 150 Box 559. 3258/76. fol. 11.

49 MNL OL C 66 Dossier 479. 1847 F 31. No. 14056/1847. July 20, 1847. fols. 87r–v.

to future alienists, who would plan and manage such an institution – and the best means to do so would be through a European tour.[50]

Eventually, with the decree no. 85/85 of 1847 of the Hungarian Court Chancery, the two doctors could begin their tour through Europe, and this journey would come to play a significant role in the process of psychiatric institutionalization in Hungary – although not exactly aligning with the original plans outlined by the official authorities and the narrow circle of doctors taking part in the planning process.[51]

Schwartzer and Pomutz did not receive a detailed instruction on how and what to observe and record during their travels; in this regard, they had to rely on their own professional experiences and theoretical knowledge. The only requirement was to compile a detailed journal which could be used during the planning process of a new, purpose-built curative asylum.[52] In the end, Schwartzer was forced to complete his journey alone, as his companion, Pomutz had fallen ill in Vienna. His route can be considered a "classical" one by contemporary standards, visiting both older, more prestigious, state-run institutions and smaller, newer, private ones: he began his journey in the Habsburg Monarchy visiting Vienna and Prague; thereafter went to Germany (Pirna-Sonnenstein, Berlin, Siegburg, Sachsenberg, Achern-Illenau, Winnenthal), Belgium (Ghent, Bruges), England (Bedlam, St Luke's Hospital, Hanwell), and France (Salpêtrière, Bicêtre, Charenton, Vanves).

Schwartzer's final report was submitted to the Ministry of Agriculture, Industry and Commerce set up in 1848. The thorough and detailed report, which was well received in the ministry, applies a similar approach to describing each asylum Schwartzer visited, discussing the location, structure, therapeutical practices (moral therapy, somatic therapies), the special tools and restraints used in everyday practice, the members of the staff, the proportion

---

50 The petition of Ferenc Schwartzer and Konstantin Pomutz to Archduke Stephen, MNL OL C 66 Dossier 479. 1847 F 31. without number, August 25, 1848.

51 Schwartzer's study tour and its personal and professional experiences exerted a significant impact on the structure and operation of his private asylum opened in 1850 in Vác and relocated to Buda in 1852. More on the management of the institution see: Lafferton, *Hungarian Psychiatry*, 101–146.

52 See the documentation of the study tour: MNL OL H 1848/1849-i Levéltár [Archives of the 1848/1849 Ministries] 52 Egészségügyi Osztály [Department of Health] 29. kútfő [record], 5. tétel [item], 4220/490–1848. Upon his return, Schwartzer did not only enclose the travel journal; he supplemented it with several attachments, such as model case histories, questionnaires used at admission, tables used to register the daily activities of the patients and doctors of institutions, and the regulations of the asylum in Pirna-Sonnenstein, Winnenthal, and Siegburg.

of the nursing staff and patients, and the finances of the asylum.[53] What is more, it discusses the evolution of psychiatric care in other countries providing a thorough historical account of the mental health reform in England.[54] Schwartzer's detailed analysis of the English model inserted into his travel journal is noteworthy, as it demonstrates that he was aware of the main reform tendencies and pursuits initiated within the English institutional context. This exerted significant impact on psychiatric institutionalization in several parts of Europe – including the Habsburg Monarchy and Hungary in particular.[55]

In April 1848, when the idea of remodeling the Ludoviceum in Vác had already been dismissed by Archduke Stephen, Palatine of Hungary, the plans of a new, purpose-built asylum for 180 patients were ordered,[56] and Ferenc Schwartzer was commissioned to draw up a proposal based on his European journey completed between April and July 1848. Schwartzer handed in his proposal to the Ministry of Agriculture, Industry and Commerce on November 2, 1848.[57] However, when drawing up his final plans for a new, purpose-built asylum for Hungary, despite his appreciation for, for example, Hanwell, which he considered one of the most progressive institutions in Europe, being a pioneer in introducing the non-restraint system propagated by John Conolly,[58] he opted for choosing a model he considered more viable and more suitable within the context of the Habsburg Monarchy. Although the idea of using the plans of the Prague asylum – the building of which was extended from the 1820s to be able to cater to the needs of an increasing amount of patients

53 Cf. MNL OL H 52, 29. kútfő [record], 5. tétel [item], 4220/490–1848, fols. 188–296. In addition to the description of the institutions, Schwartzer also attached the plan of some asylums (such as Prague, Glasgow, and Sachsenberg).

54 He discusses the history of the regulations between the last third of the eighteenth century and the 1840s, including the so-called "trade in lunacy" and the operation of private asylums, their compulsory inspection by parliamentary committees from 1774, the 1808 County Asylums Act which enabled each county to establish an asylum, and the 1845 Lunacy Act which made it compulsory for the counties to establish an asylum, resulting in a significant increase in their numbers until the turn of the century. On the lunacy reform in England see: Scull, 1993. 46–174; on private asylums see: Parry-Jones, *The Trade in Lunacy*. Smith, *Private Madhouses in England*.

55 Cf. Kovács, Elmebetegügy.

56 MNL OL K 150 Box 559. 3258/76. fol. 11.

57 Schwartzer's proposal was published in its entirety by Nándor Horánszky in 1963. The original documents are held in MNL OL H 52 6268/698, The report of Ferenc Fekete (formerly Schwartzer), surgeon-physician's report to the Ministry of Industry, Commerce, and Agriculture concerning the national asylum, November 2, 1848. Throughout the text, I use Horánszky's edition of the text (hereinafter referred to as Horánszky, Schwartzer Ferenc javaslata, 257–269).

58 MNL OL H 52, 29. kútfő [record], 5. tétel [item], 4220/490–1848, fol. 258.

and transformed into a therapeutic asylum during the premiership of Josef Gottfried Riedel[59] – as a potential model had come up in earlier discussions, as part of, for example, the report commissioned by Archduke Stephen to reexamine the plans of the Vác asylum,[60] it was Schwartzer whose proposal first built solidly on the structure and therapeutic practices of Riedel's institution, taking it as its model.

In the introduction to his proposal, Schwartzer, echoed the most modern and contemporary medical ideas on the necessity of building asylums. He also highlighted that even though by the nineteenth century mental problems had undergone medicalization and had eventually been accepted as *illnesses*, he defended his opposition against those voices that argued for the "home treatment" of the people with mental disabilities. In the debate "home treatment versus institutionalization", he opted for institutional treatment, because, although a homelike environment was considered fundamental to healing, it should be provided in an "artificial" form, within the walls of an institution, where the patients were sealed from their families that, in many cases, caused their illnesses in the first place.

What is more, patients were often not aware of their mental and physical conditions, which was hard to handle without medical knowledge and experience. In a well-organized asylum, characterized by security, expertly care, a well-structured building, and a good location, where the most important task of the physician was to heal and reintegrate his patients into society, the chances of getting better were higher than in a home environment. According to the approach of moral therapy,[61] a view followed and propagated by Schwartzer, mental illness was curable, because these conditions did not affect individuals as "moral beings", and the soul was merely a "tool" that was prone to illnesses, but at the same time, it was curable.[62]

A second burning question, characterizing earlier Hungarian debates on asylums as discussed above – eventually derailing the institutionalization process by the late 1840s – concerned the location and type of the building. In this regard, Schwartzer proposed two solutions, considering that only a centrally located mental asylum could serve the purposes of healing and clinical instruction, which was fundamental to solidifying psychiatry as a discipline and training the next generation of alienists. In the case of reconstructing an earlier existing building – the good examples of which are the German asylums

59 Chaloupková, *Správa a fungování*, 23–42.

60 MNL OL C 66 Dossier 479. 1847 F 31. No. 31.357/847, July 10, 1847. fols. 90r, 93r.

61 Horánszky, Schwartzer Ferenc javaslata, 259–260.

62 Horánszky, Schwartzer Ferenc javaslata, 257–259.

in Winnenthal, Sonnenstein, and Siegburg –, he proposed that the old monastery in Kiscell in Óbuda (Budapest's 3rd district today), which were used as a military depot and hospital for injured soldiers, would be the most suitable. It was relatively cost-effective to turn it into an asylum, because it was situated in a picturesque environment with clear air and the building could host 450 patients. It had three courtyards (two bigger and a smaller) along with a farm and a vineyard.

Furthermore, the corridors and rooms were long, vaulted, narrow, and bright – a factor most beneficial to mentally ill patients. The necessary reconstruction works – all serving the purposes of moral therapy – included the extension of the single-story wings with an upper story, a new building for the "furious insane", new courtyards and gardens, and mounting the upper-story windows with bars to prevent accidents.[63] This latter factor also signified a shift in perspective: in earlier discussions, window railings were included in asylum buildings to prevent escapes and protect society at large from the mentally ill[64] – in this case however, their primary function was the protection of the patients.

Yet, even though the reconstruction of the Kiscell monastery could have been more cost-effective in the short run, the opening of a new, purpose-built asylum seemed a more substantial and forward-looking project. According to Schwartzer's plans, the ideal location of a new asylum would be in Buda, as Pest, on the left side of the Danube was too plain and windy, and the natural environment was less spectacular than the hilly areas of Buda. On the right side of the Danube, four options came up in the discussions: Kamaraerdő (in today's 11th district), Ferenc-halom (or Ferencdomb in Schwartzer's text), Szépjuhászné, and Lipótmező (all three of them in the 2nd district of today's Budapest). In Schwartzer's assessment, Lipótmező – which had already been offered by the Buda city council as a possible location for the royal national asylum in 1829 free of charge – was the best suited to the purposes of a therapeutic asylum, because it was close to the city and easily accessible.[65] It was

63 Horánszky, Schwartzer Ferenc javaslata, 259–260.

64 See more on the most characteristic discourses on "managing" the mentally ill and the idea of protecting society in the late eighteenth- and early nineteenth-century Habsburg Monarchy in: Kovács, Elmebetegügy.

65 Although Schwartzer (and Riedel) believed that Lipótmező could be a suitable location because of its vicinity to the Medical Faculty, not long after the Royal National Asylum was opened, already in 1873, when the idea of establishing a university department for psychiatry came up at the faculty, it was found that the only clinic – Lipótmező – that could provide adequate patient material for the purposes of clinical instruction was too far from the city and students could not afford to travel there three times a week. Consequently,

also protected from northern winds by the surrounding hills, it had "nice vistas",[66] and the nearby wells could supply enough water to cater to the needs of the patients. Schwartzer highlighted that his plans are merely a "skeleton" based on professional, expertly insights and an architect's vision is needed to bring them to life.[67]

The structure and aims of the asylum – following the Prague model explicitly – lay great emphasis on the approach of moral therapy. The focus was not only on its location in a picturesque area, but also on its ideally homelike appearance (a "bourgeois home" instead of a castle, a monastery, or a workhouse[68]). The plan prescribed the separation of patients not only according to gender, but also their rank and intellectual abilities, conditions and state. It accommodated the staff – especially the nursing and medical staff responsible for monitoring patients from central apartments –, and underlined the harmonious organization of gardens, rooms, and common areas.

Along the lines of moral therapy, Schwartzer paid great attention to creating spaces for various (communal) activities considered fundamental for a successful therapeutic environment, such as common rooms for games (card, billiard, domino, chess), a piano room, therapeutic gardens, workshops for tailors, cobblers, carpenters, turners, or plaiters. In addition to leisure activities, men were expected to work in the gardens and in the fields, while women were expected to do domestic work.[69] Reflecting on contemporary ideas on the role and function of hospitals,[70] which from the turn of the eighteenth and nineteenth centuries pursued the *healing* of patients rather than merely *keeping* them, Schwartzer's plan proposed the separation of curable and incurable patients. The incurables – the elderly, those who suffered from stupidity

---

establishing a separate department for psychiatry was postponed for nearly a decade. Cf. Lafferton, *Hungarian Psychiatry*, 202.

66 Spectacular views and beautiful vistas formed a significant part of the approach of moral therapy, following the Lockean theory of association, in the context of which mental illnesses could be viewed as a chain of wrong associations that could be healed with therapy and the sufferer could be (re)integrated into society. Consequently, beautiful natural views, such as hills or forests, the perception of which invokes positives thoughts in the onlooker could bring forth positive associations and have a healing effect. See more on this in: Hickman, *Therapeutic Landscapes*, 2013, 426–428.

67 Horánszky, Schwartzer Ferenc javaslata, 260–261.

68 Horánszky, Schwartzer Ferenc javaslata, 262.

69 Horánszky, Schwartzer Ferenc javaslata, 262–267.

70 During the reconstruction and extension of the Prague asylum at the time of Riedel's premiership, the premises of the former monastery became a ward for the incurably mentally ill, while the new building became a modern therapeutic asylum, one of the most modern facilities of its kind in contemporary Europe. Cf. Chaloupková, *Správa a fungování*, 33.

(*Blödsinnigkeit*) either from birth or as a result of madness, and those who suffered from "general madness" (unspecified by Schwartzer) – were to be placed in a separate institution where they could spend the rest of their days. Those who were assessed as curable were placed in the therapeutic building/wing, where they would receive ample care.[71]

Nevertheless, even though Schwartzer's approach allowed as much freedom to the mentally ill as possible and considered humane treatment the most viable option, the question of security was woven into his text with the aim of securing a proper therapeutic environment and preventing escapes and accidents. In the refectory, only spoons and blunt knives were to be allowed, while forks were only to be allowed for patients who did not pose danger either to themselves or others; the doors had to be made strong and durable, only to be opened and closed by the nursing staff; and the gardens had to be organized in a way so that patients can be monitored all the time (no large bushes, pavilions, or places where they could hide). The rooms for those patients who were excluded from the community (the furious and the unclean) had to be located on the ground floor, their windows had to be built in a way that they could not reach them, less furniture was allowed than in "normal" rooms, and in these isolated wards, the rooms of the nurses had to be located centrally, so that they could monitor patients all the time. Furthermore, patients were allowed to take their own clothes to the asylum so that a homelike ambience could be created.[72]

Schwartzer's 1848 plan, however, due to a variety of factors – external, such as the years of retaliation following the Revolution and War of Independence in 1848–1849; internal, such as the disinterest of the medical community; and financial[73] – was also dismissed by the official authorities and the building of the asylum was postponed for an indefinite time. The events of 1848–1849 halted not only the asylum project, but also the operation of the most important associations and forums of the medical community that could have lobbied for its continuation.[74] Only from the second half of the 1850s were two

71 Horánszky, Schwartzer Ferenc javaslata, 268.

72 Horánszky, Schwartzer Ferenc javaslata, 268.

73 According to the 1869 report, which details the history of the struggles of building an asylum between 1808 and 1848, the main reason behind the failure was primarily financial: the plans all relied on the national asylum fund (supplemented with donations and bequests) which could not cover the reconstruction and/or building costs. MNL OL K 150 Box 559. 3258/76. fol. 11.

74 The last issue of the first medical journal in the vernacular, *Orvosi Tár* was published in 1847. From among the two medical associations, only the Royal Budapest Medical Society could resume its operation in the 1850s, but, as demonstrated by their internal

new medical journals allowed to be published in Hungarian: *Orvosi Hetilap* (*Medical Weekly*) from 1857 and *Gyógyászat* (*Medicine*) from 1861. From this point onwards, the discourse on mental illnesses and the need to establish an asylum became "denser". However, between 1857 and 1868, the actual planning and construction process were determined in and controlled from Vienna. The Hungarian medical community had to come to terms with its own unpreparedness for the opening of an asylum and the professional challenges such an institution brought.

3 The Decades-Long Struggle Comes to an End: Planning a New Asylum for Hungary

From an official point of view, the cause was picked up again after the k. k. Statthalterei ("Helytartóság") was set up in Hungary in 1851. In a report issued in 1852 (no. 28154), it was declared that besides the national asylum fund, state funds should also be used when planning and building the asylum for Hungary. The initial negotiations were limited to the size of the building, the admission of patients, and their placement within the institution.[75] However, for a few years, no steps were taken towards realizing these goals, even though, already in December 1852, Michael Viszánik, the chief physician of the Viennese asylum had urged the Statthalterei to act. Besides echoing the ideas circulating in the decades-long discourse on establishing asylums (the necessity of choosing a central location, a purpose-built asylum versus a remodeled building), he, from the perspective of both an insider (he was born and educated in Hungary) and an outsider (he had been working in the Viennese asylum for decades by this time), employed a rather critical tone towards the authorities and the medical community, whom he accused of impeding the asylum project.

In his petition to Franz Joseph I, Emperor of Austria and King of Hungary, Viszánik analyzed the reasons for the decades-long, unsuccessful attempts to establish a mental asylum in Hungary. He blamed the impotence of both local authorities and the imperial government for the situation. He insisted that the

---

documents, their work was rather fragmented and haphazard. Cf. SOMKL I. Budapesti Királyi Orvosegyesület, Boxes 3–4. (1849–1860). The first itinerary congress of the Society of Hungarian Physicians and Naturalists was held in 1863 and they could only publish the proceedings of the 1847 congress held in Sopron in this year, containing Ferenc Bene's lecture on the importance, methods, and models of asylum care for the mentally ill. Cf. Bene, 1863.

75 MNL OL K 150 Box 559. 3258/76. fol. 11.

establishment of a specialized institution for the mentally ill would benefit the affected individuals (the patients and their environments) and the state, thus advancing the cause of the (medical) sciences in Hungary. He added that the institution would only be the first step towards a solution: it could act as a central body within a network of smaller asylums in the country, as local institutions would be established that could cater to the needs of patients whose transport to Buda or Pest poses difficulties.[76]

As for the financial side of the matter, he proposed varied funding for the new Hungarian asylum based not only on the national asylum fund, but also other donations and the profits of a national charity lottery.[77] In general, Viszánik propagated the model he devised based on his travels[78] for the Lower Austrian Provincial Asylum (Niederösterreichische Landesirrenanstalt) in Brünnlfeld[79] under construction at the time. The new asylum was planned to serve not only the purposes of healing, but also theoretical and practical clinical instruction. Furthermore, he urged the establishment of an association for the patients discharged from institutions, a similar organization led by him in Vienna.[80]

Despite voices urging the continuation of the asylum project in 1852, the issue of its establishment was not on the agenda again until 1856–1857. This was the moment when the actual planning process began as the available funds (which by this time grew to 733,427 gulden) were assessed and the potential location identified. The locations that had emerged earlier in the discussions[81] were re-evaluated. The committee set up by the Statthalterei – supporting Schwartzer's original project – decided that Lipótmező would be the most suitable site for building a hospital, as it was in a picturesque environment and

---

76 In the 1860s, the same idea was brought up by Károly Bolyó, the secondary physician of the Schwartzer asylum after travelling across the Habsburg Monarchy and Western Europe visiting mental asylums. He argued that opening the Lipótmező asylum was only a first step, a network of affiliated asylums was needed to cater to the needs of patients from all walks of life – Bolyó contends that an agricultural worker cannot be healed in the same environment as, for example, an intellectual. Cf. Bolyó, Miként lehetne.

77 Later in 1857, the planning and building of the Royal National Asylum in Nagyszeben in Transylvania was funded by the profits of a national charity lottery. Later, the psychiatry ward in the general hospital in Miskolc in northwestern Hungary also received parts of the funds collected via lottery. Cf. Pándy, *Emlékkönyv*, 18–19.

78 Cf. Viszánik, *Die Irrenheil- und Pflegeanstalten.*

79 Gabriel, Psychiatrische Einrichtungen. Ledebur, *Das Wissen der Anstaltspsychiatrie*, 31–33.

80 MNL OL D 2 Box 168. 5512/301–853. Michael Viszánik, Doctor der Medicin, Primararzt der k. k. Irrenheilanstalt, m. Decan der Wiener mediz. Fakultät. Wien am 10ten Dezember 1852.

81 Káposztásmegyer, Kamaraerdő, Szépjuhászné, Ferenc-halom, the fields near the military hospital in Pest, and Lipótmező.

could supply enough water to the institution. Partly honoring the 1829 agreement, when the Buda city council promised to consign the 45-acres ground for the purposes of the asylum, they sold it for a relatively small sum of 16,000 gulden along with other smaller plots.

According to the original plans, the asylum was to be built for 800 patients, which seemed sufficient, as in the five administrative districts of Hungary,[82] altogether 1025 individuals were counted who were suffering from milder forms of mental disturbance ("bárgyu [stupid], nehéz nyavalyás [epileptic], and elmegyenge [weak minded]"). Additionally, 1438 individuals were listed who were considered "valóságos elmebeteg (real insane)".[83] However, the methodology of the survey and the accuracy of the data is not discussed in the report. To be able to make the necessary calculations, the plans of the asylums in Brno and Prague and the Lower Austrian Provincial Asylum were sent to the Statthalterei so that they could be informed on the ideal composition staff along with the nurse per patient ratio, and estimate the amount to be allocated for furniture and other equipment, the salary of the staff, and the price to be paid by the different classes of patients. Eventually, their calculations amounted to roughly 825,000 gulden, which was financed partly by the national asylum fund and partly by a further 300,000 gulden allocated personally by Franz Joseph I for the project.[84]

The professional plans of the therapeutic institution were produced by Josef Gottfried Riedel, by then the foremost expert of asylum psychiatry and moral therapy in the Habsburg Monarchy.[85] In twentieth-century Hungarian medical historiography, Ferenc Schwartzer is often regarded as an important councilor who took a significant part in the planning process, and whose earlier proposal is strongly reflected in the final plans of the institution.[86] However, so far, research has failed to take into account that Schwartzer's proposal written in Hungarian was built largely on Riedel's earlier publication, his personal visit to the Prague asylum in 1848, and the plans sent to Hungary from Prague and Brno in 1848, after the asylum project in Vác fell through.

Therefore, although it is true that there are overlaps between Schwartzer's 1848 and Riedel's 1857 plans and that they both reinforce the same ideal – a therapeutic asylum following the basic principles of moral therapy – it was

82 Pest, Pozsony (Bratislava, today in Slovakia), Sopron, Kassa (Košice, today in Slovakia), Nagyvárad (Oradea, today in Romania).

83 MNL OL K 150 Box 559. 3258/76. fols. 12–13.

84 Ibid., fols. 14–18.

85 He was responsible for the large asylum projects in, for example, Nagyszeben, Venice, Brno, Ybbs an der Donau, Agram, and Lemberg. Cf. Chaloupková, *Správa a fungování*, 39.

86 Horánszky, Schwartzer Ferenc javaslata, 268; Fekete, Intézetünk megalapítása, 68–69.

Schwartzer who (explicitly) copied the Prague model. His proposal was probably not taken into consideration by Riedel when outlining his own program.

Riedel's plans,[87] produced after his personal visit to the grounds, were completely tailored to both the features of the 45-acres land in Lipótmező and the financial possibilities laid out by the Statthalterei earlier in 1857. He devised a plan for 800 patients, 300 of whom were to be placed in the hospital for therapy, while further 500 incurable patients were to be taken care of in the nursing institute, keeping the option of further expandability in mind.[88] Following Riedel's program developed in Prague, the structure of the building reflected the aims of moral therapy: the fundamental principles to be taken into account by the architect were simplicity, cheerfulness, a homelike ambience, and harmony which had to be mirrored not only in the style of the building, but in all minor details and aspects from its accessibility and permeability (so that each patient can have access to all spaces dedicated to them easily), in the layout of the rooms and corridors (light, airy, spacious), in the organization of the different spaces within the building (corridors had to have a view to the courtyard, while the rooms and common areas to the surrounding hills).[89]

Furthermore, the architect had to consider that the features built into the asylum serving the purposes of security – such as high windows, bars to prevent escapes and suicide, heavy windows, lavatories designed especially for patients unable to control their bodily functions, gardens and courtyards in which patients could be monitored all the time – could not remind the patients that they were isolated and taken out of their home environment. As part of the moral therapeutical approach, Riedel also paid careful attention to the feasibility of work therapy. In the name of security, Riedel also added – since his proposal was written as an expertly instruction for an architect – some non-negotiable components, such as the careful isolation of patients. He applied the usual guidelines for separating them (according to gender, condition, and class), stipulating that a significant emphasis had to be put on planning the ward for furious and/or unclean patients, placing it in a separate, remote part of the building so that their noise would not bother other patients. This ward had to be on the ground floor to prevent accidents, all patients had to have their own rooms, and their corridor had to have direct access to the

87 Programm für den Bau der Landes-Irrenanstalt auf dem Leopoldfelde bei Ofen. ÖstA AVA Inneres MdI Präsidium A Teil 1 1045 7215/1857.

88 In 1884, as a third public asylum was opened in Hungary after the centrally important Lipótmező and the locally relevant Nagyszeben in Transylvania; its role was originally to alleviate the pressure on Lipótmező due to overcrowding and to admit incurable patients.

89 ÖstA AVA Inneres MdI Präsidium A Teil 1 1045 7215/1857. fols. 1–10.

enclosed gardens. Additionally, the staff had to be able to monitor all rooms from a central post.[90]

All in all, Riedel's plans followed the general and most popular guidelines for purpose-built therapeutic asylums in the mid-nineteenth century, however, its architectural implementation did not come without challenges. Initially, the plans elaborated by the Department of Architecture in Buda (K. K. Landes Baudirections Abtheilung zu Ofen) were found insufficient. Thereafter, the Austrian Ministry of Interior ordered a separate committee to review the plans, accepting the proposal of Austrian architect, Ludwig Zettl on August 16, 1859,[91] with decree no. 9916. Since neither these nor other plans had taken into account the geographical features of the area properly, the space for patients within the asylum had to be significantly reduced, from 800 patients to 500 patients. Eventually, construction began in March 1860, and, according to the initial plans, the building was supposed to be finished by May 1864.[92]

Although reconstructing the entangled history of the building process would be beyond the framework of this chapter, it must be noted that, as early as 1861, the contractors entrusted with stonemasonry, József Mayer and Mátyás Wessely (Mayer and Company), went bankrupt and had to be taken off the project. According to the 1869 report, this is one of the main reasons for the failure to finish the construction until 1864. Work was temporarily suspended in April 1861, and a committee made up by the delegates of the Statthalterei[93] was ordered to monitor the building process. The committee was divided into subcommittees (a mechanical-architectural one and a medical one), which were responsible for the restructuring of plans, considering the financial possibilities and limits.

The medical subcommittee recommended lowering the number of patients to be admitted from 800 to 500 and the number of extra cells for "the furious insane" (*Tobzellen*) from 64 to 32. Furthermore, the mechanical-architectural subcommittee criticized the construction of walls, the materials used by the contractors, and the stability of the building. The committee reprimanded the inspectors of the building operations, János Krausz and the architect Ludwig

90 Ibid., fols. 6–7.
91 See the final layout of the hospital in the Appendix.
92 MNL OL K 150 Box 559. 3258/76. fol. 21.
93 The delegation included László Korizmics and Károly Sztankovics; architectural inspector Vilmos Fest; chief architect Jakab Óhegyi; Ignác Sauer, the protomedicus of Hungary and royal councilor; Ferenc Schwartzer, director of the Schwartzer private asylum; the engineer Adam Clark, and the architect József Diescher.

Zettl and terminated the contract with Mayer and Company in 1863. The Statthalterei made a new contract with Mátyás Zitterbarth (who had already been a contender for the management of the asylum project in Vác in the late 1840s) in April 1863, and construction work resumed with a detailed schedule for each year, with the opening of the asylum predicted to 1866.

Despite the idealistic plans, the opening was significantly delayed again, when Mátyás Zitterbarth went bankrupt in 1864. The project was eventually delegated to Heinrich Drasche, a Viennese land- and factory owner, who was only able to finish the building by May 1868 and the minor construction works by December 1868.[94] The building was finally opened to the public on December 6, 1868, however, as the Hungarian medical community was largely left out of the planning process and the discourses around constructing, equipping, and staffing the asylum, anxieties, and doubts had quickly arisen on the feasibility of such an institution already in the early 1860s.

4 Preparing for the Opening of an Asylum: Technological Travels and Reform Plans

While the discourse on the necessity of opening an asylum for Hungary intensified with the launch of the two new medical forums in the vernacular and with Ferenc Schwartzer as a private tutor holding theoretical lectures at the Medical Faculty of the University of Pest, offering his private asylum for the purposes of clinical instruction, the Hungarian medical community had still been thoroughly unprepared for operating an asylum. Realizing this, upon his own request, the Locumtenential Council (set up again in 1861 after its operation was halted between 1848–1860) sent Emil Schnirch – a physician from Borsod County in northeastern Hungary and later in Fejér County in central Hungary, who successfully set up a small psychiatric ward in the general hospital of Miskolc[95] – on a two-years long mission to learn about new technologies and methodologies in asylum management and therapy.[96] Schnirch, who had already spent five years as a secondary physician in the Viennese asylum next to Viszánik entered into a contract with the medical department of the Locumtenential Council, promising to take up the directorship of the newly

94 Ibid., fols. 30–82.

95 On the earlier training and experiences of Schnirch, see: MNL OL D 217. IV. Egészségügyi kútfő [Medical records], Box 340. 375778/1862, fols. 537r–540v.

96 MNL OL D 217 IV. Egészségügyi kútfő [Medical records], Box 340. 4625/1861, fol. 554r.

established asylum in Lipótmező, a position which – although with a detour to Nagyszeben between 1863–1868 – he eventually occupied.[97]

The aim of his travels was to receive thorough training and experience in asylum management to be able to take responsibility for the day-to-day operation of the Royal National Asylum. Similarly to Schwartzer, Schnirch did not receive detailed instructions regarding the criteria and methods of observation; this was left to his discretion based on his previously acquired professional knowledge. His journey was financed from the national asylum fund, with two conditions. Firstly, he had to send a detailed report to the Locumtenential Council in every three months. Secondly, after completing a practical year at the Lower Austrian Provincial Asylum, he had to visit four institutions determined by the medical department of the Locumtenential Council. These included the asylums in Halle and Achern (Illenau), the Salpêtrière in Paris, and the Bedlam in London, thus, in addition to the well-established but by then considered somewhat older and "outdated" asylums, he also had to visit two newly established German institutions. The institution in Achern opened in 1842, while the Halle asylum opened in 1844. The location and design of both asylums already reflected newer therapeutic principles, such as withdrawal to a natural environment and the use of the building as a therapeutic tool.[98] At that time, Heinrich Philipp August Damerow, one of the most influential psychiatrists of the first half of the nineteenth century, headed the Halle institution and welcomed Schnirch to the institution.[99]

Nevertheless, Schnirch did not strictly follow the prescribed route.[100] Based on the directions of his travels, the institutions he visited, and especially the structure of the reports on each institution, it can be inferred that he might have been familiar with Ferenc Schwartzer's travel account from 1848 or could have consulted with the psychiatrist before embarking on his journey. However,

97 Initially, when Schnirch signed the contract in 1860, it was planned that the Royal National Asylum in Lipótmező would open earlier, where he would be able to occupy the post of director. However, as the asylum project was severely held back, he was forced to accept the premiership of the Nagyszeben asylum in Transylvania (which was not part of Hungary administratively until 1867) as a temporary solution. Cf. Horánszky, A magyar elmegyógyászat, 51.

98 Cf. Collins, *The Architecture and Landscape of Health*, 98–124.

99 Damerow was a co-founder of one of the most significant professional forums in German psychiatry (*Allgemeine Zeitschrift für Psychiatrie*) and a major advocate of a holistic approach combining somatic and psychological approaches to the treatment of mental illnesses.

100 See the documentation of Schnirch's journey in: MNL OL D 217 IV. Egészségügyi kútfő [Medical records], 1862–1867, 13. tétel [Item 13], Box 340. 71245/1863. fols. 487–557 and Box 341. 71245/1863. fols. 561–721.

Schnirch's route and the number of institutions he visited were much more extensive. This can be justified by the duration of his travels (Schwartzer was on the road between early April and late July 1848, while Schnirch traveled for nearly a year) and the increased number of institutions opened or became accessible after 1848. Schnirch's journey included not only well-established and newer, larger, state-funded model institutions in his focus but also smaller, experimental, private, and rural institutions that were beyond the financial possibilities of Ferenc Schwartzer or were opened later in the 1850s. Accordingly, after spending a year in the Viennese asylum, Schnirch visited German (Halle, Winnenthal, Göppingen, Frankfurt, Siegburg, Aachern-Illenau, Pirna-Sonnenstein, Leipzig-Thonberg, Leipzig-Möckern, Munich, Werneck, Eichberg), French (Salpêtrière, Bicêtre, Charenton, Maréville, Châlons-sur-Marne, Stephansfeld), Belgian (Ghent, Gheel), English (Bedlam, St. Luke's Hospital, Colney Hatch, Hanwell) institutions, and some of the asylums in the Habsburg Monarchy (Hall, Ybbs an der Donau, Linz, Salzburg, Brno, Prague).

Schnirch's reports on the various asylums followed the structure outlined by Schwartzer (primarily in terms of the practical management technologies of institutions, the composition of institutional staff, and quantitative data). However, what distinguishes Schnirch's accounts is the meticulous description of the material culture of contemporary psychiatry, lacking in the systematic, analytical approach to developing reforms that are observable in the accounts of other contemporary (mental) health professionals. Nevertheless, as Schnirch was the first director of the Hungarian Royal National Asylum in Lipótmező, the insights he gained during the two years might have fundamentally influenced the institutional practices during the asylum's initial period until 1884. It is crucial for current research to recognize the challenges in accessing and exploring hospital materials that shed light on the nature and quality of care, given the limited availability and accessibility of the records. Exploring how Schnirch's acquired knowledge was practically applied, in what form, and within what constraints presents a challenging task due to the restricted accessibility of hospital materials illuminating the nature and quality of care.[101]

---

101 Currently, the records of the asylum's operation are preserved by the National Hospital Directorate of Hungary. However, due to the lack of expert archival management and proper archival guides, researching these records is extremely challenging and can only produce fragmentary results. Partial insights into the functioning of the asylum can be deduced from the Ministry of the Interior's documentation, with a larger number of documents primarily related to the maintenance of the asylum building held in the Hungarian National Archives. In contrast, relatively few and fragmented documents (such as reports and protocols) are available concerning the internal operations of the asylum.

Adding another layer to the discourse on the uncertainties of asylum management and the Hungarian medical community's unpreparedness for managing the institution, another prominent physician embarked on a European journey to observe technologies and methods of care. Károly Bolyó, the secondary physician at the Schwartzer asylum and later, from 1868, the chief physician and director of the Lipótmező asylum between 1899 and 1906, began his Western European journey around the same time as Emil Schnirch. However, a significant difference lies in the fact that by this time, Bolyó had several years of experience in Hungarian psychiatry serving in its leading institution. Equipped with the most advanced theoretical knowledge he set out with substantial criticism regarding the adaptability of numerous Western European technologies in Hungary.

Bolyó's travels represented a step forward in the Hungarian discourse on mental health from several perspectives. Bolyó did not only share his observations in the form of travel accounts. Instead, he presented scientifically underpinned, analytical articles encouraging the medical community to take action. While the manuscript travel accounts of Schwartzer and Schnirch did not gain much publicity beyond the reviews of physician-counselors, Bolyó published and debated his experiences and plans on multiple platforms. He discussed his travel accounts, experiences, and related plans, along with critiques of the current situation in Hungary, in presentations at monthly and annual meetings of the Royal Budapest Society of Physicians and the itinerary congresses of the Society of Hungarian Physicians and Naturalists.[102] Bolyó also based his articles on these discussions,[103] making them accessible to a wider audience through publications in the main forums of the Hungarian medical community.

Bolyó undertook his first European tour in 1861–1863. He periodically sent travel reports, appearing with significant delays, approximately a year later, highlighting tools and medical technological innovations (such as syringes for subcutaneous drug administration effective in treating mental patients[104])

102 See for example: Bolyó, Utazási napló-töredékek, 724–727. The same text was published in the proceedings of the 1866 congress of the Society of Hungarian Physicians and Naturalists: Bolyó, Az elmebetegek, 25–30.

103 See for example: SOMKL I. Budapesti Királyi Orvosegyesület [Royal Budapest Society of Physicians], Box 5, 2: 1864 és 1866 közötti iratok [Documents: 1864–1866], 2.1. Jegyzőkönyvek [Reports], 1864–1866, A buda-pesti kir. orvosegylet 864ki October 14kén tartott évi nagygyülésének jegyzőkönyve [The report of the Royal Budapest Society of Physician's grand assembly held on October 14, 1864].

104 Bolyó, Utazási napló-töredékek, 726.

and non-medical technologies (such as steam washing[105] or sewage systems[106]) that he deemed useful for operating an asylum. However, he also critically reflected on practices to be avoided based on his own experiences. For instance, he extensively discussed the construction of isolation chambers for violent mentally ill patients, emphasizing that the careful execution of these rooms was required for maximum efficiency. As Bolyó's detailed analyses indicate, even in institutions with more serious therapeutic traditions, this posed a challenge.[107]

Furthermore, Bolyó's choice of direction and destinations indicates a shift and a higher level of awareness compared to Schwartzer's journey in 1848. He partly followed the route taken by Schnirch, but was more selective in the number, type, and quality of institutions he visited. Schnirch primarily employed the method of meticulous observation rather than analytical contemplation, considering spaces and practices in the asylums he visited along similar lines. In contrast, Bolyó consciously selected aspects to focus on. In his published reports, he provided brief descriptions of institutions he considers less innovative, such as those in Vienna, especially the Döbling asylum operated by Max von Leidesdorf and Heinrich Obersteiner from the 1860s. However, he offered detailed reports on German asylums, which he perceived as more modern and exemplary, along with technologies he deemed adaptable for use in Hungarian asylums, from places like Pirna-Sonnenstein, Halle, Berlin, Siegburg, Bendorf, Eichberg, Achern-Illenau, and Munich.

It is of great importance that Bolyó did not only disseminate his therapeutic experiences gained during his medical practice in the Schwartzer asylum and in foreign asylums and his reform plans in written form but also gave professional lectures at narrower medical forums. This opened up the possibility for debate. In his presentations, Bolyó emphasized the necessity of institutional psychiatry and highlighted the rights of the mentally ill individuals in society. He also advocated for a broader legal-medical discourse on the subject and argued that patients from different social environments required different approaches to healing in varied institutional settings.

105 Bolyó, Utazási napló-töredékek, 766.

106 Bolyó, Elmebetegeinket, 45.

107 In July 1861, Bolyó sent a report from the psychiatric department of the Charité in Berlin, analyzing both commendable and undesirable isolation practices. He discussed possible improvements in the design of chambers for the violent patients, recognizing the challenges even in institutions with more significant therapeutic traditions. Bolyó, Utazási napló-töredékek, 725.

He proposed the establishment of medically supervised "family care" (the so-called heterofamilial system) that he observed in Belgium and France for those not served well by central asylums, such as agricultural workers. He also recommended, in addition to a central asylum responsible for overseeing the whole network, the creation of affiliated asylums near urban public hospitals or psychiatric wards to extend patient care, an idea partially implemented after the Austro-Hungarian Compromise in 1867 and the opening of the Lipótmező asylum in 1868: the psychiatric wards of the public hospitals in Miskolc and Pozsony and the hospitals of the Brothers of Mercy in Eger and Buda, as well as the Nagyszeben asylum were in close contact with the Lipótmező asylum.[108]

5 Conclusion

The early history of psychiatric institutionalization in Hungary was characterized by obstacles, setbacks, and conflicts which left a lasting mark on the history of mental health care and the fates of mentally ill patients in the country. In the decades between the 1790s and the 1860s, characterized by several unrealized and failed plans, a number of correlating factors were at play that hindered the process of institutionalization from the shortages of theoretical and practical education (in Pest, the introduction of medical psychology/psychiatry courses were in an almost 20-years delay as compared to Vienna and Prague), which significantly limited the number of those physicians, who could have taken part in the institutionalization process, produce viable plans, and lobby for suitable treatment options for mentally ill patients.

As the analysis of the medical discourse (or rather the lack of it) pursued via different forums and means, such as medical journals, congresses, and meetings has shown, until the late 1850s and 1860s, the question of psychiatric institutionalization surfaced in a rather fragmented and unfocused form within the broader medical community. The intensification of discussions on institutionalization occurred only later, concurrently with the planning and building process of the Lipótmező asylum directed from Vienna. Nevertheless, the chapter has also pointed out that only bureaucrats, councilors, and only a handful of physicians in higher positions could contribute in a

108 See the admission documents of these wards and asylums in: MNL OL K 150 IV. 20. kútfő [record]: Tébolydák, tébolydai felvételek [Asylums, admission to asylums].

meaningful way. The most important obstacle for a successful asylum project was the lack of ample financial means to fund the project. Relying solely on the national asylum fund consisting of donations and bequests could not guarantee a reliable source for either the remodeling of a preexisting building or the construction of a new one.

In addition to the financial burden of the project, finding a suitable location close to the medical faculty where clinical instruction could also take place posed further challenges and limits to the project. And even though by 1848 a viable plan was conceived by Ferenc Schwartzer based largely on the Prague model and the experiences of his European travels, the political turmoil of 1848–1849 and the subsequent retaliation in the early 1850s halted the process completely. However, after the mid-1850s, the Hungarian asylum project could not be postponed any longer, partly because the agreement on the admission of Hungarian patients to the asylums of the Monarchy ceased in the 1850s, and partly because the already existing infrastructure in Hungary (smaller wards in public hospitals and the hospitals of the Brothers of Mercy, as well as the Schwartzer asylum) could not cater to the needs of an increasing number of patients.

From the late 1850s, when the measuring, planning, and building process had begun and the financial matters and shortages were settled with the personal donation of Franz Joseph I after his visit to Hungary, a decades-long struggle seemed to have come to an end. And while the actual building process lasted almost a decade, severely delaying the placement of patients in a proper public asylum in the territory of Hungary, further issues paralyzed the institutionalization process. Due to the limits in medical education and within the medical community, the history of psychiatric care in Hungary did not witness an "organic development" and therefore, already during the building process, both bureaucrats and physicians had been forced to realize that care could not be provided without doctors trained thoroughly in this branch of medicine. Therefore, a hurried process of preparation and (re)training had begun with, for example, the assignments of Emil Schnirch and Károly Bolyó to travel to Europe to learn about the current trends in asylum management and therapy in Europe. The ensuing accounts by both doctors and the reform plans produced and disseminated highlighted the anxieties and uncertainties surfacing within the medical community concerning the feasibility of an asylum (and in fact, a network of asylums and psychiatric wards) without well-trained medical staff. This had serious implications for the operation of the asylum on both shorter and longer term. The unfolding of this discourse and the problems caused by the unpreparedness of the medical community for the task has already been dealt with by earlier research based mostly on printed material,[109] therefore the task of future of future research will be to examine the day-to-day operation and care of the Lipótmező asylum and other affiliated institutions (public hospitals, the hospitals or religious orders, and the asylum in Nagyszeben after 1867) relying on their archives to gain a clearer image of how the delayed and conflict-ridden institutionalization process and the unpreparedness of the community of physicians impacted the therapeutic prospects of psychiatric patients.

Appendix

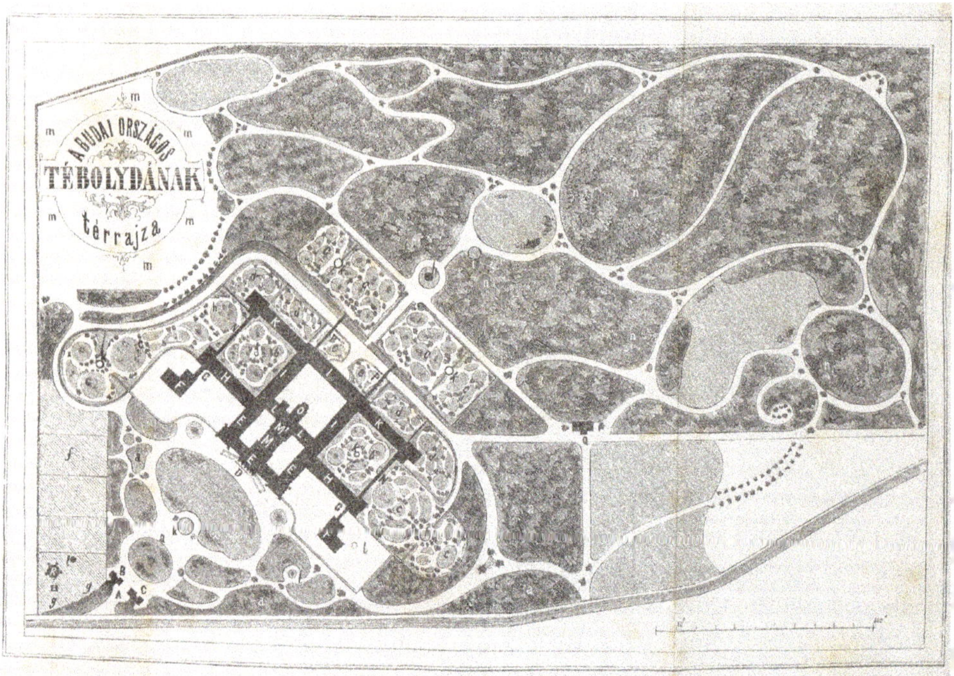

FIGURE 7.1 The ground plan of the Lipótmező asylum. In Lipót, Grósz. *Emlékirat a hazai betegápolási ügy keletkezése, fejlődése, s jelenlegi állásáról, különös tekintettel a betegápolási költségekre.* Buda: A Magyar Királyi Tudom. Egyetemi Nyomdából, 1869, 145

109 On the operation of the Lipótmező asylum under four directors until the early twentieth century, see: Lafferton, *Hungarian Psychiatry*, 147–191.

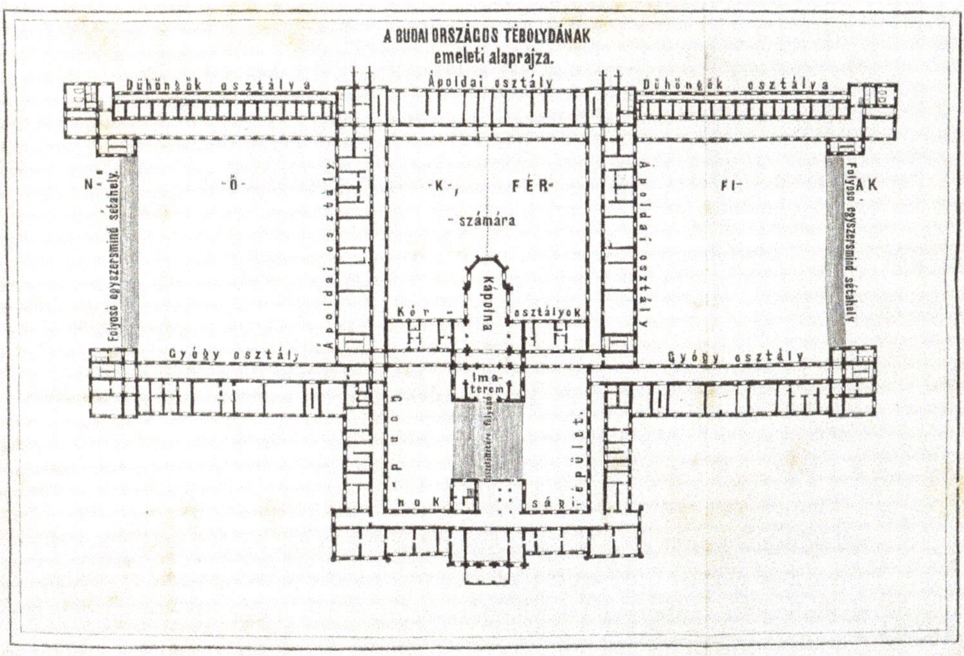

FIGURE 7.2 The floor plan of the Lipótmező asylum. In Lipót, Grósz. *Emlékirat a hazai betegápolási ügy keletkezése, fejlődése, s jelenlegi állásáról, különös tekintettel a betegápolási költségekre.* Buda: A Magyar Királyi Tudom. Egyetemi Nyomdából, 1869, 147

Acknowledgement

Research was supported by the National Research, Development and Innovation of Office of Hungary, project number: OTKA PD 142913.

CHAPTER 8

Between Religious and Imperial Scrutiny: Continuity and Change in the Operation of the Vilnius General Hospital, 1799–1804

Martynas Jakulis

The opening of the General Hospital in Vilnius (Wilno) on 16 June 1799 was a significant event, marked by the conspicuous participation of the elite. The ceremony was attended not only by Jan Nepomucen Kossakowski, the Bishop of Vilnius, who delivered a sermon on charity,[1] but also by the Governor of Lithuania Ivan Friezel and other high-ranking representatives of the imperial administration, as well as numerous noblemen, officials, and other distinguished guests. The events that took place in the Church of St. James and St. Philip in the suburb of Lukiškės (Łukiszki), which at that time was quite far from the heart of the city, were mentioned in the local newspaper *Kuryer Litewski*[2] and attracted the attention of diarists who documented the highlights of the life in city.[3] Above all, however, this ceremony signaled both the birth of a new charitable institution – the first in the former capital of the Grand Duchy of Lithuania after the end of the Polish-Lithuanian Commonwealth (1795) – and the final transformation of the almost three-century-old network of numerous almshouses and hospitals.

The newly founded General Hospital replaced six almshouses, and a hospital and took over their funds and bequests.[4] Contemporaries understood this as a necessary step, as the old health care and poor relief institutions were, in their view, inadequately funded, poorly managed, unsuitable for inmates and patients and simply dangerous to the environment. These facilities were seen as incompatible with the demands of a growing city. Hospital staff, under the direction of a professional doctor, were to provide adequate medical care for patients and constant care for the disabled and other inmates who were housed in the spacious wards of the general hospital.[5]

1 Kossakowski, "Kazanie Jana Nepomucena Korwina Kossakowskiego," 418–32.
2 "Z Wilna V. S. 8 N. S. 19 Czerwca," *Kuryer Litewski*, June 19, 1799, 1.
3 Tekieliński, *Opis dzienny szkół wileńskich*, 99.
4 Kurczewski, *Biskupstwo wileńskie*, 362; Korybut-Marciniak, *Dobroczynne Wilno*, 55.
5 Janicka, *Kultura higieniczna*, 55, 227.

 HTTPS://DOI.ORG/10.1163/9789004755062-010

The initiative to establish a general hospital was fully supported by the imperial administration, but local actors – prelates, representatives of religious orders, urban elites and medical professionals – played a decisive role as well.[6] Earlier experiences and attempts to reform charity were also of great importance. In the early 1760s, a general hospital was founded in Warsaw. The years between the 1770s to the mid-1790s were characterized by continuous, albeit only partially successful, endeavors to reorganize, secularize, centralize and bureaucratize the health care and poor relief institutions in the Grand Duchy of Lithuania and especially in Vilnius.[7] These processes reflected the far-reaching European-wide reforms inspired by the Enlightenment, populationist and mercantilist concerns.[8]

Despite the significance of these changes, the establishment of the General Hospital, its organization, financing, operation and other related topics remain largely on the margins of research. In mostly Polish historiography, which has focused on the history of the Catholic Church or healthcare and poor relief in late eighteenth-and early nineteenth-century Vilnius, the general hospital has received little attention. Therefore, it remains unclear what kind of institution the general hospital was, to what extent it resembled the old institutions of health care and poor relief, and how it differed from them. Considering this, the article argues that the general hospital was neither a completely novel institution nor a facility that functioned in a way that was characteristic of the old almshouses and hospitals.

This chapter uses the protocols of the most important administrative body, the Lithuanian Hospital Commission (*Kommissia Szpitalna Litewska*; hereafter referred to as the Commission), which cover the period from 1798 to 1804.[9]

6 Rosiak, *Prowincja Litewska Sióstr Miłosierdzia*, 250.

7 Małudzińska, *Próżnowanie stało się powszechnym nałogiem*, 230. Gordziejew, *Komisje Porządkowe Cywilno-Wojskowe*, 161–62, 167–68, 170; Srogosz, "Próby reform szpitalnictwa," 403–13.

8 Risse, *Mending Bodies*, 231–278; Lindeman, *Medicine and Society*, 175–176.

9 Protocols of the Lithuanian Hospital Commission (hereafter, Protocols) (1798), Lietuvos valstybės istorijos archyvas (Lithuanian State Historical Archives, Vilnius; hereafter, LVIA), f. 390, ap. 135, b. 2; Protocols (1799), LVIA, f. 390, ap. 135, b. 3; Protocols (1800), LVIA, f. 390, ap. 135, b. 4; Protocols (1801), LVIA, f. 390, ap. 135, b. 5; Protocols (1802), LVIA, f. 390, ap. 135, b. 6; Protocols (1803), LVIA, f. 390, ap. 135, b. 7; Protocols (1804), LVIA, f. 390, ap. 135, b. 9. Note: although the Commission was officially disbanded in 1808, however, due to the illness of its chairman bishop Jan Nepomucen Kossakowski, its activities ceased in 1805. Moreover, the Board of Public Care (*Prikaz obshchestvennogo prizreniya*) took over the general hospital in 1808, and it was eventually transferred into the hands of the Sisters of Charity in 1809. For more, see Aurimas Andriušis and Tadeusz Srogosz, "Litewska administracja opieki," 31. Rosiak, *Prowincja*, 253.

These sources shed light on the circumstances under which the general hospital was established and the challenges that characterized the first years of its existence. According to the original idea, the Commission was to be responsible for the general supervision of the hospital. However, due to ongoing difficulties in managing the facility and other problems, the Commission had to deal with various issues related to the organization, financing, and operation of the general hospital. What makes these sources particularly useful is the fact that they contain not only the decisions and deliberations of the Commission itself, but also its appeals to the civil authorities, courts or local police, as well as data on the financing of the general hospital or the number of patients.

1 Attempts to Reform Charity in Vilnius before 1795

The Vilnius General Hospital opened its doors almost four years after the third partition of the Polish-Lithuanian Commonwealth. However, the local context and the endeavors that took place during the reign of Stanisław August Poniatowski, the last King of Poland and Grand Duke of Lithuania (1764–1795), are significant when trying to understand and explain the circumstances of the establishment of this institution.

This period was characterized by several attempts to reform the system of poor relief and health care at both state and local level.[10] The first clear step was the establishment of the Commission for the Hospitals in the Kingdom of Poland and the Grand Duchy of Lithuania (*Kommissia nad szpitalami w Koronie, y w Wielkim Xięstwie Litewskim*) in 1775 at the so-called Partition Sejm (1773–1775). Despite being forced to sanction the first partition of the Commonwealth, the Sejm attempted to implement transformations aimed at reorganizing education, government, and other areas of public life, including healthcare and poor relief.[11] The Commission's statute, drafted by the Bishop of Poznań, Andrzej Stanisław Młodziejowski, expressed the desire to fundamentally reform the existing system of poor relief and healthcare, regulate beggars and provide the population of the provinces with access to medical and obstetric care. The most important goal, however, was the establishment of a general hospital (*szpital generalny*) at the center of each voivodeship.

---

10 For more, see Witecki, "Healthcare and Catholic Enlightenment," 150–72.

11 *Volumina Legum*, 109–11. For more on the Partition Sejm, see Šmigelskytė-Stukienė, Brusokas, Glemža, Jurgaitis, Rakutis, *Modernios administracijos tapsmas*, 145, 157–219. Butterwick, *The Polish-Lithuanian Commonwealth*, 122–27; Małudzińska, *Próżnowanie*, 245–51.

These new facilities were supposed to replace the old hospitals and almshouses, especially those that were not sufficiently funded. The latter institutions were to be closed and their resources, together with their patients and inmates, transferred to the general hospitals. Contrary to the usual practice of the hospitals being run by the secular or regular clergy, the Commission proposed that the general hospitals should be administered by a lay procurator (*prokurator*) who was subordinate to the chief doctor (*doktor*) and the chaplain (*kapelan*). The main administrative body responsible for the general hospitals was the Commission, which consisted of four bishops with the physiocratically oriented proponent of the Catholic Enlightenment Ignacy Jakub Massalski, the Bishop of Vilnius, as chairman, and eighteen secular dignitaries of the Grand Duchy of Lithuania.[12] The statute thus testified to the efforts to centralize and bureaucratize poor relief and healthcare in the Grand Duchy of Lithuania.[13] However, the Lithuanian side of the Commission did not even hold a single meeting and these grandiose plans were never realized.

It should be noted that the General Hospital of the Infant Jesus (*Szpital generalny Dzieciątka Jezus*) in Warsaw had been in operation since the early 1760s. This multifunctional institution was supervised by a commission made up of both laymen and clergy.[14] Although this particular hospital is not mentioned in the Statute of 1775, it undoubtedly also served as an example for the organization of a general hospital. Another wave of reforms took place during the period of the so-called Four Years' Sejm (1788–1792).[15] Its resolutions expressed revolutionary aspirations for change in many areas of public life, including the care for the poor and sick. However, the idea of establishing general hospitals was abandoned, and the Civil-Military Order Commissions (*Komisje Porządkowe Cywilno-Wojskowe*) established in each voivodeship primarily endeavored to bring order to the existing charitable institutions.[16] As Jerzy Gordziejew noted the efforts of the Civil-Military Order Commissions led to certain results and reflected the first – and to some extent fruitful – attempts

12 Witecki, "Healthcare," 153, 155, 159–61.

13 *Volumina Legum*, VIII, 109–11. Note: as was usual in the Polish-Lithuanian Commonwealth, the commissions functioned separately in the Kingdom of Poland and the Grand Duchy of Lithuania. For more on the Commission in the Kingdom of Poland, see Małudzińska, *Próżnowanie*, 248–56.

14 Małudzińska, *Próżnowanie*, 230–33.

15 Butterwick, *The Polish-Lithuanian*, 206–300.

16 For instance, see The Inspection of Almshouses and Hospitals in Vilnius (1790), Lietuvos mokslų akademijos Vrublevskių bibliotekos Rankraščių skyrius (The Manuscript Department of the Wróblewski Library of the Lithuanian Academy of Sciences; hereafter, LMAVB RS), f. 43, b. 3641.

to reform healthcare and poor relief.[17] These efforts were continued by other short-lived institutions.[18] None of them, however achieved tangible results.[19]

The efforts to reform the charitable institutions in Vilnius were also accompanied by the more general aim of improving the city's environment, which was in line with the measures taken by many other European municipalities as described in detail by James C. Riley.[20] These initiatives resulted in the city council spending more money on sewerage, drainage and paving of streets to ensure better ventilation of enclosed spaces. These concerns were later also voiced by imperial officials.[21] Thus, earlier attempts to reform the charitable institutions in Vilnius were ambitious on paper, but remained largely unrealized for financial, administrative and legal reasons.[22] Nonetheless, these largely unsuccessful endeavors prepared the ground for the establishment of the general hospital and the reform of the existing poor relief and health care system.

2 The Establishment of the General Hospital in Vilnius

The earlier experiences of attempted poor relief and health care reform in Vilnius before the Third Partition was indeed indicative of the institutions that the imperial regime created for the same purpose. On November 23, 1795, the Governor General of Lithuania Nikolai Repnin established the Hospital Commission (*Kommissia szpitalna*) and declared that it would take over "all the documents of former hospital deputations and all other [institutions] dealing with charitable foundations".[23] It is no coincidence that the Commission of 1775 and its statute – which was rarely, if ever, used before 1795 – served as a model for the Lithuanian Hospital Commission, which operated from 1797 to 1808. Although this connection has been pointed out in previous research,[24]

17 Gordziejew, *Komisje*, 161–62, 167–68, 170.

18 The Vilnius Hospital Deputation (*Deputacya szpitalna wileńska*), the Vilnius Hospital Commission (*Kommissya szpitalna wileńska*) and the Vilnius Voivodeship Commission for Hospitals (*Kommissya szpitalna województwa wileńskiego*).

19 Jakulis, *Špitolės Vilniuje: labdara, gydymas ir skurdas XVI–XVIII a*, 293.

20 Riley, *The Eighteenth-Century Campaign*, 89–110.

21 Żytkowicz, *Zburzenie murów obronnych Wilna*, 26.

22 Srogosz, "Próby," 404.

23 The Act of the Establishment of the Hospital Commission (1795), LMAVB RS, f. 43, b. 20447, fol. 1.

24 Kurczewski, *Biskupstwo*, 362.

there have been no comprehensive attempts to explore this topic in more detail.

What is of great importance here, is the composition of the Commission. Hitherto, historians have portrayed this institution as a kind of depersonalized entity, although Stefan Rosiak rightly noted that the administrative bodies created by the imperial regime from 1795 onwards "were composed of local actors."[25] The Commission was no exception. In 1800, for example, it consisted of eight laymen (two mayors, three chamberlains, a professor from Vilnius University, and two lower-ranking dignitaries) and eight representatives of the Catholic clergy. These included the aforementioned Bishop of Vilnius Kossakowski, who chaired the Commission, the prelates of the Vilnius Cathedral Chapter Ignacy Houwałt and Walenty Wołczacki, as well as Fathers Balkiewicz, Kaspar Wróblewski, Marcin Poczobut-Odlanicki, Andrzej Pohl, and Paschalis Woydag.[26]

Based on their experience, the latter four commissioners have undoubtedly provided useful insights into the reform of the local charity. Wróblewski was the former provost of St. Roch's Hospital, while the ex-Jesuit Poczobut-Odlanicki had been provost of the Holy Trinity Almshouse for many years.[27] Pohl, the then Visitator of the Lithuanian Province of the Congregation of the Mission was not only responsible for the almshouse run by the Lazarists, but also for two hospitals kept by the Sisters of Charity. He had also been working on the reform of charity in Vilnius since 1792.[28] Woydag, the Provincial of the Lithuanian Province of the Brothers Hospitaller of St. John of God as well as the superior of the local convent and hospital of the Holy Cross, was also very well informed about the intricacies of running such an institution. As in other Central European provincial capitals, former and current members of the religious orders were involved in the urban healthcare system.[29]

These details may explain, at least in part, why the Commission relied so heavily on local practices, and in particular on the Statute of 1775, which served as a guide for the reforms in the former Polish-Lithuanian Commonwealth, rather than mechanically implementing the measures that had already been enacted in the Russian Empire during the reign of Catherine II.[30] The connection between the Commission of 1775 and the Lithuanian Hospital Commission

25 Rosiak, *Prowincja*, 250.
26 Protocols (1800), fols. 157v–158.
27 Jakulis, *Špitolės*, 92, 284, 288.
28 Rosiak, *Prowincja*, 51; Jakulis, *Špitolės*, 279.
29 Rosiak, *Bonifratrzy*, 47.
30 Hartley, "Philanthropy in the Reign of Catherine the Great," 167–202. Lindenmeyr, *Poverty is Not a Vice*, 33–36. Jahn, "Health Care and Poor Relief in Russia, 1700–1856," 161–164.

was emphasized both in the protocols of the Commission and in the brochure on the organization of the general hospital written by its member, the physician Elias Einholm, in 1800.[31] In his preface, he remarked:

> In every corner of the world and in every country, there were benefactors who endeavored to alleviate human misery. There were quite a few of them in Lithuania. They listened to the voice of nature and religion and shared their wealth with their poor neighbors. The funds grew from day to day, and eventually, the Government recognized the need to establish a Commission to oversee and manage these [foundations]. Thus, the Commission was established in 1775 in accordance with the [Sejm's] constitution. Although it was composed of the most exceptional persons who had the public good at heart, [the Commission] encountered difficulties in its work due to the constant unrest in the country. The hospitals were in extreme misery, the city [of Vilnius] was flooded with beggars, the foundations were reduced in size, and a considerable number of them were neglected. In 1797, the Hospital Commission was reinstated and, with the support of the government, was given full authority. Slowly the funds returned and reached such a level that [the Commission] was able to build the general hospital at the church of Saints Philip and James, the Apostles.[32]

The comparison between what the Commission of 1775 sought to achieve and what the Lithuanian Hospital Commission achieved – and in what way – shows the significance of the earlier reform efforts. The Commission not only adopted the idea of a general hospital, but also used the Statute of 1775 to define its organization, tasks and means of funding.

At its meeting on June 18, 1798, the Commission decided, on the basis of the Statute of 1775, to close six Catholic and Uniate[33] almshouses[34] and St. Roch's Hospital and to transfer their endowments, together with their inmates and

31 For instance, see Protocols (1803), fols. 82v–85; Protocols (1804), fols. 45, 61v–68.

32 Einholm, *Organizacya dla szpitala*, 1–2.

33 In accordance with the constitution of 1775 that confirmed the establishment of the Commission of Hospitals in the Kingdom of Poland and the Grand Duchy of Lithuania (*Volumina Legum*, VIII, 110), the intended reforms were aimed only at Catholic and Uniate poor relief and health care institutions. According to Catherine II's will, the non-Catholic (then referred to as Dissident) almshouses and other charitable institutions were to remain in the hands of various confessional (Orthodox, Lutheran, Calvinist) and religious (Jewish) communities. For more on the Russian Empire's policy towards the Orthodox and Protestants in the Polish-Lithuanian Commonwealth, see Butterwick, *The Polish-Lithuanian*, 95–106.

34 The almshouses of St Mary Magdalene (founded in 1518), Holy Trinity (1535), Spaski (Savior) (Orthodox, later Uniate, 1560s), St Peter (1620), Sts Joseph of Arimathea and Nicodemus (1631), Sts James and Philip (1723).

patients, to the General Hospital.[35] However, the reason for this decision was not only to secure the financing for the General Hospital. The Commission pointed out the inadequate living conditions in the old and, in their opinion, dilapidated almshouses and the insufficient support for their inmates. In addition, St. Roch's Hospital, the second largest medical facility in the city, which was intended for the treatment of patients suffering with venereal diseases, was to be closed as it was located "in a low place, and not in the open air".[36] The commissioners thus clearly invoked the neo-Hippocratic theory of miasma, arguing that such a hospital, which was surrounded by the still existing city walls, emitted dangerous "airs," and should therefore be closed and relocated to the suburbs.

It should be noted that this was the very first case in which charitable institutions were deliberately closed. Previously, many almshouses had ceased to operate after losing income and property due to major fires or other disasters. The deliberate closure of almshouses and hospitals, some of which had been in operation for nearly three centuries, was a bold and unprecedented move that reflected changing attitudes towards the organization of healthcare and poor relief.

It was also the first time, that the location for a hospital was deliberately chosen and the facility was built in the suburb of Lukiškės, far from the city center of the time, near the Dominican monastery and the Church of Sts. James and Philip. In the early modern period, almshouses and hospitals were built without thinking about their location beforehand, and in most cases they were simply established near existing churches.[37] It was only by chance that some of them emerged near the city walls or the city gates, and this had little to do with the incentive to strengthen the fortifications or to isolate the poor and sick from the rest of the population. Some of the buildings of the Dominican monastery and the almshouse were conveniently integrated into the structure of the General Hospital. However, the main reason for building the hospital in this particular location was to remove those who were considered dangerous to society – patients suffering from sexually transmitted diseases and beggars – from the densely populated areas of the city.[38] It was no coincidence that Bishop Kossakowski preached in his sermon at the opening ceremony:

> The swarms of beggars that roam this city, who sit in the streets, at the gates, in the churchyards and by your houses, have disappeared from your sight; you no

35 Protocols (1798), fols. 78v–80.
36 Protocols (1798), fol. 78v.
37 Jakulis, *Špitolės*, 47–82.
38 Korybut-Marciniak, *Dobroczynne*, 228.

> longer see the shameful image of misery, sorrow, wretchedness and the wailing Lazaruses, most of whom seem to be swindlers rather than [true] wretches.[39]

Moreover, the General Hospital was built as such, unlike most of the older almshouses and hospitals, which were set up in simple houses or palaces that were later converted into charitable institutions. The only exception before 1795 was the Infant Jesus Orphanage and Foundling Home, which was built specifically as such an institution.[40] The General Hospital buildings, designed by the Italian architect Pietro de Rossi, expressed the desire to create a new type of hospital with spacious, well-ventilated wards, accommodation for staff, domestic buildings and warehouses.[41]

The construction of the General Hospital, supervised by Father Wróblewski and the prior of the Dominican monastery Father Jacek Misiewicz, lasted from January 1798 to February 1799, despite many difficulties caused by insufficient funds and the lack of building materials.[42] Already at the meeting on March 1, 1799, the Commission decided to transfer the poor from the almshouse of St. Mary Magdalene,[43] while the patients of St. Roch's Hospital were transferred to the new facility on June 11.[44] In the following months, especially after the grand opening ceremony on June 16, the wards of the General Hospital filled up with paupers from other closed almshouses as well as beggars detained by the local police.

The establishment of the new institution in Vilnius could simply be seen as a direct attempt to create a more suitable hospital run by the civil authorities and medical professionals. The new regime's interest in the social conditions in Vilnius is evidenced by the fact that for almost two years (1798–1799) the local intendant Zakhariy Serebrenikov collected monthly data on the number of people in the still existing almshouses and other institutions (mainly Catholic monasteries) that cared for the poor.[45] This data may probably have influenced the planning of the General Hospital. Thus, a large hospital has been seen as a solution to the pressing social problems.

39 Kossakowski, "Kazanie," 418.

40 Rosiak, *Prowincja*, 201, 229.

41 Rosiak, *Prowincja*, 251. Einholm, *Organizacya*, 5.

42 Protocols (1798), fols. 11, 41v; Protocols (1799), fols. 27v–28.

43 Protocols (1799), fols. 27v–28.

44 Materials on Hospitals and Almshouses in Vilnius (1599–1828), LVIA, f. 694, ap. 1, b. 60, fols. 41v–42.

45 Zakhariy Serebrenikov's Reports to the Lithuanian Hospital Commission (1798–1799), LMAVB RS, f. 43, b. 20458.

In addition, the Commission saw the foundation of the General Hospital as a way to simplify and organize the administration of welfare.[46] It was undoubtedly much more convenient to oversee just four hospitals than a whole network of almshouses linked to numerous benefactors and several centers of power (most notably, the cathedral chapter and the city council). All these developments, especially the partial secularization, the centralization of charity and the considerable involvement of the state in this area were similar to the reforms carried out by Catherine II in the Russian Empire in the 1770s, as well as other measures previously introduced by Enlightenment rulers, such as the Archbishop of Würzburg or later by Maria Theresa and Joseph II in the provincial towns of the Habsburg Monarchy.[47]

Besides these factors, other incentives should also be considered, because, as Sandra Cavallo noted, "existing studies tend to prioritize arguments based on demand, and this prevents the exploration of other types of explanations that are relatively independent of the needs of the poor, but rather related to the multiple meanings that charity had for benefactors."[48] The opening ceremony of the General Hospital was marked by the bishop's sermon, a solemn mass, and a banquet. However, the event focused not on the Commission, which was primarily responsible for founding the new institution, but the imperial administration, headed by the Governor Friezel, and the then Russian Emperor Paul I.[49] According to an anonymous diarist, the ceremony culminated in prayers "for the health and happiness of His Grace the Emperor".[50] A few months later, in the preface to his brochure on the organization of the general hospital, Einholm praised Friezel as the one whose efforts made the poor "forget their misery and the sick, regain their health, while he wiped away their tears".[51]

This reflected a clear shift in emphasis from private benefactors and their will as an essential factor in the establishment of a charitable institution to the representatives of the regime and thus the monarch himself. It is important to note that, with few exceptions, the former rulers and/or the state did not play a significant role in the establishing or supporting of almshouses and

46 The Documents of the Lithuanian Hospital Commission (1797–1808), LMAVB RS, f. 43, b. 20457, fol. 42: "Once order had been established the Hospital Commission, only four hospitals remain in the city of Vilnius."

47 Hartley, "Philanthropy," 180; Lindenmeyr, *Poverty*, 33–34; Grell, Cunningham, "Health Care," 8–10.

48 Cavallo, "The Motivations of Benefactors," 51.

49 "Z Wilna," 1.

50 Tekieliński, *Opis*, 99.

51 Einholm, *Organizacya*, A2.

hospitals in Vilnius and the private initiatives of the nobility, the clergy or the citizenry were the main forces in the development of charity. The General Hospital could therefore also be seen as an expression of the imperial regime's desire to assume, at least in part, the role of the main benefactor responsible for supporting the poor. It was no coincidence that during his short stay in Vilnius in early July 1802, Alexander I visited not only the university and other important institutions, but also the three largest charitable institutions, starting with the General Hospital, and "complimented each of their overseers on their diligence."[52]

3 Administration and Organization

Before 1799, the hospitals and almshouses were overseen by various entities, most of which were closely linked to the Church. Two of the closed institutions were run by Catholic religious orders, while others were overseen by a provost or a parish priest. The remaining two Catholic and Uniate almshouses were supervised not only by priests, but also by lay overseers elected by the city council.[53] After 1799, some Catholic charitable institutions were still run in the spirit of their founders, but with the establishment of the General Hospital, a new type of administration emerged with the Lithuanian Hospital Commission at its head. In a way, its composition still reflected the former administrative system with the bishop, the representatives of the cathedral chapter, the local clergy and the city council in its ranks. However, its composition also reflected significant changes in the perception of who should be responsible for overseeing a charitable organization.

Although hundreds of decisions from the years 1797–1808 are recorded in the protocols of the Commission, they are usually only signed by the chairman, and the names of the Commissioners are only known in a few cases. These lists, albeit rare, give an indication of who, the regime' thought, should be responsible for the supervision of the General Hospital. As the list from 1801 shows, the Commission consisted mainly of secular commissioners – doctors, professors, mayors and lower-level officials.[54] Although the local clergy

52 Tekieliński, *Opis*, 113.

53 Jakulis, *Špitolės*, 84–103.

54 Protocols (1801), fol. 68v: 1. Jan Nepomucen Kossakowski, the bishop of Vilnius and chairman; 2. Elias Einholm, counselor, inspector of Lithuanian doctors, member of the Vilnius Academy; 3. Andrzej Malczewski, the chief archivist of the Lithuanian Supreme Court, 4. Szymon Malewski, counselor of the former Polish court, professor of logic, law, nature and nations; 5. Ignacy Żałkowski, chamberlain of the Polish court; 6. Father Andrzej Pohl,

had dominated the charity for centuries, they played a diminished, but still significant role in the early 1800s. As seen in Pest, Zagreb and Prague, fewer members of the clergy were involved in poor relief – either as direct overseers or as benefactors.

Furthermore, after many charitable institutions were closed, the clergy lost the limited financial benefits. The establishment of the Commission and the subsequent erection of the General Hospital therefore transformed not only the way almshouses and hospitals were maintained, but also the circle of people who oversaw charitable activities. Those traditionally involved in the care of the poor were eclipsed, at least in numbers, by those who had previously played virtually no role in this area. In many ways, the Commission resembled the Russian welfare boards, but as the clergy retained a not inconsiderable influence, it could not simply be equated with the Russian laity dominated institutions.[55] Thus, the Commission embodied a fusion of imperial and local approaches to how the main administrative body should be composed.

The Commission was primarily responsible for funding of the General Hospital and represented it in court, especially when benefactors were in arrears with their payments. Unsurprisingly, legal disputes of this kind made up for a considerable proportion of the protocols each year.[56] Only rarely did the Commission deal with other issues, such as the staff of the General Hospital,[57] or the admission of certain people to the hospital.[58] The Commission met regularly several times a week and dealt with various matters together, but only one commissioner, the commissioner-on-duty (*kommissarz dežurny*), was directly responsible for the daily supervision of the General Hospital.[59]

The General Hospital was directly supervised by the Commission, which, however, did not hold unlimited power. The hospital's organizational structure,

---

the visitor of the Lithuanian province of the Congregation of the Mission; 7. Father Kaspar Wróblewski, the vice-chancellor of the Vilnius cathedral, canon of Livonia; 8. Father Paschalis Woydag, the provincial of the Lithuanian province of the Brothers Hospitaller of St. John of God; 9. Aloizy Karner, the burgomaster of Vilnius; 10. Karol Szwartze, the burgomaster of Vilnius; 11. Józef Doroszko, the regent of the Commission; 12. Kazimierz Lenkiewicz, the chancellor of the Commission.

55 Lindenmeyr, *Poverty*, 34–35.

56 For instance, see the protocol for the meeting on 9 September 1801. Protocols (1801), fols. 75–78.

57 E.g., at the session of July 24, 1803, the Commission established modified regulations to the then overseer of the hospital Franciszek Misiewicz (Protocols (1803), fols. 56v–56av).

58 At the session of November 9, 1800, the Commission decided to admit nine disabled poor persons to the general hospital and forbade five healthy women to beg in the streets of Vilnius (Protocols (1800), fols. 151v–152).

59 Einholm, *Organizacya*, 14–15.

its financing and other similar matters therefore had to be submitted to the civil government for decisive approval. For example, the Commission's considerations regarding the need to reorganize the General Hospital's structure were addressed to the then Governor Mikhail Kutuzov, who ultimately had to decide on the matter.[60] Such an approach represented a significant change, as until then (with a conditional exception for the early 1790s) no representatives of the government had any influence on the decision-making process and each institution retained a high degree of autonomy. In this respect, the Commission resembled the Russian welfare boards, which were made up of representatives from different social classes but were dominated by the provincial governors.[61]

The General Hospital itself consisted of four organizationally and spatially separate departments: (*i*) the department for venereal diseases, or the "secret hospital" (*szpital sekretny*), (*ii*) the department for the terminally ill and the poor (*szpital niewyleczonych i ubogich*), (*iii*) the department for obstetrics (*szpital kobiet rodzących*), and (*iv*) the office of the wet-nurses (*kantor mamek*). A multifunctional institution of this size therefore required a staff of almost thirty people, who were not only responsible for the patients, the lying-in women or the poor, but also for the economy of the institution, which, like the old hospitals, functioned as a largely self-sufficient economic unit. The General Hospital as a medical facility was supervised by an unpaid chief doctor (*główny doktor, główny medyk*), who was accountable to the Commission.[62] His subordinate, the supervisor of the hospital (*prowizor szpitalny*), was responsible for the hiring of house staff (cooks, laundresses, and other laborers), supplying provisions, and other matters related to the economy of the institution.[63]

Although professional doctors regularly treated patients in the hospitals before the reform, they were never an integral part of the organizational structure. As they were not part to the monastic communities that maintained the hospitals and were employed on an annual or monthly basis, they remained subordinate to the superiors of the convents.[64] The general hospital was therefore not only the first medical institution to be run by a physician, but also the first hospital with a large and permanent medical staff (see Table 8.1).[65] This reflected, at least on a formal level, the broader developments in

60 Protocols (1801), fols. 59–59v. The governor's reply remains unknown.

61 Lindenmeyr, *Poverty*, 34; Hartley, "Philanthropy," 190.

62 Einholm, *Organizacya*, 18, 28.

63 Ibid., 15–17.

64 Jakulis, *Špitolės*, 221–22, 234, 241–42.

65 For comparison, in 1788, the staff of the St. Roch Hospital was composed of eight Merciful Brothers, a cook with an assistant, a tailor, a cobbler, three laborers, two female laborers,

TABLE 8.1 Medical staff of the Vilnius General Hospital. In Elias Einholm. *Organizacya dla szpitala generalnego wilenskiego*. Wilno: w Drukarni Akademickiey, 1800, 18–29

Office	Responsibilities	Salary (in rubles)
Chief doctor (*główny doktor*)	Daily inspection of the general hospital; methods of treatment	Unpaid
Hospital's doctor (*doktor szpitalny*)	Daily rounds; surgeries; prescription of diet and medication; supervision of the hospital's dispensary	300
Subsurgeons (2) (*subchirurg, podlakar*)	Assistance to the hospital's doctor in operations and other procedures	100 (each)
Feldsher (*felczer*)	Treatment of the poor and the incurables	30
Chief warden (*dozórca starszy*)	Supervision of caregivers; maintenance of the patients' clothing and bedding; general order in the hospital wards	50
Caregivers (10, male and female) (*stróży, dozorujące, pilnujące*)	Caring for the patients and the poor; maintaining order in the hospital wards	54 (six females) 48 (four males)

healthcare provision in eighteenth-century Western and Central Europe. As already argued in the Zagreb case, it was primarily about the medicalization of hospitals and the "expansion of the role that had hitherto been assigned to medical professionals".[66]

The medical staff was assisted by the senior warden (*dozórca starszy*) and ten male and female caregivers (*pilnujący, dozorujący, stróży*), who were responsible for the order and cleanliness of the wards and other daily tasks.[67] As these services did not require any special medical knowledge, these workers received half the wages of the doctors, with the exception of the feldsher, whose sole task was to alleviate the suffering of the poor and incurable.[68] This

two caregivers attending to the lying-in women, nineteen persons in total. See the Report on the Status of the St. Roch Hospital (1788), LMAVB RS, f. 43, b. 20590, fol. 1.

66 Risse, *Mending Bodies*, 237. See also Lindeman, *Medicine and Society*, 158.

67 Einholm, *Organizacya*, 22–23.

68 Ibid., 29.

numerous medical staff reflected the main mission of the general hospital: it was first and foremost a medical institution, even if 120 poor and incurable people were to be accommodated in its wards.

Adequate remuneration must have been an incentive for the medical staff to accept a position in the General Hospital and provide better care, which was one of the main motives for the establishment of this institution. The fact that the most important position of chief physician remained unpaid shows that it was perceived as a kind of honorary post, a *noblesse oblige*, from which the individual could have benefited in other ways (career opportunities or building up relationships of interests and business).[69] However, unlike other general hospitals, the Vilnius General Hospital did not seem to have served as a place for bedside teaching and clinical training, at least in the early days. Perhaps because of the main function of the General Hospital (treatment of venereal diseases), medical professors such as, Joseph Frank preferred to teach in the Sawicz Hospital run by the Sisters of Charity.[70]

In some respects, however, the organizational structure of the General Hospital still resembled the pre-reform institutions, and the Commission still relied on some traditional patterns of maintaining charitable institutions. In the first year, the hospital's economy was supervised by Father Misiewicz (later Father Aleksy Henrych), the prior of the nearby Dominican monastery, who was familiar with running an almshouse.[71] In addition, the Dominicans were also responsible for the spiritual care (*posługa duchowna*) of the patients and the poor.[72] Although the General Hospital was founded as a secular healthcare and poor relief facility, it remained closely linked to the local clergy, at least initially. However, for unknown reasons, Father Misiewicz was replaced as early as May 1800 by a previously unknown Bandomer, and until 1809 the economy of the General Hospital was supervised by lay overseers.[73]

Such a multi-level organization, characterized by a clear chain of command and division of tasks, appears quite balanced. In practice, however, the organization seems to have had some shortcomings. As early as June 3, 1801, the Commission approached the governor with a request for approval (*aprobata*) for a fundamental redesign of the institution's organizational structure. The Commission argued that the existing administration was not performing its

69 Cavallo, "The Motivation," 52.

70 Risse, *Mending Bodies*, 238, 252–53. See also Frankas, *Atsiminimai*, 79.

71 Protocols (1798), fol. 41v.

72 Protocols (1800), fols. 50v–51. Also see Rosiak, *Prowincja*, 250–51.

73 Protocols (1803), fol. 25v.

duties properly, the commissioners were burdened with additional tasks and were unable to fulfill their main task of supervising all the almshouses and hospitals operating in the Lithuanian Governorate. It was proposed that the General Hospital be placed in the hands of the Sisters of Charity, "who are known for their diligence and ability to oversee the [charitable] premises."[74]

Six months later, the Commission again appealed to the governor, this time arguing that the hospital's administration, which was supposed to be responsible for finding new sources of revenue, was unable to increase the facility's income at a time of "overwhelming influx of patients and the poor".[75] In such a situation, burdened with additional responsibilities, the Commission again recommended that the hospital be placed into the hands of the Sisters of Charity, who "properly maintain other similar institutions in the city".[76] It is not known whether the Commission received a response from the governor.[77] It was not until 1809, that the general hospital was finally placed under the control of the Sisters of Charity.[78]

What these discussions, decisions and eventual actions regarding the organizational structure of the hospital show is that the Commission returned to structures and patterns that were developed and used before the reform. Despite attempts to create an institution run by secular officials, the Commission was initially forced to turn to more experienced actors. The fact that the General Hospital remained in the hands of the Sisters of Charity from 1809 to 1867, when they were ultimately removed from the institution in the wake of the repression following the January Uprising, demonstrates the persistence of both old and new structures and the regime's inability to create a fully secular medical institution. In this respect, the Vilnius hospital was like the medical facilities in Zagreb, Prague, Brno and Kraków, which employed members of convents for their operations at least until the 1860s.

4 Funding

Securing sufficient funding for health and poor relief institutions remained an important issue in the process of charity reform in the late eighteenth century.

74 Protocols (1801), fol. 59.
75 Protocols (1801), fol. 104v.
76 Protocols (1801), fol. 105. The sisters ran the Sawicz hospital from 1748 and the foundling and orphan home of Infant Jesus from 1791.
77 Rosiak, *Prowincja*, 253.
78 Ibid.

As usual, charitable institutions received funding from a variety of sources: traditional donations, legacies and collections.[79] The institutions also relied on some novel sources of income, such as new taxes or voluntary contributions from the better-off citizens.[80] Apart from the one-off grant of 63,275 rubles received from the Emperor Paul I, the General Hospital was financed in a similar way. Although the new institution inherited the assets of the closed charitable institutions, it is clear from the protocols that the Commission sought new sources of income over the years, especially after the General Hospital was gradually burdened with additional tasks (e. g. the treatment of prisoners and army recruits).

The foundation of a General Hospital must have consisted mainly of land and funds (sums, bequests) belonging to six almshouses and St. Roch's Hospital. Moreover, the foundation was supplemented by real estate: houses in Vilnius and the buildings of the closed institutions themselves, which were rented or sold by the Commission,[81] as well as a bridge over the river Neris (Wilia), that had belonged to the almshouse of the Holy Trinity since the mid-sixteenth century and which was rebuilt and rented by the Commission.[82]

In addition to the possessions of the old charitable institutions, the General Hospital and the Commission also had to contend with the chronic problems of collecting money from debtors. However, numerous decisions recorded in the protocols demonstrate that, unlike the previous overseers, the Commission was able to rely not only on its authority but also on the courts and the local police. At the meeting of January 10, 1800, for example, the Commission decided to ask the police for help in recovering a meager sum of 20 guldens belonging to Ewa Skurewiczowa, who passed away in the General Hospital.[83] On October 2, 1803, an appeal was made to the lower court in order to obtain the much larger sum of 10 silver rubles.[84]

Although the General Hospital relied on various sources of revenue that guaranteed a substantial annual income (see Table 8.2), the Commission was constantly striving to improve the institution's financial situation. Therefore,

79 Dross, "Health Care Provision and Poor Relief in Enlightenment and 19th Century Prussia," 87.

80 Stolberg, "Health Care Provision and Poor Relief in the Electorate and Kingdom of Bavaria," 119.

81 The list of ten houses that were owned by the charitable institutions were rented by the Commission, as well as the buildings of the St Mary Magdalene and the Savior (Spaski) almshouses and the hospital of St. Roch that were sold. See Protocols (1804), fol. 46v.

82 Protocols (1804), fols. 41v–42v.

83 Protocols (1800), fol. 4v.

84 Protocols (1803), fol. 82.

TABLE 8.2 Annual income of hospitals in Vilnius (1800) (in guldens – złotys). In protocols of the Lithuanian hospital commission (hereafter, Protocols) (1800), Lietuvos valstybės istorijos archyvas (Lithuanian State Historical Archives, Vilnius; hereafter, LVIA), f. 390, ap. 135, b. 4, fols. 89–102v

Hospital	Number of patients	Annual income
Holy Cross (Brothers Hospitallers of St John of God)	24	4,316
Sawicz hospital (Sisters of Charity)	158	12,346
Infant Jesus (Sisters of Charity)	120	20,577
General Hospital (Lithuanian Hospital Commission)	204	52,263

the first years were marked by endeavors to supplement the income from the properties of the old facilities with revenues from previously unused sources. A good example of this is the Commission's proposal to build a brickworks (*fabryka cegły*) near the hospital to support not only itself but also the city's other charitable institutions.[85] However, it seems that this plan was never realized.

Other initiatives reflected the Commission's aspirations to encourage wider civic involvement in charitable activities, like the provincial welfare boards in the Russian Empire.[86] And this was not to be limited to traditional bequests from the deceased or spontaneous donations inspired by the Christian doctrine of good works. One of these measures was the introduction of a fixed annual contribution. At the meeting on February 17, 1800, the Commission appealed to thirty-two people of different social status and geographical origin – from bishops, canons or academics to ordinary municipal and government officials living in various towns and villages of the former Grand Duchy of Lithuania – and reminded them of their "voluntary obligation" (*dobrowolna ofiara*) to donate to the Commission (and thus to the General Hospital).[87] The amounts of between 6 and 300 guldens per year show that the benefactors could decide for themselves how much they wanted to donate.[88] These donations were to

85 Protocols (1803), fols. 89–89v.

86 Lindenmeyr, *Poverty*, 33; Hartley, "Philanthropy," 178, 190–91.

87 Protocols (1800), fols. 24–30v.

88 This practice differed significantly from the obligations of the knights of the Order of Saint Stanislaus to the orphan and foundling home of Infant Jesus, since they had to

bring a considerable sum of more than 1,100 guldens per a year into the Commission's coffers. However, twenty-one of the thirty-two benefactors were four or five years in arrears with their contributions, so this source of income was hardly reliable. In 1802, for example, the General Hospital received only 382 guldens.[89]

Other funding measures were based on the participation of local society. Early on, the Commission decided that part of the income from the sale of theatre or opera tickets, and the proceeds from balls should be used for charitable purposes.[90] Lotteries organized by local entrepreneurs and the sale of tickets for the public garden were also considered as possible sources of income.[91] However, the profit from the sale of cards, which were produced in the state factory in St. Petersburg, provided a steady, albeit modest, stream of income. As early as the second half of the eighteenth century, the monopolized sale of cards was seen as one of the measures for financing charitable institutions in the cities of the Russian Empire.[92] A separate accounting record shows that the Commission received 5 kopeks from every ruble raised through the sale of cards. Between 60 and more than 200 rubles flowed into the Commission's coffers every two months to support all charitable organizations.[93] In 1803, for example, 287 rubles of the total annual income of 12,489 rubles was paid into the hospital's treasury.[94]

Although these new sources of revenue, which the Commission itself labelled as "occasional", were not as profitable and reliable as the ordinary ones, their introduction shows certain shifts in the general perception of charity. They allowed, at least in part, a wider range of individuals to support the charities in different ways. Compared to the other three hospitals (Holy Cross, Sawicz, and Infant Jesus), the General Hospital received the highest annual income (see, for example, the data for 1800 in Table 8.2). A similar trend continued in later years.[95] However, at least in the period covered in this chapter,

donate a fixed sum of 80 guldens every year. For more on charitable duties of the knights of the Order of Saint Stanislaus, see Jeziorowski, "Order Świętego Stanisława Biskupa i Męczennika 1765–1795," 87, 103–4.

89 Protocols (1802), fol. 44.

90 For instance, 1,884 guldens came from the sale of tickets to a masquerade in 1801, while the performance of an opera in 1802 raised 1,083 guldens. See Protocols (1802), fols. 3v, 44.

91 Protocols (1803), fols. 13, 43, 85.

92 Hartley, "Philanthropy," 174.

93 Accounts Book Detailing the Expenditure and Income from the Sale of Cards (1803–1807), LVIA, f. 390, ap. 135, b. 8.

94 Protocols (1804), fol. 66.

95 For example, see the figures for the year 1801. Protocols (1802), fols. 34v–44.

all the Commission's efforts to secure sufficient funding for the General Hospital were only partially successful. As evidenced by the numerous complaints in the protocols, the Commission was unable to tackle the chronic financial problems that had plagued the superintendents of the charitable institutions long before the reform. Even five years after the opening of the General Hospital, overdue payments for almshouses and hospitals that had already been closed were still a cause for concern.[96] These complaints show that it was a challenge to provide adequate heating, especially after the General Hospital took on additional responsibilities.[97] It is therefore understandable that the Commission not only tried to wring the much-needed money out of debtors who owed even the smallest amounts, but also, despite rather insignificant returns, monitored the sale of cards and spared neither time nor effort to ensure sufficient funding.

5 Functions

Before the establishment of the General Hospital, there were more than ten Catholic and Uniate poor relief and health facilities in Vilnius. Without obvious intervention by the state or the Church, three hospitals gradually took over certain functions in the local medical market, and the city's inhabitants received specialized medical assistance from various institutions. Those suffering from venereal diseases were treated at St. Roch's Hospital, while patients ill with other ailments, such as various "fevers" were treated at the Holy Cross Hospital or Sawicz Hospital.[98] The almshouses only provided basic care for the poor and were not intended for inmates from certain social or professional circles.[99] Nevertheless, these institutions played an important role in the religious and social life of the city. They were closely associated with the churches to which they were attached, with the priests who looked after the almshouses and their inmates, and with certain neighborhoods.[100]

---

96 For instance, at the session of 12 April 1804, the Commission was notified that interest from the sums bequeathed earlier to the almshouse of Sts. Joseph of Arimathea and Nicodemus and the hospital of St. Roch were still late. See Protocols (1804), fol. 19.

97 Protocols (1803), fols. 27–27v, 100v–101, 106–106v; Protocols (1804), fols. 27v–29, 69–69v, 70v–71.

98 Only after the reform, mental patients from all over the Lithuanian Governorate were systematically admitted to the Holy Cross hospital.

99 The only exception was the almshouse run by the Lazarists, which was intended primarily for impoverished nobles.

100 Jakulis, *Špitolės*, 298–99.

The reform carried out by the Commission significantly changed the system of charity that had evolved over almost three centuries. Many charitable institutions, which reflected the will of particular benefactors and provided medical assistance and/or support to thousands of people over the years, were replaced by four hospitals designed to meet the diverse needs of the city inhabitants. An undated document, probably issued by the Commission at the end of 1799, shows that a centralized network of specialized institutions was indeed the intended outcome of the reform:

> After the Hospital Commission had established order, there were only four hospitals left in the city of Vilnius. The hospital for fever patients and sick people suffering from other illnesses is run by charitable nuns [i. e. the Sisters of Charity]. The Infant Jesus Hospital for orphans and foundlings is also run by the charitable nuns. The hospital for the mentally ill men is run by the Fatebenefratelli [i. e. the Hospitaller Brothers of St. John of God]. The General Hospital for the disabled people, the poor, male and female patients with venereal diseases, and lying-in women is run by the Commission.[101]

It is important to note that the hospitals, which were mainly concerned with medical care, rarely admitted the poor and incurable, as they considered them a burden on their finances. The almshouses, in turn, did not have the resources to provide consistent medical care.[102] Therefore, it was an unusual decision in Vilnius to deliberately assign the functions of a hospital and an almshouse to the General Hospital (this was, however, characteristic of the Infant Jesus General Hospital in Warsaw or the *Allgemeine Krankenhaus* in Vienna).[103] In comparison to other hospitals in the city, the General Hospital was not only the largest institution but also fulfilled many more functions (see Table 8.3).

First and foremost, the General Hospital served as a medical facility where mainly men and women with venereal diseases were treated. This was not really a novelty, as the General Hospital simply continued the work of St. Roch's Hospital, even if the patients were not treated by the merciful brothers, but by the medical staff of the General Hospital. It also admitted lying-in women, thus continuing the work of St. Roch's Hospital. Nevertheless, there were some novelties in the activities of the General Hospital as a medical institution. From

101 Documents of the Lithuanian Hospital Commission (1797–1808), LMAVB RS, f. 43, b. 20457, fol. 42.

102 Jakulis, *Špitolės*, 158, 212, 238–41.

103 Małudzińska, *Próżnowanie*, 233. Risse, *Mending Bodies*, 260.

TABLE 8.3 Hospital patients in Vilnius (23 January 1803). In protocols of the Lithuanian hospital commission (hereafter, Protocols) (1800), Lietuvos valstybės istorijos archyvas (Lithuanian State Historical Archives, Vilnius; hereafter, LVIA), f. 390, ap. 135, b. 4, fol. 11

Hospital	Admitted in 1802	Released	Dead	Remain in the hospital
1. General hospital	1071	750	119	205
a. *Venereal patients (male)*	*159*	*130*	*1*	*28*
b. *Venereal patients (female)*	*165*	*139*		*26*
c. *Lying-in women*	*56*	*46*	*2*	*7*
d. *Prisoners and recruits*	*241*	*205*	*4*	*36*
e. *Poor and incurables (both sexes)*	*450*	*230*	*112*	*108*
2. Holy Cross (mental patients)	240	201	19	20
3. Infant Jesus	258	59	63	135
a. *Foundlings (both sexes)*	*143*	*55*	*61*	*26*
b. *Children attending school*	*115*	*4*	*2*	*109*
4. Sawicz hospital	1623	1293	179	151
a. *Male patients*	*702*	*541*	*95*	*66*
b. *Female patients*	*921*	*752*	*84*	*85*

September 26, 1799, it systematically treated sick prisoners and recruits to the imperial army.[104] The introduction of this undesirable obligation contradicted the institution's originally defined mission and put a strain on its already limited finances. The Commission therefore repeatedly appealed to the governors to provide additional funds, as it believed that the cost of treating these surplus patients put the hospital at risk of "eventual closure".[105]

Since the General Hospital was set up in place of six almshouses, it also provided relief. On the surface, not much has changed: the poor, who had previously been housed in several charitable institutions, were simply moved to a single one, which was supposed to offer better living conditions (eight spacious wards for 120 women and men) and constant care.[106] However, this move

104 Protocols (1804), fol. 68.
105 Protocols (1804), fol. 68v.
106 Einholm, *Organizacya*, 31–32.

changed the situation of the poor considerably. Not only were they moved to another institution, but they were also isolated from the rest of society. This severed the links between the poor and the churches associated with the charitable institutions.[107] These churches played a significant role in the lives of the poor who lived in the almshouses. They had to attend daily mass, take part in other religious ceremonies such as the baptism of infants and to ensure cleanliness. In addition, the prayers they could offer to benefactors attracted new donations and bequests from different strata of local society.[108]

Such a way of life was very different from life in the General Hospital. The founders of the General Hospital were aware that closure of the charitable institutions and transfer of their endowments to the new hospital was against the will of the benefactors. Therefore, even before the hospital was built, the Commission decided to put up a board with the names of all the donors "so that [the poor] would know their benefactors and offer them their daily prayers".[109] This initiative was a traditional way of praising the generosity of the donors.[110] It also shows that the Commission expected the poor (and possibly the patients) to behave like the residents of the old charities. However, attending specific religious services does not seem to have been such a crucial part of their everyday in the General Hospital. Probably not coincidentally, Einholm does not mention any specific religious "duties" of the poor, but focuses primarily on their material well-being, living conditions and other similar issues.[111]

While the poor who lived in the old almshouses could move around the city quite freely and even beg for themselves, the inmates of the General Hospital were forbidden to collect alms and could only leave the institution of their own free will with great difficulty. The decisions recorded in the protocols show that leaving the General Hospital was a rather complicated procedure, as the inmates wishing to return home had to apply for passes.[112] Although neither the Commission nor the local police were able to confine all the paupers in the General Hospital, the mere fact that at least some of the poor living in

107 Three churches associated with almshouses and hospitals (St. Mary Magdalene, St. Roch, Sts. Joseph of Arimathea and Nicodemus) were closed and demolished in early 1800s.

108 Jakulis, *Špitolės*, 174–83, 255–66.

109 Protocols (1798), fol. 79v.

110 Cavallo, "The Motivation," 55; Hartley, "Philanthropy," 174.

111 Einholm, *Organizacya*, 31–32.

112 For instance, on July 4, 1801, the Commission decided to issue a passport to Jan and Teresa Krupowicz and their daughter Brygida who asked to be "released" (*uwolnieni*) from the General Hospital and to be allowed to return to their relatives, see Protocols (1801), fols. 70–70v.

almshouses were no longer to be found in certain places significantly altered both their status and the social and religious relations between them and the wider society.[113]

Furthermore, the functions of the General Hospital were not limited to those of a charitable facility, but in rare cases, it also served as a place of punishment. For example, a peasant woman, Marjanna Szurpowa, who had been convicted of theft, was sentenced to life imprisonment in the General Hospital (*na posługę wieczną w jeneralnym wileńskim szpitalu*).[114] This shows that, despite the Commission's objections, the General Hospital was seen by the local law enforcement officials as a particularly suitable means of solving at least some of the city's pressing problems.

6 Conclusion

The – albeit mostly negative – experiences with welfare reform in Vilnius and the Grand Duchy of Lithuania before the Third Partition of the Polish-Lithuanian Commonwealth in 1795 played a decisive role in the founding of the Vilnius General Hospital. The Statute of the Commission for Hospitals from 1775 served as a source of inspiration and a guidance for the Lithuanian Hospital Commission. Although the General Hospital was founded under a new political order, local actors, some of whom had already been involved in the reform of the welfare system before 1795, had a major influence on the process.

The organization of the General Hospital differed considerably from that of the old charitable institutions. The main administrative body responsible for the management of the Hospital, the Lithuanian Hospital Commission, was accountable to the local civil authorities. Moreover, the Commission was composed not only of representatives of the local Catholic clergy, who traditionally dominated this field, but also of laymen, who had previously been largely absent from decision-making in the field of healthcare and poor relief. The General Hospital was under the supervision of a medical professional who led a permanent team of physicians and male and female caregivers. Although the General Hospital was initially run by lay people, it was eventually handed over to the much more experienced Sisters of Charity due to constant problems with the administration. This proves once again how important local experiences and institutions were for the maintenance of the General Hospital.

---

113 Praspaliauskienė, *Nereikalingi ir pavojingi*, 23–24.

114 Protocols (1803), fol. 72.

Although the General Hospital had inherited the properties (donations, bequests, houses, etc.) of the closed charitable institutions, the first years of its activity were characterized by the Commission's constant efforts to find additional sources of income. Analysis of the protocols revealed that, in addition to income from the usual sources, the General Hospital was also supported by regular voluntary donations and income from ticket sales, the lottery and the monopolized sale of cards. These new sources not only provided an income, albeit limited, but also enabled wider circles of society to participate in charitable activities and support the General Hospital in more diverse – and essentially secularized – ways than just through traditional bequests, donations or spontaneous alms, closely associated with the Christian doctrine of neighborly love.

The General Hospital functioned as both a hospital and an almshouse. As a medical institution, it primarily continued the work of St. Roch's Hospital and systematically admitted patients suffering from venereal diseases and provided care for lying-in women. However, the new institution significantly changed the status of the poor who had previously been housed in the city's numerous almshouses. Firstly, they were physically separated from the rest of society. Moreover, life in the General Hospital led to a decline in their role in the social and religious life of the city, severing their ties to certain churches, local clergy, neighborhoods and communities. Finally, those who had been perceived as victims for centuries were gradually recognized as the embodiment of a threat to social order.

CHAPTER 9

Interlocking Interests: State Building and the Administration of St. Lazarus Hospital in Kraków, 1780–1939

Piotr Franaszek and Zdeněk Nebřenský

The St. Lazarus Hospital in Kraków developed into one of the foremost medical institutions in Galicia and attained the status of a so-called provincial hospital. Its historical trajectory was closely interwoven with the political landscape of the city. The hospital's origins date back to the adjustments made to urban welfare during the Enlightenment and are linked to the gradual abolition of convent hospitals, which had been Kraków's pre-eminent caregiving facilities since the Middle Ages. Following the Enlightenment policies, the primate of the Kraków diocese dissolved the religious orders, but the convent hospitals were continued and remained under church administration. After several years of desolate existence, some of the hospital wards merged with academic clinics and the joint institution moved to new premises. St. Lazarus Hospital was founded by the Kraków archbishop and run by the Sisters of Mercy, but medical treatment was provided by professors of medicine from the Kraków Academy. These interlocking relationships increasingly began to diverge, and committed people pushed their respective interests.

As in many other Central European cities, the church authorities in Kraków continued to exert a strong influence on the running of health facilities even after the great wave of expropriation of ecclesiastical property had subsided. The religious orders were eventually dissolved and their assets confiscated, although their members were encouraged to continue their service in the hospitals on an individual basis.[1] The unsold property was later returned and some of the losses were partially compensated, but the hospitals were placed under the municipal control, what made already convoluted administration even more complicated.[2] In Catholic regions, the church representatives also exercised supervision over the universities. During the French Revolution, these ties were loosened, and the supervisors could be liberal-minded clerics. After Napoleon's defeat, they were replaced by supporters of the counter-revolution.

1 Rosen, Hospitals, Medical Care and Social Policy, 142.
2 Mitchell, Politics in the Service of Knowledge, 205.

 | HTTPS://DOI.ORG/10.1163/9789004755062-011

In the academic clinics, the interests of the overseers of the university and the church administration of the hospitals overlapped.[3]

The involvement of church representatives in hospital administration was based on post-Tridentine religious orthodoxy, which emphasized the Catholic mission in the poor relief and education for work.[4] Hospitals were, as their name suggests, renewed as an institution of Christian charity, dedicated to providing shelter, spiritual comfort and treatment for the sick poor. Many were kept beyond convalescence by the religious nurses, who employed them to wash and clean in the infirmaries themselves in return for room and board.[5] The location, design and operation of the hospitals, which had previously been converted from ecclesiastical structures, were not left to expediency, for everything contributed to the healing of the patients – citizens on whose labor the strength and wealth of the nation depended.[6] The humanitarian reform the health institutions in which the sick were incarcerated came from enlightened scholars and civic-minded philanthropists, while men of power insisted on the observance of discipline.[7]

It has already been explained that in Würzburg the city rulers – the Catholic bishops themselves – repeatedly wanted to confiscate the hospital revenues, which were used to pay for institutional provision. The administrative structures in the Hungarian lands were not yet linked to institutionalized treatment, and the healthcare facilities in cities such as Buda and Pest were still largely dependent on the charitable activities of the Church and religious orders. In Zagreb, representatives of the higher church hierarchy supported the establishment of a modern hospital, although the provincial officials had previously taken over some religious foundations. In Prague and Brno, convent hospitals still played an irreplaceable role in the treatment of long-term patients until the second third of the nineteenth century. The presence of religious orders in hospitals was a continuation of tradition in a time of increasing secularization. It was viewed as a competitive response to the rising popularity of hospitals, aiming to retain the faithful through charitable work.[8]

It is obvious that the involvement of church representatives in the administration of hospitals was quite common in Central and Eastern Europe. Sometimes it was a double surveillance. Within the Tanzimat reforms, Ottomans

3 Ackerknecht, *Medicine at the Paris Hospital*, 39–40.
4 Jones, Sonenscher, The Social Functions of the Hospital, 176.
5 Greenbaum, "Measure of Civilization", 51–55.
6 Greenbaum, Thomas Jefferson, the Paris Hospitals, and the University of Virginia, 610.
7 Gillispie, *Science and Polity*, 244–245.
8 Golden, Long, *The American General Hospital*, 25–27.

decided not to remove non-Muslims' hospitals from the jurisdiction of their religious authorities. In Istanbul, both the Catholic and Protestant churches offered medical treatment as part of their missionary activities. The Armenian Catholics, for example had maintained two hospitals in Istanbul since the eighteenth century. As both were in poor condition, new hospitals were built in 1832 and 1834 thanks to imperial support.[9] The situation in Kraków was somewhat more complicated, as the university was the center of the Enlightenment education and Polish scholarship was flourishing. Some of the priesthood embraced progressive ideas and were politically inclined towards liberalism. University representatives, supported by the Galician clergy and aristocracy, opposed imperial control of educational and religious foundations. Their intention was to maintain the sovereignty of education and strengthen the position of the university.[10]

Like the rural Franks, the Moravians, the Slavonians and not least the Galicians still preferred folk medicine and natural healers, to which the church and secular authorities who set up modern healthcare facilities had to adapt. The pre-modern convent hospitals that existed in the Galician (and of course also in Bohemian, Lithuanian and Hungarian) cities and parishes were not very popular, as they were a source of contagion, they had a very charitable mission, and the long-term sick filled them to the ceiling. When people had enough money to see a doctor, they preferred to be treated at home. If there was a medical academy in the city and the doctors were not employed in the hospitals, they could simply turn to private practice. Somewhat more successful were the doctors' surgeries where patients could be treated and sent home to recover. Home health care for paying patients evolved to heal the sick in an accessible, safe place. It responded to the community's urgent need for personal services that families could not provide.[11]

Female religious orders directed their work in hospitals because they believed that institutional care of the sick was less costly than home treatment, that provided a haven for patients, and that it was less stressful and more efficient for nurses. Aside from the mere existence of the new health facilities, the very innovative and interesting aspect of their development was the idea of nursing education. The search for an economically feasible and acceptable way for middle-class people to receive treatment preoccupied academic physicians

9 Ueno, *Managing Religious Diversity*, 54–55, 73.

10 Vushko, *The Politics of Cultural Retreat*, 43–45.

11 Imhof, The Hospital in the 18th Century, 453. Golden, Long, *The American General Hospital*, 25–27. Surman, *Universities*, 127.

at this time.[12] In urban areas, women could receive obstetric and gynecological treatment at home from midwives (graduates of midwifery courses).[13] However, some midwives were perceived as subservient agents of the state. There is evidence that urban women were reluctant to use their services in the case of extramarital or illegitimate pregnancies because they feared that they might be recorded.[14]

In the United States and Europe, including Galicia and Bukovina, nursing and midwifery education were founded relatively early. Charitable organizations and women's clubs in the cities were aware of the importance of this education and emulated the training in religious orders. It was often regimented and thoroughly disciplined. The heads of nursing education assumed parental authority over the nursing students. Most of them were women from the countryside. Bedtimes, meals, days off, lessons and patient care duties were specified in detail. The student nurses took over the daily care in the hospitals and learned a skill that enabled them to make them self-supporting. The nurses were recruited with apparent ease. It seemed better than working in agriculture, the life in city was also tempting.[15]

Using the example of St. Lazarus Hospital in Kraków, the chapter examines how the disputes over the administration of the hospital and the management of scarce financial resources drove the development of modern medicine promoted by academic physicians. The chapter attempts to place the case of St. Lazarus Hospital in the comparative history of modern hospitals. After an introduction to the history of St. Lazarus Hospital from its foundation in 1788 to the Kraków Uprising of 1846, the chapter traces the influence of administrative and legal changes in Galicia on the construction of medical facilities in Kraków from the mid-nineteenth century to the outbreak of the Second World War. Finally, the chapter reflects on the significance of the political framework of the Habsburg Monarchy, the post imperial transition and renewal of Polish statehood for the institutionalization of healthcare in a provincial capital.

1 Enlightenment Hospitals in Kraków

In January 1780, by decision of the Commission for National Education (Komisja Edukacji Narodowej, KEN), the first Polish Ministry of Education, the

12 Golden, Long, *The American General Hospital*, 27–28.
13 Hilber, Obstetric Expertise in the Austrian Periphery, 663–688.
14 Rose, Implications of the Spanish Influenza Pandemic, 659–660.
15 Golden, Long, *The American General Hospital*, 29–30.

Hospital of St. Barbara was founded in Kraków. The hospital became the first clinical hospital where medical students from the Kraków Academy (later Jagiellonian University) received practical training. This small health facility was built in the former Jesuit building and had only 16 beds, an anatomy lecture hall and a pharmacy. The limited space did not allow for further development, so the Kraków Academy and Primate Michał Poniatowski, the administrator of the Kraków diocese, took steps to acquire larger premises for clinical teaching. In August 1787, the Primate bought the building with the church for 20,000 gulden from the Barefoot Carmelites, who were plagued by severe financial difficulties. The premises were located at Kopernika Street in the Wesoła district of Kraków.[16]

This purchase laid the foundation stone for the establishment of the St. Lazarus municipal hospital. The act of incorporation signed on April 9, 1788, did not create a new institution, but merely transferred St. Barbara Hospital, together with the maternity ward and the facility for abandoned children from Holy Spirit Hospital to the new St. Lazarus Hospital. As a result of these measures, St. Barbara Hospital ceased to exist after only eight years of operation. The St. Lazarus Hospital was built in place of the Carmelite monastery in Kopernika Street. The new institution was modern for its time and served as a clinical hospital for the Academy. It included residential buildings for the physicians and medical students. The estate and a mill on the Prądnik River were donated for their upkeep. By resolution of the Provincial Diet, the hospital foundation was extended to include three other villages.[17]

According to the provisions of the founding deed, the hospital became a church institution and could not be part of the Kraków Academy, which was a secular institution. Therefore, the Academy was completely removed from the founding act. It did not acquire ownership rights to the assets of the new hospital, nor did it have any influence on its administration. The formal basis for its presence in the hospital was not specified. The control and staff turnover of the hospital were entrusted to the Congregation of the Sisters of Mercy. Some formulations in the founding deed even suggested the Congregation as the sole owner of the hospital. Obviously, according to the Sisters' statements, the Academy clinic was at best a guest in the hospital.[18]

This created a very precarious situation for the future, as the Academy had no legal claim against the building. It was the professors of the Academy who

---

16 Wachholz, *Szpitale krakowskie*, part II, 20–21.

17 Franaszek, *Zdrowie publiczne*, 64.

18 Franaszek, "O początkach szpitalnictwa krakowskiego," 24–25.

understandably took the lead in the hospital's medical service.[19] The hospital's funds were administered by a prosecutor specially appointed by the university. Medical care for patients was provided by doctors and nuns, who were entrusted with all economic matters. This division of roles was not precisely defined and quickly triggered a debate about the scope of responsibilities. The long-standing tensions could not be contained, and an open conflict between the church authorities and the Academy ensued.[20]

The professors recognized the impending danger and undertook a strategic initiative within the Commission for National Education to achieve the formal transfer of the hospital's management into the hands of the Academy. Unfortunately, in 1791, the Police Commission in Warsaw appointed Father Jerzy Mieroszewski, a representative of the ecclesiastical authority, as administrator of the hospital. In protest to this decision, the Academy engaged the politically active professors Franciszek Kostecki and Jan Śniadecki to stand up for its rights. They wrote a memorandum addressed to both the Police Commission and the Commission for National Education, in which they asked for the Academy's governance by the institution. At the same time, the Sisters of Mercy congregation launched a counterargument refuting the Academy's unfounded claims. After lengthy negotiations and disputes with the church authorities, especially the Sisters of Mercy, the Kraków Academy's supremacy over the hospital was restored. Nevertheless, the police commissioners did not give to the Academy's demands for the removal of Mieroszewski as administrator and the transfer of the Sisters to another facility.[21]

This period marked a turbulent chapter in the annals of Polish history. Efforts to reform the public administration were met with a conservative response from a faction of the nobility, bolstered by Russian military aid. The nobility allied itself with Russia and founded the Targowica Confederation, whose decisions had an unexpectedly favorable effect on the Academy. A delegate from the confederation handed over all the hospital's documents and assets to the representatives of the Academy, which resulted in the transfer of hospital administration to the Academy and the dismissal of Mieroszewski. The Grodno Sejm of 1793, which sanctioned the Second Partition of Poland,

19 Professor Jędrzej Badurski was appointed the physician, the chief medical officer, while also leading the internal medicine clinic. The representative of the Commission of National Education in the hospital was the so-called deputy. The first to hold this position was Professor Franciszek Kostecki.

20 Franaszek, *Zdrowie publiczne,* 50–52.

21 Franaszek, "O początkach szpitalnictwa", 23–24.

approved the status of the hospital as a provincial institution (instytucja krajowa), which was integrated into the Academy.[22]

As a result, the hospital took on a secular character, which was important for its later development when Austrian troops occupied Kraków in 1796, and the Polish Kingdom was divided between Austria, Russia and Prussia. The threat of military occupation of St. Lazarus Hospital by the Austrians prompted the Sisters to suspend their dispute with the Academy. They feared that the hospital, which was recognized as a religious institution, could suffer the same fate as the convent of the Sisters of the Holy Spirit, which had been converted into a military hospital. Despite the Sisters' reluctance, the hospital and the associated academic clinics lost the financial support they had previously received from the Commission for National Education and found themselves in an extremely precarious financial situation.[23] In his report of 1801, Antoni Baldacci, a court councilor of the Galician chancellery who had been commissioned to assess the conditions in the newly acquired Polish territories for the Viennese authorities, attested to the hospital's extremely poor state. As there was a shortage of beds, patients had to be accommodated in corridors and cramped rooms due to overcrowding in the wards while others had to be turned away. The lack of medical instruments and therapeutic resources, as well as the inadequate nutrition of the patients further exacerbated the situation.[24]

Despite initial reservations, the Sisters of Mercy endeavored to reassert their influence in the hospital under the auspices of the newly established authorities. Consequently, the Austrian administration withdrew control of the hospital from the Academy and placed it back under the management of the Sisters of Mercy. The role of the clinical professors was limited to the admission and treatment of patients. The Sisters persistently tried to undermine the reputation of the academic teaching staff, focusing particularly on Professor Franciszek Kostecki. In response to the Sisters' petition, Kostecki received a reprimand from the Kraków Governor's office in July 1802 for "negligent performance of duties" and a veiled threat of resignation. Kostecki then resigned from his post as the "hospital physician."[25]

In accordance with the policy of the Viennese court, which at this time filled important provincial offices in Galicia with loyal bureaucracy, the supervision of the hospital and its medical department was transferred to the provincial chief physician of Austrian descent, who considerably extended the authority

22 Franaszek, "O początkach szpitalnictwa", 24.
23 Wachholz, *Szpitale krakowskie* part II, 36–42.
24 Gryglewski, "Trudne początki," 163–164.
25 Gryglewski, "Trudne początki", 164.

of the Sisters of Mercy in the administration of the hospital.[26] The religious assembly even gained exclusive privileges in the admission of patients. In view of these circumstances, the members of the academic faculty began to look for alternative accommodation for their clinic. Unfortunately, it was not possible to acquire a new building for financial reasons, so that the professors were forced to endure a longer stay in the barren confines of St. Lazarus Hospital. In view of the unpleasant conditions, some of them decided to give up their academic positions.[27]

In the transitional period between 1804 and 1805, the hospital comprised the monastery building and the ecclesiastical structure. Internally, three clinics were in operation: the medical department for internal diseases, which accommodated six men and six women; the surgical department for twelve patients and the maternity department coupled with a foundling ward. St. Lazarus Hospital joined the ranks of health facilities in Prague, Brno, Pest and other European principal cities where wards devoted to the care of abandoned children existed for several decades. This was much earlier than in London, where the establishment of a genuine foundlings' hospital was hampered by hostility towards illegitimate offsprings. There were also differences with the English Poor Law, which only placed responsibility for the care of abandoned babies to the parishes where they were found.[28]

During Napoleonic Wars and the incorporation of Kraków into the Duchy of Warsaw in 1809, Prince Józef Poniatowski set up a new administration and promulgated a decree regulating the operation of the Kraków Academy. The decree retained the basic organizational framework that had previously been introduced by the Austrian authorities. At the same time, German and Austrian faculty members were ousted from the medical chairs and replaced by Polish colleagues. Professor Kostecki regained control of the medical clinic. The Sisters of Mercy attempted to capitalize on the uncertain political environment by seeking comprehensive control over the hospital while separating it from its clinical departments. Ultimately, the central authorities of the Duchy of Warsaw took over the management of the hospital, but the Sisters of Mercy persisted oversight of its daily functions.[29]

Upon the establishment of the Free City of Kraków at the Congress of Vienna in 1815, a Commission was convened to reorganize the Academy and regulate relations between the Academy and St. Lazarus Hospital. The Commission

26 Vushko, *The Politics of Cultural Retreat*, 46–82.
27 Wachholz, *Szpitale krakowskie*, part II, 24–26.
28 Outhwaite, Objects of Charity, 497–510.
29 Franaszek, *Zdrowie publiczne*, 65.

confirmed the Sisters of Mercy's ownership rights to St. Lazarus Hospital, and its foundations. Moreover, it proposed the relocation of the clinical facilities from the hospital. The academic clinics could move to the premises of the dissolved monastery buildings or, alternatively, acquiring another property. In 1818, the Commission gave the hospital a new charter that entrusted the supervision of the hospital to an "Economic Council", which was charged with planning and supervising the hospital's activities. In practice, however, the management of the hospital remained firmly in the hands of the Superior of the Sisters of Mercy.[30]

Western hospitals run by religious orders were not always able to offer medical services. Instead, they emphasized the safety and respectability of the faithful to whom a small number of nurses provided care, accommodation and food. The organizational plans were simple and the work in hospitals undifferentiated. Nuns looked after the patients, did the laundry, cleaned, prepared food and medicines and helped with operations.[31] Under the administration of the Sisters of Mercy, the development of academic clinics in Kraków was restricted and conflicts between the academic faculty and the nuns escalated. Concurrently, local and sanitary conditions deteriorated rapidly. The sisters who ran the hospital faced numerous obstacles: the building needed renovation, the financial resources available to them were severely limited and the mortality rate of patients rose sharply. According to the urban denizens, the hospital was turning into a "refuge for the incurable and a burial ground for its sick inhabitants." Considering this catastrophic situation, Professor Maciej Brodowicz, head of the medical clinics, tried to separate himself from the hospital, especially in the backdrop of a typhoid epidemic that was spreading within the hospital premises.

In Western hospitals, the founders employed a variety of strategies to solve the problem of care. They often relied on nuns and their assistants to care for the sick. The autonomy of the nuns contrasted with the control that hospital administrators exercised over lay women. The fact that the nuns retained control over internal management, including the admission of patients, collecting money and membership of the medical staff, limited the efforts of the doctors.[32] Comparatively, the Kraków City Commission set up in 1818 proved ineffective in defusing the escalating tensions between the Sisters of Mercy, who administered the St. Lazarus Hospital, and the Jagiellonian University (before 1817, the Kraków Academy). As the conflict intensified, the university professors

30 Wachholz, *Szpitale krakowskie*, part I, 6–10, 54–86, 100–105, 108–110.

31 Golden, Long, *The American General Hospital*, 27–28.

32 Golden, Long, *The American General Hospital*, 29.

decided in November 1827 to move university clinics out of the hospital. They found new accommodation in a building at Kopernika Street 7, which had previously housed one of the city's masonic lodges. However, the facilities were so cramped that the surgical and maternity clinics together had only ten beds.[33]

Although the St. Lazarus Hospital and the clinics administered by the Faculty of Medicine of the Jagiellonian University officially parted, their premises were adjacent, and some wards were shared or transferred between the university clinics and St. Lazarus Hospital. Such proximity offered the opportunity to expand the area of clinical observation and to supplement the existing teaching material. As it soon became apparent that the adapted buildings of the former masonic lodge were insufficient and had to be expanded, three new buildings were acquired in a spacious English-style garden. The largest of these, which was centrally located, served as a medical facility, housing rooms for diagnostics and therapy, rooms for lectures and surgical courses. A smaller pavilion near the entrance was used as the residence of the complex's administrator, while the building within the garden was converted into a dissecting room and mortuary.[34]

Meanwhile, the Sisters of Mercy administration at St. Lazarus Hospital was struggling with serious problems related to overcrowding, exacerbated by deteriorating sanitary conditions and rising mortality rates.[35] Despite the Sisters' opposition, the obstetrics ward moved from university clinics to St. Lazarus Hospital, as the cries of the babies were considered disturbing to other patients.[36] In response to these challenges, the Senate of the Free City of Kraków undertook the planning for the construction of a new hospital. The existing building would be converted into the hospital's administrative headquarters, a maternity ward and a home for abandoned children. After lengthy negotiations and the presentation of highly interesting proposals, including one by the Italian architect Francesco Maria Lanci, the City Council withdrew from the entire undertaking, citing insufficient financial resources as the main obstacle. In November 1836, the Council decided not to erect a completely new building, but to add a story to the existing hospital. This change was intended to extend the hospital by 120 beds.[37]

This arrangement made it possible to combine theoretical knowledge and practical experience in medical training under one roof. At the same time,

33 Franaszek, "O początkach szpitalnictwa," 26.
34 Bęczkowska, "Gmach kliniczny przy ul. Kopernika 7," 46–47.
35 The average annual mortality rate rose from 33% to 61% in 1831.
36 Bęczkowska, "Gmach kliniczny przy ul. Kopernika 7," 48–49.
37 Bęczkowska, "Gmach kliniczny przy ul. Kopernika 7", 52–54.

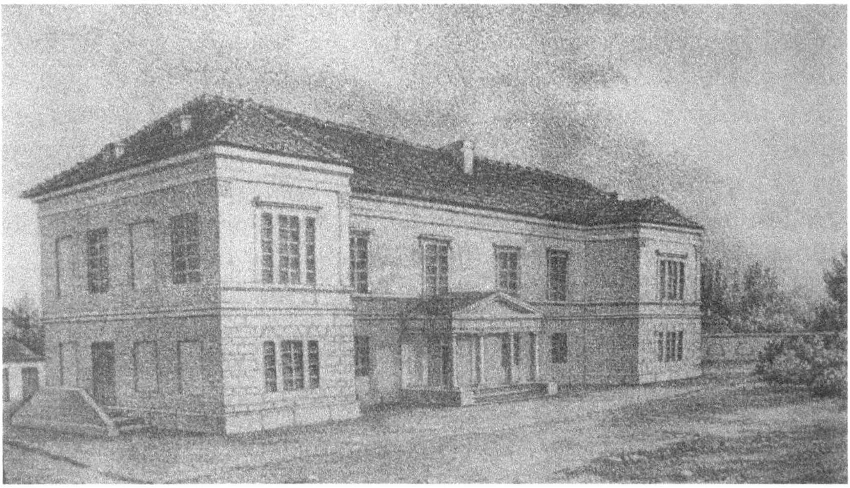

FIGURE 9.1 Clinical facility of the Jagiellonian University. In *Rys Historyczny Zakładów Klinicznych przy Uniwersytecie Jagiellońskim przez Profes. Dra Józefa Brodowicza. Dyrektora Kliniki lekarskiej*. Kraków w drukarni Uniwersyteckiéj 1845

construction work on the extension of the medical clinics continued and was finally completed in September 1843. As a result, the clinic building, which originally had a rectangular shape, was slightly raised and enlarged with two additional wings at right angles. This expansion provided the surgical clinic with new scientific and teaching facilities and increased capacity from eight to fifteen beds. It also doubled the size of the medical department, which could now accommodate twenty-four patients. Like the Bohemian, Moravian, Galician and Hungarian hospitals that had adopted the Viennese model, the patients' rooms were modest and equipped with the bare necessities. Next to the iron bed stood a stool and a cupboard with a bell, as well as a card on which the patient's name, state of health, prescribed medication and dietary instructions were noted.[38]

2 St. Lazarus Hospital on the Way to Autonomy

In February 1846, the uprising of the Polish nationalist nobility and university professors against Habsburg rule broke out in Kraków. The uprising was

38 Bęczkowska, "Gmach kliniczny przy ul. Kopernika 7," 50–51.

quickly suppressed, the Austrian forces annexed the city and its surroundings, which were incorporated into Galicia. Months of repression, trials and punishment followed. Death sentences were the order of the day.[39] The central administration achieved and extended imperial authority in many towns and villages. The Habsburg bureaucracy sought to manage state-funded progress and improve public health. Provincial institutions became increasingly dependent on officials nominated by the Ministry of the Interior and appointed by the emperor. Their budgets were expected to fulfil the state's goals.[40]

Notable examples were the ministerial decrees of March 6, 1855, which ensured the financial aspects of hospital treatment in the Galician provincial fund, and the decree of April 10, 1857, which laid down the payment principles for hospital care.[41] In the 1850s, the imperial governance renewed the tensions between the paternalism of the central state and the autonomy of the provinces, whether it was Bohemia, Moravia or Galicia. Provincial and municipal administration was strictly rationalized, universities with medical departments and clinics were exposed to state influence.[42] The Viennese government initiated a comprehensive review of the Galician bureaucracy, and the new governor ordered the appointment of a commission to investigate the functioning of the various branches of the administration.[43] The Council of St. Lazarus Hospital, in which professors and doctors were represented and which was involved in the administration of the hospitals together with representatives of the City Council, the Catholic Church and esteemed citizens, was dissolved. St. Lazarus Hospital was placed under the direct control of the Viennese government, particularly the Ministry of the Interior. The Ministry had originally planned to resume Maria Lanci's project and rebuild hospital premises. Yet, the provincial governor, representing an extension of state authority to the regional context, took on responsibility for construction plans in Kraków.[44]

The provincial governor was responsible for all state affairs, including the monitoring of sanitary conditions and the oversight of public and private healthcare facilities. He also implemented ministerial directives and orders regulating the erection of clinics, hospitals and dispensaries. He gradually took

39 Osterkamp, Imperial diversity, 732–733. Vushko, *The Politics of Cultural Retreat*, 219–222.

40 Magocsi, *The Roots of Ukrainian Nationalism*, 74–75. Deak, *Forging a multinational state*, 99–106, 113–116. Judson, *The Habsburg Empire*, 225–226. Surman, *Universities*, 67–71.

41 Kasparek, *Zbiór ustaw administracyjnych*, 1202–1207.

42 Deak, *Forging a multinational state*, 107–112, 130–134. Surman, *Universities*, 52–53. Osterkamp, Imperial Loyalties, 864–865.

43 Vushko, *The Politics of Cultural Retreat*, 224–229. Polonsky, The Revolutionary Crisis, 443–469. Wollf, *The Idea of Galicia*, 194.

44 Franaszek, "Publiczna ochrona zdrowia w Galicji," 133–134.

control of St. Lazarus Hospital and placed it under a unified administration. Under the direct supervision of the provincial and city authorities, St. Lazarus Hospital underwent a comprehensive restructuring that led to the demarcation of three different departments. Initially, the medical department took care of all patients, apart from those with psychiatric disorders and chronic skin diseases. The second department specialized in surgery. The third department focused on obstetrics. Increasing the number of hospital beds, improving hygiene and reducing the average mortality rate to 10% were remarkable successes that completed the advance in medical treatment. Professor Józef Teofil Kwaśniewski, who headed a maternity ward, was the first in Kraków to use chloroform for anesthesia during childbirth.[45]

Austria's defeat in the war with Piedmont and France in 1859 revealed the weakness of the "bureaucratic form" of the Bach's government, which did not consider the subjects of the multinational state.[46] The ruling circles in Vienna began reform efforts to prevent the collapse of the monarchy. The imperial administration was balanced by representative provincial and municipal bodies that derived their power from limited elections. Sanctioned statutes for the provinces secured them the right to decide on matters concerning their monies, welfare and health without interference from the central state. From this point onwards, intensive measures were taken to achieve autonomy. A large part of the regulatory framework in Galicia itself emanated from the Provincial Diet (Sejm Krajowy), the highest legislative body based in Lviv.[47] The contours of public policy were expressed in legislative acts such as the Provincial Statute of the Kingdom of Galicia and Lodomeria (Statut Krajowy) of 1861, Laws on County Representation and on the Organization of Municipalities of 1866. These legal frameworks served as the cornerstone for hospital administration in general and St. Lazarus Hospital in particular. They underlined the paramount importance attached to provincial healthcare. They influenced the complex interplay between central and provincial regulatory initiatives and shaped the dynamic landscape of medical institutions.[48]

The number of public hospitals in Galicia rose from 25 to 39 during the period of autonomy, and the total number of beds in all public hospitals increased systematically.[49] Between 1873 and 1909, it reached an average of

---

45 Franaszek, "O początkach szpitalnictwa," 25–26. Gryglewski, "Trudne początki," 166–167.

46 Deak, *Forging a multinational state*, 132.

47 Magocsi, *The Roots of Ukrainian Nationalism*, 73–74. Deak, *Forging a Multinational State*, 146–151, 155–156. Judson, *The Habsburg Empire*, 251–252. Unowsky, The Plunder, 28–29.

48 Osterkamp, Cooperative Empires, 134–135. Surman, *Universities*, 115. Bęczkowska, "Rozbudowa szpitala powszechnego," 76–79.

49 Franaszek, "Szpitale galicyjskie," 129–130.

3,381 beds. The lowest cumulative number of hospital beds was recorded in 1884 (2,511) and the highest number in 1909 (4,875). The increase in these indicators was largely due to the establishment of new hospitals. The so-called provincial hospitals occupied a special position, as they had the largest number of beds and clearly outnumbered all other hospitals. Together with the general hospital in Lviv, St. Lazarus Hospital had the largest bed capacity.[50] In 1875, the hospital had around 360 beds and cared for a total of 3,372 patients who underwent treatment over a period of 89,350 days. Two decades later, the capacity had grown to 766 beds, which corresponded to 9,920 hospitalized persons, and 266,132 days of treatment. In 1916, the hospital reached 943 beds and 324,683 days of medical care.[51]

The supervision of the hospitals became the responsibility of provincial authorities, especially the Provincial Health Council (Krajowa Rada Zdrowia), which acted primarily as an advisory body to the governate on healthcare matters and assessed the health state of the Galician population. The Council was chaired by the provincial health commissioner, assisted by six members officially appointed by the Ministry of the Interior and two others delegated by the Provincial Committee. The term of the Council members lasted three years. The implementation of the official instructions was supervised by the provincial hospital inspector. The management and administration of the general hospitals was subject to sanitary and police supervision.[52]

While some hospitals were explicitly founded as public healthcare facilities, others, which initially functioned as district or municipal hospitals, were later granted the status of general hospitals through special legislation enacted by the Provincial Diet. To qualify for this status, hospitals had to meet several conditions, which were standardized throughout the monarchy by ministerial regulations, including guidelines on the admission criteria for terminally ill patients. The financial resources of the hospital included the hospital's own funds, reimbursements for treatment costs, subsidies from the provincial fund and other sources. By the 1870s, St. Lazarus Hospital was unable to meet all ministerial requirements and Galician representatives had to negotiate repeatedly with the imperial authorities, because a new obstetrics department and a midwifery school were urgently needed.[53]

The authorities attempted to transfer St. Lazarus Hospital to the administration of the Kraków municipality to obtain the financial means for further

50 Franaszek, "Krajowy szpital powszechny," 133–134.

51 In 1885, the number of hospitalized individuals rose to 6,816, amassing 165,302 days of hospitalization. See Wachholz, *Szpitale krakowskie*, part II, 60–61.

52 Franaszek, "Wybrane problemy publicznej ochrony zdrowia," 159–168.

53 Franaszek, *Zdrowie publiczne*, 63–64.

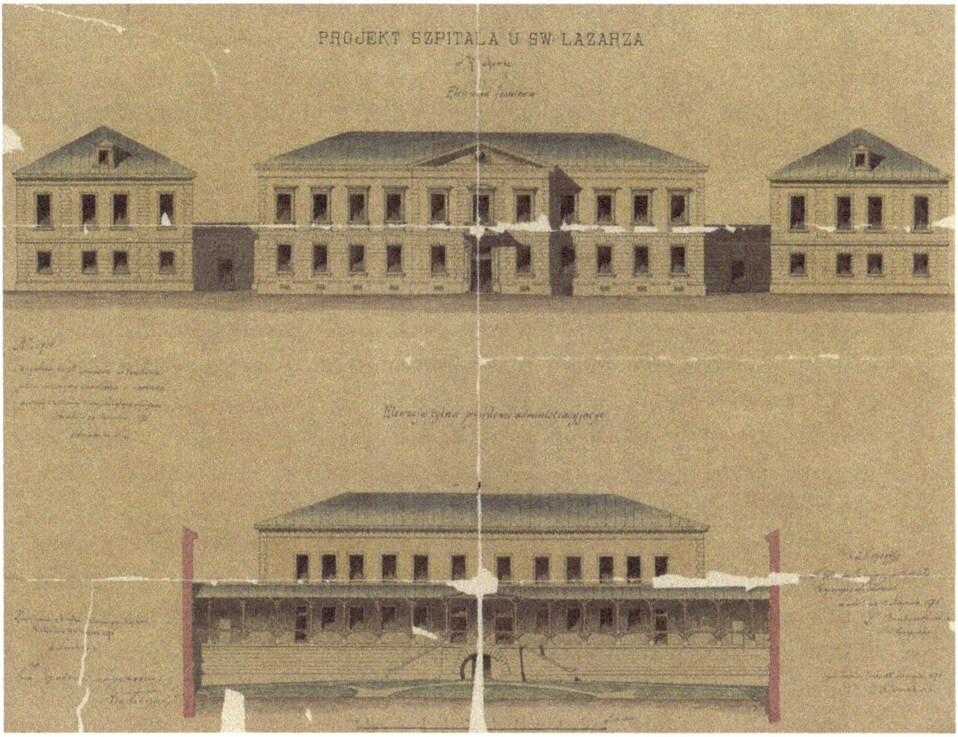

FIGURE 9.2 Project for the pavilions of the Department for Internal Diseases, around 1875. In Elżbieta Waszczyszyn. The 19th century Medical Clinic of Collegium Medicum of the Jagiellonian University in Kraków. An outline of conservation problems in the light of requirements of a modern university hospital. *Wiadomości Konserwatorskie/Conservation News* 27/210, 51–66

expansion. However, the negotiations proved unsuccessful. As a result, the Provincial Diet decided to take control of St. Lazarus Hospital and recognize it as a single institution, despite its various locations within Kraków to streamline its management.[54] This allowed St. Lazarus Hospital to renovate the old premises and add a planned second floor for surgery. The renewed Health Council has also decided to construct new hospital wings. The central building was designated for hospital administration, while two flanking pavilions housed internal medicine, one for women and one for men. The psychiatric ward was located at the back of the site, overlooking the garden, offering peace and quiet to patients.[55] Construction was completed in 1878, and the new facilities were inaugurated on January 1, 1879. The cost of the project exceeded the original

54 Kopytko, *Służba zdrowia w Galicji doby autonomicznej*, 3.
55 Bęczkowska, "Rozbudowa szpitala powszechnego," 76–79.

estimate due to the need to extend the building plot and create ancillary facilities. Economic and sanitary facilities were improved. The department of internal medicine has comprised 90 beds in ten rooms. The psychiatric institute accommodated patients transferred from other hospitals. The departments of obstetrics-gynecology and venereal diseases occupied the entire area on the lower floors. The surgical ward was refurbished.[56]

At the time, in hospitals in Western Europe, surgery developed into a first-class method of treating diseases. Surgery and hospitals became inextricably linked. Surgeons operated in a new suite equipped with an amphitheater in which tiles, metal and glass replaced wood as the material for floors, beds, tables and instrument stands. Teams of doctors and nurses assisted the surgeons and administered the medical instruments. Medical students gathered in the operating theaters to observe the procedures at close range under bright gas and electric lighting. Antisepsis and anesthesia became standard. Most surgical patients were given either chloroform or cocaine.[57]

In 1889, on the initiative of university professors, a surgical clinic in Kraków was established at Kopernika Street 40, colloquially known as the "White Surgery." On the first floor of the main building, two separate wards were set up for female and male patients, each with between twelve and fourteen beds. The surgical operating rooms were housed in the wing of the building at the end of which was the amphitheater lecture hall.[58] The expansion continued with the removal of the older caregiving facilities. The City Council decided to demolish the buildings of St. Spirit Hospital, and the same fate befell the former St. Spirit church. The buildings, which had previously housed healthcare facilities, became municipal property. This allowed the Provincial Committee to decide on the construction of a new building for the surgical clinic. The new surgical pavilion with 120 beds was opened in the fall of 1893. Due to its brick construction, the building was colloquially known as the "Red Surgery."[59]

3 St. Lazarus Hospital at the Height of Modern Nation Building

In the late nineteenth century, the administration of public hospitals in Western Europe petitioned city councils to build health facilities and expand

56 Wachholz, *Szpitale krakowskie*, 102, 111–112.
57 Badertscher, A New Wishard Is On the Way, 352–353.
58 Bęczkowska, "Budowa nowych gmachów dla kliniki," 106–108.
59 Franaszek, *Zdrowie publiczne*, 66.

hospital premises. Sometimes however local administration was unable to provide sufficient capital. The challenge of closing the gap between tax appropriations and necessary funding would eventually require the cooperation of local philanthropists. Some of them bequeathed many of their assets to the cities for the expansion of hospitals. They specifically earmarked their donation for the construction of "modern" wards for patients who were unable to pay for their treatment. This represented a significant improvement in the old facilities, even though not all the necessary departments were set up. In the Habsburg Monarchy, the central government struggled with nationalist centrifugal claims.[60] In order to at least somewhat mitigate their severity, the government made additional funds available to the provinces for the renewal of infrastructure, including health facilities. At St. Lazarus Hospital, the provincial treasury and the hospital's internal funds, shared the financial responsibility for building new units, adapting the premises, managing the hospital and ongoing maintenance, with part of the charges also being levied on patients. A not insignificant amount of help came in the form of philanthropic contributions from nationally conscious Kraków citizens.[61]

At this time, nursing and midwifery education was gradually integrated into hospital departments. Young women attended specialized courses, completed their training and were then usually employed as nurses and midwives in hospitals. They were qualified to take on tasks that went far beyond cleaning the wards, bathing patients and changing dresses. They administered medication when doctors were unable to do so due to time and work constraints. While many people felt that upstanding lay women should avoid working in hospitals, in the decades that followed, nursing evolved into a legitimate profession for women to pursue.[62] Nursing education brought prestige to the city. Trained nurses and midwives working for health of the nation became a matter of national pride. Under the protective wing of a constitutional monarchy that protected "the health of the nation" and supported the flourishing of "national medicine", the vacated premises of St. Lazarus Hospital were subsequently rededicated and made available for the Department of Dermatology and Venereology, while at the same time the Department of Obstetrics and Gynecology was expanded and developed into a training center for midwives.[63]

---

60 Magocsi, *The Roots of Ukrainian Nationalism*, 74.

61 Bęczkowska, "Budowa nowych gmachów dla kliniki," 109–110.

62 Badertscher, A New Wishard Is On the Way, 353–354. Seidman, Legitimizing the Revolution, 357.

63 Franaszek, *Zdrowie publiczne*, 67.

The scientific revolution brought the concepts of localized diagnosis, germ theory, antisepsis, and anesthesia, which contributed to the professionalization of medicine, even if this did not mean keeping pace with accelerated technological advances and the creation of new facilities. The acquisition of novel devices, such as X-ray diagnostic unit, resulted in higher costs that could not be covered with existing funds.[64] After the university building underwent extensive reconstruction, the surgical clinic at Kopernika Street was equipped with sterilization apparatus, an X-ray machine, and a photographic darkroom. There was electric light in the aseptic surgical operating room, while the other rooms were lit by gas lamps. The newly built department of descriptive anatomy had several specimens, including blood and lymph vessels, histological and embryological specimens and an extensive skull collection.[65]

Since isolation had long been the prevailing method of containing the spread of typhoid and smallpox epidemics, hospitals had maintained only outside pavilions for the contagious. In the dingy pest houses, patients lived crammed together on flimsy cots. In many western hospitals, plague houses could be as small as thirty by forty feet in size, with rooms for up to twenty patients.[66] The pervasive and serious problem of infectious diseases was also a major challenge for St. Lazarus Hospital. Patients suffering from contagious maladies were transferred to the Department of Internal Medicine. Reactive measures were taken, a separate pavilion was set up in the so-called English Garden and special rooms were allocated for patients with typhoid fever.[67] The seriousness of the situation reached its peak in 1892, when cholera was brought to Kraków from Hamburg. The patients housed in the department of internal medicine inadvertently contributed to the spread of the epidemic. As a result, the crucial decision was made to set up an isolated ward for infectious diseases, which was initially located in an outdated building outside the hospital. From 1894, the administration carried out rabies vaccinations at this location using Pasteur's pioneering method. However, the inauguration of a purpose-built building for the Department of Infectious Diseases on the hospital grounds did not take place until 1905.[68]

In the following years, development efforts culminated, when the municipality of Kraków donated a large plot of land to the Jagiellonian University for the construction of the neurological-psychiatric clinic. In 1912, new operating and

64 Badertscher, A New Wishard Is On the Way, 353, 358.
65 Rostafiński, *Krakow pod względem*, 7, 14–17.
66 Badertscher, A New Wishard Is on the Way, 359–360.
67 Bęczkowska, "Budowa nowych gmachów dla kliniki," 112–115.
68 Franaszek, *Zdrowie publiczne*, 66–67.

sterilization rooms were added to the building. The departments of psychiatry and venereal diseases were also gradually relocated to the newly constructed premises. The construction, which consisted of three pavilions arranged parallel to Kopernika Street, took five years. Shortly before the outbreak of the First World War, a barrack of the former "Red Surgery" was added for children who needed surgical help and were previously housed in the private St. Louis Pediatric Hospital.[69]

In this respect, they were no different from the American route, where independent children's hospitals had been opened at the time. These institutions were usually the result of a coalition between health care providers and social reformers. For some physicians, the hospitals provided an opportunity to gain greater medical authority as pediatrics emerged as a new specialty.[70] However, it cannot be overlooked that Kraków lagged considerably behind other European and Polish cities, especially Warsaw, where a children's hospital had already existed for more than a century. Kraków had a rather middle-class character, it was not nearly such an industrial center, so the arguments of the social reformers, who pointed out the unhealthy effects of urban society, did not apply to it.[71]

Although a psychiatric ward was part of the hospital from very early on, the neurological-psychiatric clinic was founded thanks to the city mayor, who arranged a grant from the Galician Diet and the municipality by exchanging a large and dry plot of land. The efforts of the Minister of Finance, Witold Korytowski, enabled the university to obtain additional funds for the construction of the clinic in the amount of several hundred thousand crowns. The construction, which consisted of three pavilions arranged parallel to Kopernika Street, lasted five years and the official opening took place at the beginning of 1914. With the outbreak of the First World War, however, it was quickly converted into a military hospital. It became a facility for the hospitalization of military personnel suffering from nervous and mental disorders, mainly caused by post-traumatic stress syndrome resulting from war experiences.[72]

After the renewal of Polish statehood, many hospitals were economically ruined by the war and embroiled in the ongoing conflicts with the Soviet Union, Czechoslovakia as well as by internal strife.[73] The institutions turned

---

69 Franaszek, "O początkach szpitalnictwa," 33.
70 Sloane, "Not Designed Merely to Heal", 332–334.
71 Szpak, Industrialization, 133–134.
72 Piltz, *Klinika neurologiczno-psychiatryczna*, 6.
73 Jochen Böhler, *Civil War in Central Europe, 1918–1921. The Reconstruction of Poland* (Oxford: Oxford University Press, 2022).

into breeding grounds for deadly epidemics spread by soldiers moving from battlefield to battlefield and by impoverished, starving civilians travelling away from the front lines in search of safety and a livelihood. In 1918 and 1919, the Polish health authorities reported more than one hundred thousand cases of typhus and stated that in Western Galicia, the Jewish population was hit particularly hard by the typhus epidemic.[74] In the middle of summer, influenza attacked the inhabitants of Kraków. As one local doctor put it, the epidemic soon took hold of "all combustible material", which meant that anyone without immunity fell ill.[75] Poland became the focus not only of emergency humanitarian aid, but also of longer-term medical and sanitary programs that were intended to stop epidemics on their own doorstep.[76] Parallel to the efforts to combat the epidemic, a public health system was established, and corresponding health and welfare laws were passed. The Ministry of Public Health, founded in December 1918, coordinated healthcare and set up the government's Extraordinary Epidemic Commission, which led nationwide campaigns to contain epidemics. Compulsory medical service was introduced, and physicians were made available to the Commission. The Commission's main focus was on establishing a "sanitary zone" to help prevent new epidemics from penetrating across the porous borders to "Bolshevik Russia."[77]

The Ministry of Public Health took also control over the St. Lazarus Hospital by decree of the Provincial Committee of the former Kingdom of Galicia and Lodomeria on July 28, 1919.[78] Despite the high expectations of the Medical Faculty of the Jagiellonian University and the management of St. Lazarus Hospital for post-war projects and the comprehensive modernization of the health facilities in Kraków, the financial constraints of the young Polish republic limited the realization of these aspirations. The construction of a clinic for obstetrics and gynecology in the neighborhood, which had been planned before the war, was considerably delayed. The laying of the cornerstone in 1921, which Józef Piłsudski attended, preceded the completion and official opening of the clinic fifteenth years later. The state's investment policy for St. Lazarus Hospital in the interwar period was characterized by slow progress. The only significant expansion during this period was the new pavilion for the urology department.

74 Golden, "Show that you are really alive", 132.
75 Mieszkowski, A Foreign Lady, 206.
76 Golden, "Show that you are really alive", 132.
77 Golden, "Show that you are really alive", 133–134.
78 Wachholz, *Szpitale krakowskie*, 64–65.

In 1925, the support of the Rockefeller Foundation made it possible to extend the building of the Kraków nursing school at Kopernika Street 25.[79]

The debate about the administrative merger of St. Lazarus Hospital and the university clinics resurfaced. The procedural aspects appeared to be relatively straightforward, as both institutions were under the control of state authorities, albeit different ministries – the Clinic was under the Ministry of Religious Affairs and Public Enlightenment, while St. Lazarus Hospital was under the Ministry of Public Health. Pointing out the numerous advantages of such a solution, there were proposals to merge the two institutions under the title "St. Lazarus University Hospital." However, it was not until October 1939 that a resolution was passed at one of the last meetings of the Faculty Council. It was decided to place the clinics under the administration of St. Lazarus Hospital, what paved the way for the practical merger of the two institutions.[80]

4 Conclusion

The development of healthcare facilities in Kraków was linked to the Enlightenment policies of the city's archbishop, the striving for the survival of religious orders and the university professors' quest for medical modernity, a dynamic that continued from the late eighteenth to the mid nineteenth century. The St. Lazarus Hospital was founded by merging with the older clinics of the Kraków Academy and the convent hospitals. It was located in the premises of the dissolved monasteries and became a church institution where academic doctors provided medical treatment. Apart from a short period before the Third Partition of Poland in 1795, when decisions about the hospitals were made by the professors of Kraków Academy, the hospital was administered by the Congregation of the Sisters of Mercy. According to the new statute of St. Lazarus Hospital in 1839, the Hospital Council consisting mainly of university professors, took over the hospital's administration. Secular influence over the hospital was restored and remained for the following decade within the Free City of Kraków – a political entity established at the Congress of Vienna. In 1846, Kraków once again became part of Galicia and St. Lazarus Hospital was incorporated into the hospital system of the Habsburg Monarchy.

A decisive turning point for St. Lazarus Hospital was the transformation of imperial authority in the second half of the nineteenth century, when health policy was the responsibility of the central government in Vienna,

79 Pisarski, *Sprawozdanie z działalności*, 45–50.

80 Michalewicz, *Inwentarz akt wydziałów i studiów Uniwersytetu Jagiellońskiego*, 138.

while administration of individual hospitals was delegated to the provincial bodies. This distinct dualism often proved conducive to dealing with complicated challenges, especially in times of epidemic threat. It also frequently led to lengthy and controversial discussions, as the Habsburg Monarchy attached paramount importance to the field of public health, which was underlined by the proactive engagement of the central authorities in developing both the legal and organizational framework for healthcare facilities. Their concerted efforts were aimed at ensuring the smooth functioning of these institutions.

After Galician autonomy was achieved in the 1860s, St. Lazarus Hospital in Kraków was placed under the jurisdiction of the provincial authorities. Self-governing institutions at various administrative levels, from the highest, such as the Galician Diet and the Provincial Governate, down to the county representations and municipalities, assumed responsibility for health issues. In the meetings of the Provincial Diet, its executive body, the Provincial Committee, and especially the Provincial Council for Healthcare, topics such as the containment of infectious diseases, the promotion of medical personnel, the financial aspects of healthcare and the organizational challenges associated with medical facilities, in particular the construction of new hospitals and the expansion of existing ones, such as St. Lazarus Hospital were discussed. Its operation was governed by state, provincial and municipal regulations, which primarily concerned the financial underpinnings and administration.

St. Lazarus Hospital could only be an institution whose sole purpose was to treat patients. The treatment fees were set by the provincial bodies. It was obliged to accept patients regardless of their place of residence, social origin, or religious affiliation. The latter criterion was of particular importance, as St. Lazarus Hospital had previously been allowed to refuse admission to the Jewish population, who generally sought medical care in facilities organized by themselves. In 1872, the Provincial Governate recognized the incompatibility of this provision with the state laws regulating the equal rights of all inhabitants of monarchy. Two years later, the Galician Diet passed a law that ensured the admission of Jews to general hospitals on the same terms as Christians.

In the comparative perspective, religious differences permanently caused conflicts among the faithful and religion remained an important factor in the smooth running of hospitals. The legalization of religious pluralism led to people of different faiths being brought together in hospitals. In theory, the hospital administration was supposed to ensure the practice of religion in specially designated premises or at least provide the services of suitable priests, but this was not always possible for economic and structural reasons.[81] No wonder that religious groups, not only the Jews in Galicia, spent scarce resources on founding and maintaining their own hospitals until the beginning of the twentieth century. In Protestant facilities, a single clergyman was sufficient for an entire hospital, as there was no requirement for large chapels, no altars in every ward and no convents with monks and nuns.[82]

Another important milestone was the passing of a law by the Galician Diet in January 1875, which provided free hospital treatment for the needy. This legal act stipulated mutual assumption of costs for treatment in public healthcare facilities, which also applied to spouses, (grand)parents and (grand)children. At the same time, employers were obliged to cover the cost of treatment for their employees, while the perpetrators of crimes, particularly robberies, were made financially responsible for the treatment of victims. Detailed provisions on payment principles were issued for prisoners, convicts and foreigners. However, the comprehensive financial responsibility for the treatment of the impoverished inhabitants of Kraków in St. Lazarus Hospital lay entirely with the (missing) provincial budget.

The adjustments in the administration of St. Lazarus Hospital resulted from the provincial law enacted in the late 1890s, which established hospital committees to oversee the province's general hospitals and detailed the conditions for obtaining general hospital status. Such status could only be granted by a law passed by the Galician Diet, and potential founders included local and municipal authorities or private individuals. Failure to comply with the prescribed sanitary and police conditions, which were controlled by the Governor, could result in the status of general hospital being revoked by parliamentary legislation. Although they were formally private hospitals, some of them, such as the St. Louis Pediatric Hospital, also received financial support from provincial funds. As it did not have trained staff, it worked closely with St. Lazarus Hospital and the university clinics, to which it gave part of its premises.

The delicate economic balance of St. Lazarus Hospital, which was tied to the public budgets, was upset by the First World War. The withdrawal of men to the front and the mass entry of women into the profession, including that of nurses, confronted the state authorities with the need to provide them with hospital care on a larger scale than before. The constant stream of wounded soldiers, who kept bringing epidemics of various diseases to the home front, turned the hospitals in Kraków into the kind of caregiving facilities they had been trying to escape from since the Enlightenment. St. Lazarus Hospital and

81 Rosenberg, And Heal the Sick, 438.

82 Greenbaum, "Measure of Civilization", 55.

the university clinics were certainly at the cutting edge of surgical and internal medicine. However, they treated not only physical pain, but also psychological obstacles, be it post-traumatic conditions due to war injuries or stress syndrome triggered by war experiences.

In the interwar period, investment in hospitals in the Wesoła district was cut back considerably. The adjustments mainly concerned the reconstruction and expansion of existing facilities. Some older buildings were converted into hospital wards and came under the management of university professors, who not only took control of their own medical departments, which they had already been running for previous years, but also redesigned the premises. The plans drawn up for the clinical infrastructure highlighted the building constraints in the urban centre and the challenges of integrating new medical technologies and equipment into the outdated facilities. This included the construction of new pavilions and teaching halls for the medical faculty on the outskirts of the city. Medical care for children and the provision of suitable space in the hospital for the establishment of a paediatric clinic became increasingly important, accompanied by demands for additional funds from the state budget. However, these projects were halted by the invasion of Nazi Germany and the atrocities of the war. They could only be implemented gradually over the following decades.

CHAPTER 10

Coping with Imperial Legacy: the Epistemic Community at the General Hospital in Prague, 1902–1939

Barbora Rambousková and Zdeněk Nebřenský

In his memoirs, Zdeněk Mařatka, a leading researcher in the field of gastroenterology and professor of internal medicine at Charles University in Prague, mentions statements by his older colleagues about the recruitment of medical staff at the Second Internal Clinic of the General Hospital in the first half of twentieth century. Doctors who studied medicine and then practiced in the Bohemian lands considered teaching and research at clinics to be the greatest professional achievement. Working in a clinic became the goal of many of them as soon as they graduated. Mařatka wrote that an academic career was only possible for those who had demonstrated the ability to conduct original clinical research. However, according to Mařatka,

> personal character traits, temperament, cultural and, of course, social background played a major role. All this was constantly reflected in daily mutual contact and was observed by the senior members of the clinic, who formed an unofficial governing body … It was fierce competition and a constant struggle for supremacy.[1]

This system was introduced by the chiefs of the hospital departments in the late Habsburg Monarchy and perfected by their successors in the Czechoslovak Republic during the interwar period. Medical experts carefully monitored the work of students and trainees during their studies and internships in the clinic or later, based on the positive reactions of patients to their treatment in everyday practice. As soon as a position became vacant at the hospital, experts consulted with their colleagues from this "unofficial committee", which was made up of associate professors, assistants and possibly also secondary doctors, and only awarded the position after jointly assessing the qualities of the candidates in question. The posts of assistants and secondary doctors were

1 Mařatka, *Paměti*, 76.

 | HTTPS://DOI.ORG/10.1163/9789004755062-012

filled for a specific period, usually two years. The candidate had the hope of an extension if he had proven himself and there were no other promising peers. According to Mařatka, this procedure guaranteed the scholarly quality and personnel development of the general hospital.[2]

However, the recruitment process and the appointment of new staff were criticized by the younger generation of reform-minded doctors as inhumane. As a result of that, the state authorities gradually replaced it with a limited number of paid positions in the general hospital. Employment opportunities for unpaid doctors – guest candidates for the vacant post – were abolished. Appointment based on a selection procedure was converted into a permanent post. Although the number of paid positions increased, the possibility of selecting the most qualified and motivated students disappeared. All posts were filled for a long time with doctors who could not be dismissed without serious reasons. In the meantime, many graduates with potential scientific skills left for vacancies outside the university hospital and were unable to pursue the field they were interested in. In this way, university medicine lost many talented individuals.[3]

As the testimonies of Mařatka and others emphasize, the Second Internal Clinic was a special institution – part of the General Hospital in Prague, but at the same time located at the Medical Faculty of Charles University, where students practiced. It was also an important center for clinical research, in which medical trainees and candidates were often involved. The Clinic was a prestigious place, and the work there became a destination for many medical graduates and future distinguished scholars. The Clinic was difficult to reach and a longer stay there was demanding. The Clinic was administered by individual professors who had very different approaches to running the hospital departments themselves and managing their staff.

From 1921, the Second Internal Clinic was headed by Josef Pelnář, the respected Professor of Internal Medicine and Neurology at the Charles University, who was regarded as a key figure in clinical teaching and research in the interwar period. After his retirement in 1939, the professors of the faculty and the Minister of Education authorized the extension of Pelnář's term of office to three additional years.[4] Together with Josef Thomayer, his predecessor at the head of the clinic since 1902, Pelnář unintentionally created what social scientists and historians today call an epistemic community, i.e. a network of

2 Mařatka, *Paměti*, 77.

3 Mařatka, *Paměti*, 77.

4 Masaryk Institute and Archive of the Czech Academy of Sciences (MUA AV ČR), Archive of Academy of Sciences (AAV), fond (f.) Josef Pelnář, box 1, Signature (Sign.) 1b, fol. 12.

professionals with a recognized field of knowledge who make an authoritative claim to policy-relevant expertise.[5]

Although the concept of epistemic communities gained prominence almost four decades ago and has been reconsidered repeatedly, its application in history is relatively modest. Following the original conceptual framework for international affairs, epistemic communities in the narrower sense referred to transnational networks of technicians, environmentalists or economists in a globalizing world.[6]

While in the case of medical professionals working on behalf of the health organizations in the global South, their claim to policy-expertise was beyond doubt, in the case of clinical doctors their relevance to politics and internationalism was not immediately obvious.[7] However, the doctors at the Second Internal Medicine clinic in Prague were members of the health authorities. Due to a lack of income, Josef Pelnář himself began working as an expert witness at the Provincial Criminal and Commercial Courts.[8] In the interwar period, he was involved in the activities of the National Health Council and several other bodies of the Ministry of Health.[9] As the professors of medicine treated leading politicians and party leaders with whom they were very familiar, Pelnář was also active in various committees for the promotion of international relations, which supported the official foreign policy of the Czechoslovak Republic at expert level.[10] Pelnář's political commitment to the foundation of new medical fields such as occupational medicine or endocrinology indicated role in the mutually reinforcing dynamic of co-producing knowledge and policy.

Pelnář followed in the footsteps of his predecessors, who would not have reached higher official positions without underpinning the established political order with their expertise. This did not mean that their intellectual achievements were limited to mere political schemes and the repetition of hackneyed phrases. Medical professors carried out extremely precise and rigorous analyses which, however, had effects on the existing worldview. Unlike, his disciples who were challenged by the National Socialist and Communist regimes, Pelnář did not have to formally act as an agent of a planned, ideologically conditioned

5 Haas, "Introduction: epistemic communities," 1–35. Iacob et al., State Socialist Experts, 147–152. See also Bourdieu, "The Forms of Capital", 241–58.

6 Cross, Rethinking epistemic communities, 137–160. Pașca, A Détente Equation, 160–183. Manulak, Developing World Environmental Cooperation, 103–127.

7 Iacob, Malariology and Decolonization, 233–253. Mueller, Risk on the Negotiating Table, 138–162.

8 MUA AV ČR, AAV, f. Josef Pelnář, box 1, Sign. Ia, fols. 15, 17.

9 MUA AV ČR, AAV, f. Josef Pelnář, box 1, Sign. Ia, fols. 22, 29, 38–39, 42–43, 51–53.

10 MUA AV ČR, AAV, f. Josef Pelnář, box 1, Sign. Ia, fols. 31–32, 36–37, 44, 48–49, 56.

scholarship that was inextricably linked to a project of societal change determined by a totalitarian state.[11]

The chapter examines the history of the healthcare facilities as they were perceived and remembered by its staff – former students, doctors and professors. It is necessary to point out that most of the testimonies were written by Pelnář's former students and colleagues. All come from people who not only studied but subsequently worked under Pelnář and whom he helped in their careers. In order to revise some of their uncritical views of his colleagues, an archival investigation was carried out in the personal collection of Josef Pelnář. These were mainly male scholars, although the work of women – nurses, cleaners and cooks who did the "dirty tasks" in the hospital – was essential to maintaining the hospital operation. Occasionally, the doctors' wives were also mentioned because they made their husbands' professional success possible through their economic assets, the care of the children and the household. In this respect, the testimonies are gender-specific and tell the story of a male world, although this narrative is not misogynistic.

The chapter attempts to contribute to the history of general hospitals and clinical teaching and research. It has already been argued that regional epistemic communities were synchronized with transnational dynamics. However, epistemic communities have rarely been studied in the context of a specific place such as the Second Internal Clinic in Prague. Therefore, the chapter focuses on the less explored aspects, such as the history of formal and informal selection, reproduction and sociability within the epistemic community.[12] First, the chapter traces the origins of the clinic and its connections to the general hospital. It provides an historical overview of clinical teaching at the Prague General Hospital based on the available secondary literature. The second part is based on the analysis of the memoirs and testimonies published by the Pelnář's former students and colleagues. Some of them appeared in the medical journals that dedicated special issues to Pelnář's life anniversaries.[13]

1 The General Hospital and Clinical Training in Prague

In line with European trends linking medical training with hospital practice, the beginnings of clinical teaching in Prague date back to the second half of

11 Cf. Iacob et al., State Socialist Experts, 147–148. Maingot, *Race, Ideology*, 268–292.

12 Foucault, *The Birth of the Clinic*. Ackerknecht, *La médecine hospitalière à Paris*. Granshaw, Porter, *The Hospital in History*. Vogel, The invention of the modern hospital.

13 Deyl, *Die Deutsche Karl-Ferdinands-Universität*. Surman, *Universities*. Matoušek, "The Medical School of Vienna and of Prague," 99–106.

the eighteenth century. As in Vienna, Pest and Kraków, clinical teaching was introduced as part of the Enlightenment reforms of the Habsburg monarchs. Maria Theresa's personal physician Gerhard van Swieten, a disciple of the Dutch scholar Hermann Boerhaave, who was one of the pioneers of clinical teaching at the bedside, was responsible for crucial changes in public healthcare within the Habsburg Monarchy. The number of hours of clinical teaching was increased and it became part of the medical curriculum. The emphasis was placed on practical training in the clinic, where students met face-to-face with patients and their diseases, which they had previously only known from textbooks. It was important to gain hands-on experience and graduate with practical skills.[14]

The lectures first took place at the bedside, where the students were asked to help diagnose and examine the patients. They then discussed the individual cases they encountered in the clinic with the professor in the lecture hall. Each day, the chosen diagnoses and treatments were reassessed and adjusted. In 1767, bedside lectures were introduced in Prague. From 1787, medical students learned in practice at the Hospital of the Brothers of Mercy. Only men could be admitted to this facility as inpatients, while women and children were treated as outpatients. Clinical teaching was offered there until the academic year 1791/1792, when it was moved to the new premises of the General Hospital. It became part of the final year of study, which lasted four years. Later, the medical course was extended to five years. Prospective surgeons studied for two to three years, depending on their previous training. They also completed an internship at the general hospital.[15]

The General Hospital in Prague was originally located in the older building of the Foundation of the Institute for Impoverished Noble Women. In 1787, the building was purchased for 28,619 gulden and converted into a hospital facility within two years. The conversion also included the construction of a completely new asylum for the mentally ill and a hospital chapel. The cost of the ambitious conversion was so high that a similar complex could have been built from scratch. The conversion was proposed by the professor and director of the Prague Polytechnic, Franz Anton Herget, who also supervised the construction work. The conversion was complicated due to the nature of the building, which was more than eight decades old. In the end, the hospital had

14 Foucault, *Les Machines à guérir*. Imbert, *Histoire des hôpitaux*. Geyer-Kordesch. German Medical Education, 177–205. Núñez-García, *Los hospitales docentes*, 53–77. Bernard, The Limits of Absolutism, 194–207.

15 Černý, *Lékařství*, 221–222. Hlaváčková, *Dějiny všeobecné nemocnice*, 29–30. Květ and Tinková, *Jan Theobald*, 32, 42, 48.

a total capacity of 300 beds and a further 34 beds for the staff, who shared the rooms with the patients, which was quite common at the time.[16]

The General Hospital, which became an endowment institution under the direct supervision of the provincial authorities, opened in the winter of 1790/91. The start of its activity was promulgated by an imperial decree published in Czech and German. Instead of the expected official announcement, it took the form of a rather enticing advertising leaflet:

> Every patient admitted to the care of the general sick house may expect the advice of carefully selected physicians, the assistance of skillful surgeons, good medicines, careful nursing, decent and sufficient food, and a clean bed, also, if the need requires it, clothing. This home for the sick, as an institution whose soul is love of fellow-man, from the highest director down to the lowest servant, endeavors to deal kindly with everyone.[17]

As in other hospitals in Central Europe, whether in Brno, Pest or Zagreb, where the sick were to be treated equally, the imperial decree also emphasized that patients were to be admitted regardless of status, age, language or religion. However, the level of care, facilities, and food depended on the amount paid by patients for their stay. The hospital fund was insufficient to cover the rapidly growing costs, and the hospital administration tried to claim compensation for the deficits from the Prague municipality, pointing out that the Prague residents were the most frequent patients.[18]

The staff of the General Hospital was divided into two categories – the first consisted of two doctors, two paramedics, a hospital administrator, a controller and a scribe. These positions had a fixed salary and therefore, unlike private practice, offered a degree in financial and material security. In addition to their salary, the employees were given an apartment in the hospital, wood for heating and candles for lighting. At the same time, they gained experience, which was a prerequisite for prestigious positions in health administration. The second, lower category included medical professionals such as private doctors and nurses, but also non-medical staff such as laundresses, cooks, etc. The second category offered no financial security, let alone prestige. The nurses, originally called attendants, were very poorly paid, although they had to be in the hospital almost constantly. In the course of the nineteenth century, the

16 Svobodný, Hlaváčková, *Pražské špitály*, 55.

17 Svobodný, Hlaváčková, *Pražské špitály*, 59.

18 Svobodný, Hlaváčková, *Pražské špitály*, 58. Hlaváčková, Svobodný, Bříza, *History of the General University Hospital*, 20.

nurses – originally men – were replaced in their role by women, who gradually received professional nursing training directly in the hospital.[19]

At the end of the eighteenth century, clinical teaching at the bedside became the standard for medical faculties in Central Europe that wanted to maintain their prestige and reputation. However, the institutionalization of clinical teaching did not run smoothly and there was frequent friction between the university and the hospital. In Prague, the decision to relocate clinical teaching from the convent to the general hospital was taken reluctantly and the original plans did not include facilities for the clinic. Once the move had been decided, the hospital premises had to be adapted. The clinic, originally called the "practical school" was divided into an internal and surgical ward. Each of the wards had twelve beds, six for men and the same number for women. The ward for internal medicine was housed on the ground floor and had three rooms. The two side rooms were each intended for one gender and the central connecting room was the lecture hall, which was later rebuilt into an operating theatre. The patients used for the demonstrations during the lectures were selected from the entire hospital or directly upon admission to the hospital.[20]

At the beginning of the nineteenth century, each ward was headed by a professor who was supported by an assistant appointed for two years. In May 1811, the Imperial Education Commission issued a decree confirming the role of the General Hospital in the training of university teachers and researchers. The professors of the medical faculty were to recruit from the ranks of assistants, trainees, interns and surgeons. The General Hospital became indeed a school for future professors. Unless they came from abroad, most of them started as trainees, interns and assistants. The management of the clinics was combined with the position of university professor as head of the hospital department.[21]

2 The Division of University and Its Aftermath

The development of the General Hospital and its clinics was fundamentally influenced by the Czech German national rivalry in Bohemia.[22] In the first half of the nineteenth century, German was the main language of teaching

19 Svobodný, Hlaváčková, *Pražské špitály*, 56–58, 78.

20 Hlaváčková, Svobodný, Bříza, *History of the General University Hospital*, 17.

21 Svobodný, Hlaváčková, *Pražské špitály*, 62–64, 75. Hlaváčková, Svobodný, Bříza, *History of the General University Hospital*, 23–24.

22 Svobodný, Hlaváčková, *Dějiny lékařství*, 147.

and communication at the Faculty of Medicine in Prague. With the approval of the provincial governor, the professors were also allowed to teach in Czech, whereby lectures in Czech were particularly encouraged in the training of midwives.[23] During the highly centralized rule of Alexander von Bach, Minister of the Interior in the mid-19th century Habsburg Monarchy, it was difficult to give lectures in Czech at the university. It was due to the lack of medical terminology as well as to the suppression of Czech intellectual emancipation. Jan Špott, an orthopedist who is considered a pioneer of hydrotherapy and physiotherapy, was the first to teach in Czech. However, his lectures took place in the privacy of his apartment and were optional. His younger colleague, Bohumil Eiselt, professor of surgery and pathology at the medical clinic, taught exclusively in Czech at the Faculty of Medicine after his habilitation ("second dissertation"). As head of the surgical department, he devoted himself most intensively to the development of Czech medical terminology.[24]

With the political liberalization in the 1860s, Czech scholarly circles, including physicians, promoted teaching in Czech at Prague university, so that graduates of Czech-language grammar schools could continue their studies in their native language without major obstacles. The establishment of Czech grammar schools ("gymnasia") and the teaching of the Czech language at university was not only an academic matter, but also a central demand of the representatives of the national movement. It was an attempt by Czech patriots to build an equivalent to grammar schools and university education in German. Although the argument of the need to understand and speak Czech fluently in order to facilitate communication between physicians and patients was frequently used, especially in the context of hiring doctors in hospitals, and was indeed reasonable, it did not fully explain the insistence on university lectures in Czech.[25]

An even more pressing issue was the division of the university, which arose in 1864 when Jan Evangelista Purkyně, professor of physiology and at the same time a leading poet in the Czech language, expressed his first public thoughts on the subject. After Purkyně's death, the idea of a Czech university was taken up by Bohumil Eiselt who conducted negotiations with German professors on the division of the medical faculty.[26] The division of the university took place in February 1882. The corresponding law provided for two universities to be founded in Prague from the academic year

23 Tinková, *Tělo, věda, stát*, 412–413. Černý, *Lékařství*, 277.

24 Thomayer, *Ze zápisků lékaře*, 78, 80.

25 Hlaváčková, Svobodný, Bříza, *History of the General University Hospital*, 35–36.

26 Svobodný and Hlaváčková, *Dějiny lékařství*, 148.

1883/1884 – one with German as the language of instruction and the other with Czech as the language of instruction. The university was also given a new name: the Charles-Ferdinand University with Bohemian and German sections. The reference to the medieval emperor Charles IV emphasized the antiquity and prestige of the institution.[27] It accommodated scholarly interests and played the "nationalist" card by recruiting new academic posts from state and provincial authorities.

The division of the medical faculty initially brought with it the problem that there was a lack of teaching staff for theoretical subjects in the Czech part. This shortage was remedied with the arrival of qualified scholars from the Russian Empire, mainly from present-day Ukraine. They contributed to the dissemination of scientific knowledge and to the development of Czech medical terminology. Still, the Czech medical faculty faced several obstacles in terms of material resources. Most of the premises remained with the original German medical faculty, and the two faculties had to share the clinics in the General Hospital. For example, the eye clinic was handed over without any equipment. Because of failure to transfer the individual hospital facilities, it was decided to build new pavilions for the Czech clinics.[28]

3 The Foundation of the Second Internal Clinic

In the 1880s, the first internal clinic could not cope with the influx of students attending medical lectures in large numbers. In order to comply with the parity rule, the Czech professors sought the building to house the Czech propaedeutic clinic and the second clinic for internal medicine. The propaedeutic clinic was to teach students the theoretical foundations of medicine before they began their practical training in the internal clinic. After two years of protracted negotiations, the Ministry of Education issued a decree in June 1885 approving the establishment of the Czech propaedeutic clinic. The propaedeutic clinic was responsible for treatment similar to those of the internal clinic. The problem, however, was that the teaching in the propaedeutic clinic was not equivalent, as rigorous examinations could not be held there. This undermined the academic prestige and power of teachers. Professor Eiselt therefore

27 Surman, *Universities*, 103–105. Hlaváčková, *Dějiny všeobecné nemocnice*, 50–70. Černý, Lékařství, 280–283, 336.

28 Černý, *Lékařství*, 333–334. Svobodný, Hlaváčková, *Pražské špitály*, 62–64. Hlaváčková, *Dějiny všeobecné fakultní nemocnice*, 95–96.

applied for the newly founded propaedeutic clinic to be converted into the second clinic for internal medicine.[29]

After the establishment of the second clinic for internal medicine, the question of its director immediately arose. Professor Eiselt, a respected scholar and at the same time a skillful manager, appointed his former assistant and son-in-law, Emerich Maixner, Professor of Internal Medicine, as head of the clinic. In 1902, when Eiselt died, Maixner moved into Eiselt's position and took over the management of the First Internal Clinic.[30] This also raised the question of the head of the Second Clinic, which was filled relatively quickly, as Eiselt trained several potential candidates. Maixner's successor was Josef Thomayer, a scholar with an enormous reputation and professor of internal medicine. Thomayer was the highly motivated son of a count's gardener from a village near the small West Bohemian town of Domažlice/Taus. He originally studied and passed his examinations under German professors who appreciated him for his talent and diligence. They expected him to become an assistant in surgery, but his patron died unexpectedly and Thomayer had to change the plans.[31] In his memoirs he wrote

> If Heine [German professor of surgery] had stayed alive and I had become an assistant with his help and, in a favorable case, an associate professor, I would probably be an unpaid associate professor at a German medical faculty today. I would hardly have made it as a professor at the Czech faculty. The path I took was incomparably more advantageous in material terms.[32]

The doctors judged their future careers based on which lectures they attended, who they took exams with, where they practiced medicine and, above all, which university professor they liked. A graduate of Charles University who aspired to a career in medical teaching and research worked as an unpaid assistant in the clinic. The medical students had familiarized themselves with the procedures in a clinic during their internships. The medical program at Charles University lasted five years and was divided into three strict examinations. Medical students could only apply for the second rigorous exam after they had completed their internship – more specifically, they had to spend four semesters in the

29 Hlaváčková, *Dějiny všeobecné fakultní nemocnice*, 96. Hlaváčková, *Druhá česká*, 16–17. Hlaváčková, Svobodný, Bříza, *History of the General University Hospital*, 52–53.

30 Hlaváčková, *Druhá česká*, 16–17.

31 Hlaváčková, *Druhá česká*, 18.

32 Thomayer, *Ze zápisků lékaře*, 122.

Department of Internal Medicine and the Department of Surgery and at least one semester in the Department of Obstetrics and Ophthalmology.[33]

Newly qualified doctors were faced with an important life decision that depended on their financial possibilities, as they had been without a regular income for several years. One option was to find a paid position in a hospital or to combine the university path of an unpaid academic with private medical practice. Thomayer chose the latter path during the first years after graduation: he began working without financial remuneration as an assistant in a surgical clinic and earned his living as an external doctor in the provincial institute for mentally ill. He benefited from the division of the university and settled at the Czech medical faculty in 1883 after he habilitated [submitted a second dissertation] at Eiselt's suggestion.[34] With his immense organizational, research and teaching activities, Thomayer influenced the trajectory of the Second Internal Clinic for almost four decades. During his time in office, he renovated hospital premises and acquired modern medical equipment after lengthy negotiations with university and provincial authorities in this regard.[35]

4 The Second Internal Clinic after the First World War

The organization of the medical institution was unique in that the individual institutes were both clinics of the faculty and departments of the general hospital. The clinics were administered by the Ministry of Education. From the beginning of the nineteenth century, the head of the clinic was a university professor who also headed the general hospital department and was therefore controlled by the hospital director. The assistants were employees of the clinic and thus subordinate to the Ministry of Education. The secondary doctors were employees of the general hospital. This dual administration was a constant source of discord between the secondary doctors and the assistants, who enjoyed higher professional status, longer vacations and some other benefits. The secondary doctors were ordinary medical employees as in other hospitals.[36]

After Thomayer's retirement in 1921, the Dean's Office of the Czech Medical Faculty set out to find a qualified director who would be at least somewhat

33 Černý, *Lékařství*, 280. See also Rambousková and Martykánová, *Social class*, passim.

34 Hlaváčková, *Druhá česká*, 19.

35 Hlaváčková, *Druhá česká*, 19, 30–31. Hlaváčková, Svobodný, Bříza, *History of the General University Hospital*, 76.

36 Mařatka, *Paměti*, 76.

equal to him in his work. Thomayer's successor at the head of the Second Internal Clinic was his disciple and colleague Josef Pelnář, whose biography is almost identical to that of Thomayer. He grew up in poor circumstances and attended grammar school in the small town.[37] Thanks to the financial help of various provincial funds for poor students and the material support of his wealthy, childless uncle, with whom he lived, he enrolled at Charles University in Prague.[38] It was a great relief for Pelnář to study at the Czech medical faculty, which enabled him to avoid competition from German fellow students on his way to a university career. Pelnář was an excellent student and had no difficulty learning foreign languages, including German, which had been an optional subject at the grammar school since the 1885/86 school year.[39] Like Thomayer, he benefited from a year of military service in the garrison hospital in Prague, working in a pathology institute in Lviv and completing an internship in a psychiatric clinic in Karlov.[40] In both places, he gradually worked his way up to a higher assistant position as was his wish.

A turning point in his career was Thomayer's request to appoint Pelnář to the Second Internal Clinic, where he was given the post of paid assistant for five years. Pelnář was already thirty years old at this point, five years after his doctorate, but he was still supported by his uncle, because there had not been an earlier vacancy.[41] Thomayer's recommendation enabled Pelnář to go on several study trips abroad and undertake short internship at several Western European hospitals.[42] Thomayer seems to have laid the foundation for a community of doctors that Pelnář later expanded with his students and colleagues. In addition to clinical teaching and research, he organized social and cultural events, including joint visits to Prague Castle and excursions to the countryside.[43]

Despite the friendly relations among the doctors at the clinic, there was pressure to habilitate and secure a better starting position for a well-paid professorship. It is interesting to see how Pelnář pursued his goal in this competitive environment despite Thomayer's disapproval. Thomayer tried to postpone Pelnář's habilitation so that he could remain in the position of a paid assistant, but Pelnář did not want to wait.[44] Thomayer had urged him to leave the

37 MUA AV ČR, AAV, f. Josef Pelnář, box 1, Sign. Ia, fol. 1.
38 MUA AV ČR, AAV, f. Josef Pelnář, box 1, Sign. Ia, fols. 5–6, 8.
39 MUA AV ČR, AAV, f. Josef Pelnář, box 1, Sign. Ib, fol. 5.
40 MUA AV ČR, AAV, f. Josef Pelnář, box 1, Sign. Ia, fol. 69. MUA AV ČR, AAV, f. Josef Pelnář, box 1, Sign. Ic, fol. 1–3. See also Mařatka, Hlaváčková, *Josef Pelnář*, 13.
41 MUA AV ČR, AAV, f. Josef Pelnář, box 1, Sign. Ia, fols. 7, 13–15.
42 MUA AV ČR, AAV, f. Josef Pelnář, box 1, Sign. Ia, fols. 10–11.
43 MUA AV ČR, AAV, f. Josef Pelnář, box 1, Sign. Ib7, fols. 26–27.
44 MUA AV ČR, AAV, f. Josef Pelnář, box 1, Sign. Ib7, fols. 37–39.

post at the time, claiming that it was not appropriate for an associate professor ("Docent") to perform the work of a clinical assistant.[45] Moreover, Pelnář had married and Thomayer – himself a bachelor – refused to employ married assistants. Pelnář did not agree since it would have meant that he had to leave the clinic. He finally gave in and opened a private practice in his apartment.[46]

It soon became clear that Pelnář could not support his family with the modest income from his practice. He found an improvement in his financial situation by working as an outpatient doctor for insured employees of electrical companies, a position that he received with Thomayer's help. On the recommendation of one of his patients, he was also able to work as a forensic expert witness in court. He kept in touch with clinical teaching and regularly lectured at the clinic on Saturdays to a large class of medical students.[47] At the outbreak of the First World War, he enlisted as a staff doctor on the Serbian front. His hard work earned him the directorship of military hospitals in Cejle/Cilli and Trieste/Tierst. After the end of the war, he put his management experience to good use when he was appointed full professor in 1920 and succeeded Thomayer as head of the Second Medical Clinic a year later, even though this advancement was not without its difficulties.[48]

At the beginning of the twentieth century, more than thirty members of the academic body of the medical faculty decided on the admission of professors, clinic directors and heads of hospital departments. During the war, some members died, and others left the faculty. Their places were taken by younger colleagues who gradually expressed "dissent" within the academic body. The "dissenters" consisted of a group of about twelve people. They never achieved a majority in the academic body, but they repeatedly asserted their will in secret votes against the "older gentlemen", who were also referred to as "conservatives".[49] The dissenters debated fiercely, argued objectively and tried to have personnel issues decided in favor of the faculty on the basis of the qualifications and good character of potential candidates. These groups of doctors met informally in a different restaurant in the center of Prague. In this regard, Pelnář wrote:

> Before the meeting of the academic body at which the head [of the Second Internal Clinic] was to be appointed, I learnt that the assembly in Platejz's pub had

45 MUA AV ČR, AAV, f. Josef Pelnář, box 1, Sign. Ia, fol. 16. See also Hlaváčková, *Druhá česká,* 34. Mařatka, Hlaváčková, *Josef Pelnář*, 23.

46 MUA AV ČR, AAV, f. Josef Pelnář, box 1, Sign. Ib7, fols. 32.

47 MUA AV ČR, AAV, f. Josef Pelnář, box 1, Sign. Ia, fols. 18, 21.

48 MUA AV ČR, AAV, f. Josef Pelnář, box 1, Sign. Ia, fols. 25–27. See also Mařatka, Hlaváčková, *Josef Pelnář*, 14–15.

49 Vondráček, *Lékař dale vzpomíná*, 31.

> firmly decided to nominate Hnátek ... I liked Hnátek and always respected him, but at that time Hnátek was so much less energetic that I thought it was a mistake that he ... ran the second clinic.[50]

When it came to appointing the head of the Second Internal Clinic, the conservative professors put forward their candidate Hnátek, who was strongly rejected by the representatives of the dissenting wing. Thomayer, the outgoing head of the clinic, proposed the members of a selection committee, the composition of which was considered too one-sided in favor of the conservatives. Thomayer therefore set up a new committee in which the conservatives were more strongly represented. The committee agreed on Pelnář as the best candidate when the Ministry of Education – Professor of General History Josef Šusta – who had long known Pelnář from various Prague restaurant events, promised to establish the third internal clinic to be run by Pelnář's counter-candidate Hnátek. However, this never happened. Hnátek was respected as a leader, but without his own clinic, fell seriously ill and died a few months later.[51]

Pelnář's tenure in the administration of the Second Internal Clinic was characterized by a flourishing of clinical teaching and research. A most fundamental adjustment that he made was the career advancement of the new generation of doctors, who benefited from the expansion of healthcare facilities in Prague, a process that had begun in the late Habsburg Monarchy and intensified after the establishment of the Czechoslovak Republic. At that time, the head of the clinic was in charge of three paid and three unpaid assistants.[52]

Working in the clinic was still economically demanding because only after the candidates became "official" unpaid assistants could they qualify for a remunerated position. Associate professors, external physicians, visiting academics and research students did not have a fixed salary, but they could receive various scholarships or temporary financial support from non-university funds. Of the dozens of them who started at the clinic in this way, only a few were successful, and usually only after a few years. The vast majority left the clinic after a certain time, either to practice or to find a paid position in other hospitals.[53]

---

50 MUA AV ČR, AAV, f. Josef Pelnář, box 1, Sign. Ib7, fols. 47–48.

51 MUA AV ČR, AAV, f. Josef Pelnář, box 1, Sign. Ib7, fols. 46–48. See also Mařatka, Hlaváčková, *Josef Pelnář*, 14–15.

52 Hlaváčková, Svobodný, Bříza, *History of the General University Hospital*, 68 ff. Mařatka, Hlaváčková, *Josef Pelnář*, 25.

53 Mařatka, *Paměti*, 76.

In his memoirs, Vladimír Vondráček, Pelnář's favorite student and later professor of neurology and psychiatry at Charles University, described how a young doctor's decision to pursue an academic career was not only linked to the prestige of clinical teaching and research, but also to overcoming material insecurity. Vondráček explained that he worked as an unpaid assistant at the general clinic for fifteen years.[54] As a doctor of medicine, he gained experience in patient care and medical research, but no salary. The solution was to look for another paid job, but in doing so, many had to give up their dreams. However, it was necessary to secure a regular income in order to have anything to live on at all:

> There were only a few paid jobs and assistantships anyway … getting a good and well-paid position in a clinic in Prague or even in a hospital outside Prague was not easy back then. There was a complicated patronage system, especially in the medical field, and the sons and daughters of doctors always had priority. The background was somehow decisive.[55]

Vondráček was orphaned in infancy, but his parents' inheritance ensured that he was provided for during his medical studies. Initially, he worked as an intern and unpaid assistant. Together with a close colleague, they attempted to improve the assistants' material conditions, but the state authorities, including the Minister of Health, refused to change the prevailing rules. Thanks to the encouragement of his professor, Vondráček obtained a position in the department of pharmacology.[56] Other, less cordial testimonies pointed to economic interest, which is confirmed by historical sources from the interwar period.[57] Patron-client relationships resulted, among other things, from the lack of financial security of the candidates in clinical medicine.

The lack of salary was the price for the opportunity to meet and to collaborate with university professors at the clinic. To temporarily overcome the economic hardship, the doctors opened private practices to earn money. They drew their potential patients from the hospitals – clinics where they worked. Paid senior doctors often recommended the services of younger unpaid colleagues to their patients. The other colleagues were able to work for free as a guest intern because of their solid material background. Some of them were married and supported by their wife's family in the opening of a private

54 Vondráček, *Fantastické a magické vzpomínání*, 403, 652.

55 Vondráček, *Lékař dále vzpomíná*, 36.

56 Vondráček, *Lékař dále vzpomíná*, 37.

57 Arndt, Pahl, *Capitalist Cold*, 3.

practice. They combined the public reputation of their clinical work with their experience in practice.[58]

In general, the doctors' background could limit their professional careers, as those who could not rely on the material support of their family (not necessarily their parents) were unable to concentrate fully on their work in the clinic. To build an academic career, they also needed support from their superiors. There are exceptional cases of doctors of poor origin who "made it", such as Josef Pelnář, who remained head of the Second Internal Clinic until his retirement. Although it cannot be denied that he enjoyed the protection of influential colleagues who appreciated his efforts, it was only later in his life that he achieved the highest recognition for his numerous commitments outside the official medical service.[59]

5 Second Internal Clinic as Epistemic Community

The establishment of the Czechoslovak Republic had an impact on the development of the hospital facilities. University professors appealed to the state authorities and in some cases received additional funding. The outdated diagnostic and clinical equipment was modernized. Chemical laboratories were set up and the X-ray department was expanded. The auditorium was renovated. The general change in medical care was particularly evident in the treatment of diabetics, who often died. It was not until the mid-1920s that several dozen doses of insulin were flown in from Paris at an unheard-of price, saving the lives of many patients.

The somewhat schematic division into "dissenters" and "conservatives", which was mentioned in connection with the appointment of Pelnář as head of the Second Internal Clinic in 1921, resulted from the doctors' attitude to medical treatment. Wherever possible, Pelnář appointed assistants who had completed physiological, pharmacological or chemical training. There were not many such graduates. He encouraged students to devote themselves to laboratory research. One of the Pelnář's colleague, and the later prominent professor of endocrinology, Josef Charvát recalled that

> Physiological and functional thinking was on the rise in the clinic, but nobody was prepared for it. Neither the heads nor their students. The professors had all grown up before the war, in times when percussion and auscultation were the

58 Mařatka, *Paměti*, 77.

59 Rambousková, Martykánová, *Social class*, passim.

> most important examination methods in internal medicine and when nothing else was done in the laboratory.[60]

Since there was no official procedure for recruiting well-trained and hard-working scholars familiar with the latest healing practices, Pelnář had the leeway to form an epistemic community according to his own ideas. His most important and far-reaching decision was to maintain the continuity of clinical training and research. Whereas previously doctors had to go into private practice at the end of their paid assistantships and thus lose contact with the clinic, Pelnář arranged that qualified persons were allowed to continue working in research as honorary staff. They usually came to the clinic for a few mornings a week and took part in clinical research in one of the new working groups initiated by Pelnář. They also received some money for lectures, which were compulsory and for which tuition fees were paid at the dean's office.[61]

The retrospective opinions about Pelnář highlight his fatherly attitude towards his protégés. He was a teacher and superior to whom his junior colleagues were grateful for the opportunity to devote themselves to medical teaching and research.[62] As head of the clinic, he pursued a paternalistic approach, planning the careers of his subordinates and often determining their private lives, something he had in common with Thomayer. Those who followed a similar path to success admired his leadership, describing the clinic as an exceptional academic environment for those interested in medicine.[63] Despite the warm feelings, it cannot be overlooked that these positive views were expressed in retrospect and thus distort our perspective of relations between Pelnář and his colleagues. For instance, Josef Charvát wrote:

> At the beginning, with the morning reports, it was like being in the army … he didn't tolerate much discussion, everyone reported what they had, he gave the orders, that was all and we went to work. I didn't mind. I had returned from the war as an artillery officer and knew discipline.[64]

Not only his close disciples, but also less successful pupils obtained jobs at regional hospitals because of Pelnář's connections. Others became regular doctors and reported to the Second Internal Clinic because such connection

60 Charvát, Pelnář a jeho klinika, 1565.
61 Charvát, *Můj labyrint světa*, 107.
62 Charvát, Pelnář a jeho klinika, 1564.
63 Herles, Akademik Pelnář, 1564.
64 Charvát, *Můj labyrint světa*, 127.

attracted solvent patients to their private practices. The testimonies of these underdogs, crushed under the pressure of academic and social competition, did not survive because they left clinical research or even died prematurely. Among them was a "colleague Hubáček", an outstanding student who impressed Pelnář with his knowledge of seven languages. According to testimony, Hubáček was

> a good boy who was somehow unable to cope with the turbulent ferment of the clinic ... He was replaced relatively soon by another doctor. He was an unhappy man, he didn't grow old ... somewhat shy and timid, he goes down in history as one of the first, or perhaps the first, assistant of Pelnář.[65]

Over the years, Pelnář's demeanor changed, becoming less military and more civil. One day, the assistants plucked up their courage and invited him for a coffee in the office after a long morning medical round. But he firmly refused. As he mainly worked in the clinic, he only met with colleagues regularly for short periods of time and each of the young doctors had to use the time to make their mark. He was conservative on the matter of women's advancement in the medical system. It took him two to three years to admit that nurses could not only serve patients but also assist doctors in their treatment. No wonder he was quite rude to one of the first women among the clinic's secondary doctors when she wrote a report on a patient.[66] Later in life he stopped behaving rudely toward female colleagues, this being the case not only the doctors, but also his assistants.

Together with colleagues from the First Internal Clinic, Pelnář introduced weekly seminars in which the assistants presented the latest published findings in foreign medicine, which were hotly debated and scrutinized by the seminar participants. These initiatives marked a turn from German influence to a focus on medical research in France, Great Britain and above all, the United States. North American scholars rapidly became influential among Central European doctors.[67]

When Pelnář took over the administration of the clinic a new world opened up for its students. The seminar participants had the opportunity to study abroad, e.g. some of them completed internships in Cambridge, where they came into contact with the international medical community and worked with American, Chinese or Philippine colleagues. In 1926, doctors from the

65 Vondráček, *Lékař dále vzpomíná*, 29.
66 Charvát, *Můj labyrint světa*, 127.
67 Prusík, Akademik Pelnář, 1389–1390.

Interstate Postgraduate Medical Association of North America visited the Prague clinic. Three years later Charles H. Mayo, the founder of the famous clinic in Rochester, made Pelnář an honorary member of the association in recognition of his achievements in medicine and his efforts to promote Czechoslovak-American relations.[68] The personnel of the Clinic later took part in medical congresses in Boston and Vichy.

Public speaking talent and the ability to convincingly debate at academic events and conferences were important prerequisites for a career in clinical teaching and research. Official academic sessions were often followed by a series of informal meetings organized by Pelnář throughout the academic year. Professional and personal ties intertwined at these meetings, creating an unobtrusive, feigned or deeply felt sense of belonging to the community that bound colleagues to Pelnář for many years. Pelnář created a group of people who were loyal to him. The candidates learned their roles through shared moments and rituals in the doctors' rooms, where colleagues from the clinic came together and sometimes also guests from abroad, who spent pleasant moments among the clinic staff at the end of their visit. Shared meals, even if they were just snacks with "warmed sausages" or coffee breaks, playing chess during long night shifts and debates about work issues were among the everyday practices that kept the community alive under Pelnář's leadership.[69] Although most of the doctors at the clinic stated that Pelnář guided them, it is also clear that he did not interfere too much in their work. Many of them introduced new clinical procedures and their applications through independent research, in which Pelnář was only minimally involved. They thus worked autonomously in the clinic; he, as their head, only formally supervised their work, but did not actively participate in it.

6 Conclusion

As in other Central European cities, the clinical training of students in the General Hospital became part of the study program at the Medical Faculty of Charles University in Prague at the end of the eighteenth century. The clinic itself – a hospital department that was also part of the medical faculty – was a highly distinctive workplace precisely because of this dual administration. The medical system underwent several organizational changes in the period under

68 MUA AV ČR, AAV, f. Josef Pelnář, box 1, Sign. Ia, fols. 40–41.

69 Cmunt, K sedmdesátce prof. J. Pelnáře, 1249. Herles, Akademik Pelnář, 1564. Mařatka, *Paměti*, 79.

study here, including the creation of Czech internal clinics due to the division of the university into a Czech faculty and a German faculty, as more and more scholars used the "nationalist" card as a means of pushing for additional university posts with the state authorities.

In the interwar period, Czech and German medical faculties were confronted with an influx of students due to government opening and support for higher education. The problem was that the number of beds in the patient rooms where clinical training took place did not increase. Students complained about the lack of space, as the patient rooms in some clinics were used as lecture theatres. Thanks to the pressure from medical professors, additional funds were made available and the outdated hospital facilities were gradually renovated. Old buildings were extended and new premises created. In connection with the recent development of medicine and its specializations, various research groups were set up by the leading medical professor and hospital manager Josef Pelnář after his appointment as head of the Second Internal Clinic in order to ensure the continuity of clinical teaching and research.

The Second Internal Clinic under the direction of Josef Pelnář became a phenomenon within the Czech-speaking medical community, as evidenced by numerous testimonies from former students and doctors who had worked there. Pelnář's main merit was above all the change in the recruitment of new colleagues and the way teaching and research were organized at the clinic. Instead of the direction deciding upon employment, Pelnář introduced a recruitment process involving all members of the clinic. A diploma from medical school and recommendations from respected professors were no longer sufficient, even though they still remained significant. The most important criteria now were the intellectual skills that Pelnář and his colleagues observed during the candidates' internship and research stays at the clinic.

In addition to completing their studies, candidates had to show a particular passion for the medical profession. Doctors aiming for an early career required sufficient financial support from their families. Most training positions at the clinics were unpaid, so candidates had to run a private practice, which gave them additional income but was often not enough to support their families. Some of them postponed marriage, others married women with high dowries – one of the few occasions when the doctors' testimonies mentioned women at all. Pelnář slightly modified this highly unequal method of selecting young academics by extending the paid assistantships by one and two years and allowing associate professors to fill these positions. He also looked for opportunities in non-university funds to temporarily bridge the existential uncertainty and send talented doctors on study trips abroad.

The candidates recruited by Pelnář and his colleagues joined an epistemic community – a group of interns, assistants, experienced doctors and professors who worked in specialized research groups. The establishment of this group prevented the massive migration of qualified people into private practice, as they remained in the clinic. Such socialization encouraged collaboration and created a favorable environment for individual research. New treatment methods were applied that would otherwise be difficult to achieve. It should be noted that the members of the Pelnář's community completely eclipsed the needs and feelings of their patients: they became objects of research and learning. In their testimonies, the doctors rarely mentioned the patients.

Numerous joint academic meetings facilitated academic communication by among the members of the community that developed at the Clinic. People refined their notions and adopted beliefs that emerged from their teaching and research. Yet, candidates for a post at the Second Internal Clinic not only had to prove their scholarly abilities but also demonstrate the right professional views and political opinions, which were sometimes associated with patriotic attitudes. It is probably no coincidence that four of Pelnář's close colleagues were executed during the Nazi occupation, one died in prison and one on the barricades. However, other colleagues collaborated with the protectorate government, which facilitated Pelnář's recognition even during the Second World War.[70] Pelnář formed an epistemic community cemented not only by career ladders and academic prestige, but also by shared rituals and bonds in the form of discussion seminars, informal gatherings and outdoor events. As for Pelnář's leadership qualities, his subordinates admired not only his professional skills and knowledge, but also his personality and democratic approach. Pelnář is depicted as an inspiring teacher and chief who was fair, made no distinctions between his subordinates and gave equal opportunities to all his colleagues. However, this praise and admiration from the celebratory articles stand in contrast with the personal recollections of his colleagues, who are somewhat more open and critical of Pelnář. They describe his treatment of his colleagues as paternalistic and somewhat authoritarian.

This chapter used the example of the Second Internal Clinic to demonstrate that a general hospital constituted a vibrant site of epistemic socialization. As head of the clinic, Pelnář wielded considerable power: with the support of his colleagues, he developed specific recruitment strategies of highly talented male and later also female students through informal methods, scrutiny and discreet favors. Pelnář's community focused above all on the advancement of medical treatment, though it often achieved it in a very arbitrary manner.

70 MUA AV ČR, AAV, f. Josef Pelnář, box 1, Sign. Ia, fols. 60–61. See also Vondráček, *Fantastické*, 241. Syllaba, *Vzpomínky*, 50.

Conclusion

Zdeněk Nebřenský

If one can speak of the emergence of medical modernity in Central Europe, as the individual chapters in this volume assume, its chronology and dynamics were decisive for distinguishing its specificities in comparison with established cases, such as those of the Great Britain or France. Scholars working with the idea of historical continuity may recall Henry VIII's confiscation of church property during the English Reformation and the French court reforms that restricted religious institutions. These sovereign acts placed the early modern church hospitals under secular control (for additional insight on this topic also see chapters by Kovács, Jakulis).[1] It seems that the changes in administration did not only affect the church hospitals. In Würzburg, the municipal hospital was conceived as a civic institution financed by a secular foundation. In the late seventeenth and the first half of the eighteenth century, the city's rulers from the rank of episcopate attempted to wrest control of the hospital from the town. Even though the local bishop failed, he established institutional provision only for the poor.

The factor often cited in connection with the structural adjustments in early modern hospitals, and encountered in the individual chapters of this volume, was new security concerns that shook the European continent. Many cities were inundated by a wave of vagrants and beggars coming from the countryside. The demand for charitable activities, including medical care, had increased dramatically. The provision of food, clothing and firewood on the premise that people would look after themselves and promote the welfare of the community often proved inadequate (for additional insight on this topic also see chapters by Pelzl, Kušniráková, Hajdinová, Nebřenský, Franaszek).[2] Buda became the capital of the Hungarian kingdom, which had a positive impact on the social and economic development of neighboring Pest on the other side of the Danube. In Brno, a large number of laborers arrived at the new factories emerging in the city. This workforce was repeatedly plagued by disease. As ecclesiastical bodies in Prague and Vilnius, plagued by financial

1 Lovejoy, The Hospital and Society, 545, 554. Thompson, Goldin, *Hospital,* 105–108. Risse, *Mending Bodies, Saving Souls,* 293–294. Lane, *A Social History of Medicine*, 82–83. Henderson, *The Impact of Hospitals*, 16.

2 Lovejoy, The Hospital and Society, 540–544. Bernard, The Limits of Absolutism, 196–198. Hartley, Philanthropy in the Reign of Catherine the Great, 168–171.

 HTTPS://DOI.ORG/10.1163/9789004755062-013

difficulties, were unable to bear the material burden, the rulers intervened vigorously. The hospitals were part of the poor relief and health care was an aspect of the rehabilitation of the poor. In Pest and Zagreb, these services had to be augmented by governmental and municipal monies, even if the operation of the hospitals, unlike the almshouses, could not be regarded as the responsibility of city administration (for additional insight on this topic also see chapters by Kušniráková, Hajdinová, Nebřenský, Jakulis, Franaszek).

According to the principles of cameralism, the poor were to become productive citizens in order to increase tax revenues. "Idle" people were brought into workshops; men were needed to provide soldiers and to settle the colonies. The monarchs of the Enlightenment sought to improve people's well-being and put their health under the official scrutiny. Hospitals were intended to help secure prosperity and increase the potential wealth of the state. The newly introduced medical police investigated inappropriate behavior and disciplined broad societal strata.[3] Similar to the court and municipal officials in Vienna, the authorities in Zagreb moved to push the beggars from the city and the province, the sick poor were registered and monitored. It was in the public interest to restore patients to health and fitness for work as quickly as possible. The convent hospitals and wards for the mentally ill in Prague and Brno played the role of confinement institutions and never ceased to do so. At the same time, the general hospitals in Vilnius and Kraków mainly admitted patients who, given the circumstances and the known therapeutic possibilities, had a chance of recovery or at least a significant improvement in their state of health (for additional insight on this topic also see chapters by Horbec, Hajdinová, Tinková, Nebřenský, Jakulis, Franaszek).

The income of the early modern hospitals came from a patchwork of occasional sources, supplemented by feudal rents. The caregiving institutions collected funds through various bequests and legacies. They also relied on foundations and voluntary contributions from better-off burghers. The running of such facilities remained vulnerable to fluctuating economic conditions and local crises in agriculture and handicraft production. The civic hospital in Würzburg lamented the "hard times" it had been experiencing for many years and blamed poor harvests and the resulting insolvency of the hospital's debtors and tenants for its plight. The economy of the hospital in Kraków (and Brno) was dependent on the yields of local agriculture, which meant

3 Lovejoy, The Hospital and Society, 554. Thompson, Goldin, *Hospital*, 109–113. Bernard, The Limits of Absolutism, 197. Frevert, *Krankheit als politisches Problem*. Ulbricht, The Debate about Foundling Hospitals, 211–214, 227–229. Hartley, Philanthropy in the Reign of Catherine the Great, 177–179.

that it was subject to the ups and downs of farming (for additional insight on this topic also see chapters by Pelzl, Franaszek). Rising prices and labor costs caused financial difficulties for the poorly run facilities. The health institution in Zagreb, Varaždin and Koprivnica suffered from a chronic lack of funds and the buildings could not be properly maintained. Private charitable donations steadily declined. The measures taken by the authorities in Vilnius in the form of tax exemptions and levies on consumption and lottery winnings proved to be insufficient (for additional insight on this topic also see chapters by Kušniráková, Hajdinová, Jakulis).

In most of the cities explored in the chapters of this collection, there were neither private funds nor wealthy merchants to establish and operate voluntary hospitals and larger private facilities. Market relations developed only slowly. In Prague and Pest, royal patronage dominated; nobles in Vilnius benefited from their support of humanist endeavors, which were presented to the public as a refuge for the worthy poor. Donors expected to be rewarded for their charitable deeds by grateful, pious residents. Most of the institutions in Crotian towns were small facilities with only a few beds staffed by religious caregivers (for additional insight on this topic also see chapters by Nebřenský, Franaszek).[4] Thanks to the generosity of noble men and women, who followed the example of the monarchs and invited the Augustinians, the Brothers Hospitallers of St. John of Good and the Sisters of Mercy to the provincial towns and parishes, the convent hospitals were built on the sites of former farmhouses and inns. The convents in Pest, Brno and Prague subsequently financed themselves from the interest on the endowments, from alms and from donations they received themselves, as the authorities regarded their hospitals as charitable rather than medical facilities, which was not justified (for additional insight on this topic also see chapters by Kušniráková, Hajdinová, Jakulis).

However, the sovereigns and their courtiers kept a watchful eye on the foundations and the assets of the charities. They raised the issue of centralization, which would lead to economic efficiency and financial self-sufficiency for the hospitals. In Prague, Brno and Vilnius, the foundations were dissolved, and their assets were redistributed to cover the running costs of the general hospitals, which had a complex infrastructure.[5] In the Croatian lands, the existing ecclesiastical and civic almshouses did not have rich endowments and their income was very low. Although the property of caregiving facilities in Pest and Zagreb was sold and the proceeds pooled with the money from the

4 Curtiss, Russian Sisters of Mercy, 84–100. Brooks, Reform in the Russian Army, 63–82.

5 Lovejoy, The Hospital and Society, 545, 554. Thompson, Goldin, *Hospital,* 105–108. Risse, *Mending Bodies, Saving Souls,* 293–294.

sale of other municipal assets, it was still not enough to build a new hospital. The construction of the hospitals was halted several times and dragged on for decades despite repeated fundraising campaigns. Without the support of the central authorities, the buildings were not completed, and the hospitals were not put into operation. As a result, the court officials took control of the hospital administration (for additional insight on this topic also see chapters by Kušniráková, Horbec).

Moreover, the reasons were not only economic, but also political. The government's decisions aimed at weakening the power of the former superiors over the religious communities and turning their members into state citizens. This was also seen as an extension of the new government's desire to assume the role of supreme benefactor responsible for alleviating the poor sick (for additional insight on this topic also see chapter by Jakulis).[6] The closure of caregiving facilities in Vilnius, Kraków or Brno and the transfer of their funds to new type hospitals went against the will of the benefactors. Links with certain churches and priests were cut and the role of hospitals in the cultural life of the city slowly declined. The sick poor who were housed in health facilities were isolated from the wider society, although they were previously expected to attend daily mass and participate in other ecclesiastical ceremonies. Laymen, who had previously been excluded from the decision-making process, because the field of healthcare was dominated by the (Catholic) clergy, were involved in the hospital administration (for additional insight on this topic also see chapter by Jakulis).

In the context of discussions about the gradual loss of influence of the ecclesiastical authorities on health care, the case of the hospital in Kraków is very interesting. There was no such fundamental break in the relationship between the Catholic Church and caregiving institutions. The initiator of the establishment of a new type of hospital there was the Primate together with the secular authorities. This was done at the expense of the foundations of the former church orders, but the Primate retained a decisive influence on the management of the hospital. The control and staff turnover of the hospital were entrusted to the Sisters of Mercy. While the battle over the hospital administration in the General Hospital in Vienna and elsewhere was fought between court-appointed officials and reform-minded doctors, in Kraków it took the form of disputes between the church representatives and the professors of the Medical Academy (for additional insight on this topic also see chapter by Franaszek).

6 Lane, *A Social History of Medicine*, 82–83. Henderson, Horden, Pastore, *The Impact of Hospitals*, 16.

In Prague, the religious orders endeavored to keep pace with secular challenges, entered into cooperation with the medical faculties at an early stage and converted the lecture hall in which students performed autopsies. Later, they promoted clinical teaching in surgery and provided beds for students of anatomy and internal medicine. In Valtice, sixty kilometers south of Brno, the Brothers of Mercy were even able to run a very old training facility for male nurses in the convent hospital. Some talented members of the order were able to both train at a medical school and working as physicians in the monastery. Educated members of the order were loyal servants of the state and the convent hospitals in Brno and Kraków also admitted secular patients (for additional insight on this topic also see chapters by Hajdinová, Nebřenský, Franaszek).

The Enlightenment reforms did not create a predictable and irreversible path to the secular hospital. The medical operation and, in part, the administration of the new hospital in Zagreb were entrusted to the Brothers of Mercy, who had been granted the right to care for the sick as part of their charitable work. The provincial authorities recognized these old rights and focused exclusively on the financial feasibility of maintaining the hospital. In Kraków, the Sisters of Mercy endeavored to reassert their influence over the hospital under the auspices of the newly established authorities. The Austrian administration withdrew control of the hospital from the Academy and placed it back under the management of the Sisters of Mercy. As the transfer of the general hospital to the Sisters of Mercy in Vilnius and the use of the Brothers of Mercy's premises to house the mentally ill in Brno due to lack of financial resources showed, the convent hospitals in the Habsburg Monarchy and the Russian Empire could not be replaced in institutional provision until the late nineteenth century (for additional insight on this topic also see chapters by Horbec, Nebřenský, Kovács, Jakulis).

Despite private foundations and the personal wealth of the rulers, the new hospitals became a heavy burden on the state treasury. The financial difficulties prompted the authorities to appoint their own directors, who were responsible for economic matters instead of the medical director. The institutions in Prague and Brno followed the example of the General Hospital in Vienna and the superintendent took on a crucial administrative position in the 1790s, while the chief provincial physician continued to formally manage the hospitals. In Zagreb, a special committee consisting of representatives of the authorities administered the hospital. In Vilnius, the committee for the supervision of the general hospital seemed more anchored in early modern corporate traditions. Although the episcopate dominated hospital administration for centuries, secular commissioners – doctors, professors, mayors and lower-level officials – were now mostly involved in supervision (Horbec, Tinková, Nebřenský, Jakulis).

Most hospitals in Central Europe were not self-supporting. Patrons from the provincial estates and additional income from the emperor enabled the facilities to remain solvent in the early years of their existence; without the help of the court, the hospitals could not survive. Many administrative powers were transferred to imperial and provincial authorities, who became responsible for the internal economy of the hospital, including the hiring of staff and the supply of food. Commissions even considered closing some hospitals, but the economic and logistical consequences of such a move and the lack of alternative facilities precluded this. Severe budget cuts were introduced which impacted on patient care, including reductions in nursing personnel and surgical assistants. The hospital dispensatory was overhauled, and hospital physicians were forced to limit their prescriptions to the items listed in these documents (for additional insight on this topic also see chapters by Hajdinová, Tinková, Jakulis).[7]

An important step was to regain control of hospital supplies, which had previously been provided by private contractors. Better timing of doctor' visits was intended to avoid conflicts between medical duties and the proper distribution of meals. Given its increased role, nutrition was placed under direct control, as food was to be brought in to reduce the cost of medicines and meagre rations jeopardized convalescence (for additional insight on this topic also see chapter by Nebřenský).[8] In the Habsburg Monarchy, the emphasis on food rationing was based on the statutes of the Vienna General Hospital, which were adopted by most provincial healthcare facilities and in which the daily food rations were precisely specified. In the Prague mental asylum, the daily bread rations were precisely measured, as food was an important part of the therapy. In the St. Anne's House in Brno, food for convalescents was to be bought on a budget. In Zagreb, nutrition consisted of two hot meals for lunch and one hot meal for dinner.

Due to the restrictions in medical education and within the healthcare community, the history of general hospitals and mental asylums in the Habsburg Monarchy and the former Polish-Lithuanian Commonwealth was not characterized by "organic development". During construction, both bureaucrats and doctors realized that care was not possible without trained specialists. Therefore, a process of preparation and (re)training was hastily initiated, with

7 Thompson, Goldin, *Hospital*, 109, 115. Risse, *Mending Bodies, Saving Souls*, 268.

8 Risse, Mending Bodies, *Saving Souls*, 265. Miller, Food, Medicine and Institutional Life, 200–219.

a mandate to learn about current European trends in hospital management and therapy. Prague was affected by the reforms in nearby Saxony, which had become one of the cradles of medical care in Central Europe. The person chosen to head the medical departments at the Leipzig university had an impact on the Prague environment. The Jesus Child Hospital in Paris was a model institution for many doctors in Vilnius. Some of them gained short-term work experience in Scottish, Lombard and Rhineland hospitals.

The subsequent reports of doctors and the resulting reform plans clearly show the uncertainties in the medical community regarding the feasibility of healthcare institutions based on humanity and science. Institutional provision of mentally disabled people in the Habsburg provinces was inspired by the Prague *Irrenanstalt*, but the political turmoil of 1848–1849 and the subsequent reprisals in the early 1850s brought the process to a complete standstill. From the mid-1850s, the reform of the asylums and the establishment of new psychiatric institutions could no longer be postponed, as the general consent to admit patients to the regional asylums was no longer respected and the existing infrastructure, such as smaller wards in public and convent hospitals, could no longer meet the needs of a growing number of patients.

For a long time, the central urban location was essential to the functioning of asylums, both practically and symbolically. It was common and prestigious for the planners of early public asylums to locate them in city centers, usually next to general infirmaries. Asylums were among the most prominent buildings in the town. Their architecture reflected the piety and mercy of the founders and later symbolized civic self-confidence. They were usually built on elevated ground, away from other dwellings, because it was believed that harmful fumes from within caused disease. The main windows faced south so patients could benefit from the healing power of sunlight. Proximity to a water course was important for the water supply and made waste disposal easier.[9] In Prague, negotiations on the construction of the new premises started in the late 1830s. The head of the *Irrenanstalt* who proposed the design, acquired the necessary permits and funds for the construction of a new building in the former convent garden, which was used by patients for occupational therapy. The Institute provided one-eighth of all psychiatric beds in the Habsburg Monarchy.

There was still a difference between the proposals of the medical circles, which were mainly represented by the heads of the medical departments, and those of the authorities in the Habsburg Monarchy. The doctors did not consider a mere increase in capacity to be a systematic solution. In their view, it

9 Risse, Mending Bodies, Saving Souls, 6–8.

would have been much more effective to establish specialized institutes and concentrate on care in the so-called pavilions. With later pavilion-type facilities, it was much easier to add smaller buildings or place them on the site. This type of facility could also be built and commissioned more flexibly to respond to current medical trends in Western Europe. However, the Viennese authorities rejected the pavilion-type hospital for financial and structural reasons. In Brno, the doctors had to work with the builders to mix elements of both building types and unite the hospital wings and individual wards under one roof.

The establishment of mental asylums and psychiatric wards had an impact on the perception of the mental ill in the individual Habsburg provinces. Admission to the psychiatric institutes placed certain demands on medical practitioners in smaller towns and rural areas: they were asked to watch out for persons whose behavior indicated a mental disorder, and if these people posed a danger to themselves or others, they were to assist in their hospitalization. They were also asked to take their medical history, which in practice meant talking to them with the aim to reconstruct their personal history. They could then perhaps try to categorize their undesirable behavior so that it fitted into one of the categories of 'insanity' defined by contemporary doctors. Later, a decree of the Ministry of the Interior came into force and general practitioners were obliged to register the mentally ill in their district, even those who were not under institutional care. In this way, the concept of insanity – or rather mental illness – began to enter the general discourse (for additional insight on this topic also see chapter by Tinková).

A decisive turning point for health institutions came in the early 1860s. While hospital administration in the Kingdom of Poland was restricted and, after the suppression of January Uprising, completely subordinated to the Russian imperial authorities, the general and psychiatric hospitals in the Habsburg Monarchy were taken over by the provincial bodies. This did not alter the fact that both powers attached paramount importance to public health facilities. Although, the hospitals in Galicia were the responsibility of the central officials, they were nevertheless delegated to the provincial governments and assemblies. This distinct dualism often proved conducive to dealing with complicated challenges, especially in times of epidemic threats. Moreover, the hospitals were never cut off from the local population, as their renovation showed. Medical and technical equipment was often imported from Western Europe, but most of the construction work was carried out by builders and craftsmen from the province. They joined forces to ensure the functioning of the facilities involved (for additional insight on this topic also see chapter by Franaszek).

In the late 1870s, the administration took responsibility for the health facilities at various levels, from the upper echelons, down to district representatives and municipal officials. Their operation was regulated by various ordinances, which stipulated that a public hospital could only be an institution whose sole purpose was to treat the sick. In theory, general hospitals were obliged to admit patients regardless of their religious affiliation, social background or place of residence. Religion was of particular importance, as the Galician hospitals had previously been allowed to refuse admission to the Jewish population, who had to seek medical care in facilities organized by themselves. The provincial administration recognized the incompatibility of this provision with the imperial laws on the equal rights for all inhabitants. A law was passed that ensured the admission of Jewish believers to the general hospitals under the same conditions as Christians, as was customary at the time in the healthcare institutions in Vienna, Prague and Brno (for additional insight on this topic also see chapters by Nebřenský, Franaszek).

The meetings of the provincial authorities mainly discussed topics related to the containment of infectious diseases, the promotion of medical personnel, the organizational challenges in the healthcare, and the financial difficulties of hospitals, especially in the construction of new ones. Hospitals were so overcrowded that they could not even provide adequate care for the people who had residential status in the particular municipality. Persons from different regional and social backgrounds could be treated on the recommendation of the parish priest and the district doctor. Later, patients with no fixed abode were also admitted if a respected citizen vouched for their treatment and paid for it. From the establishment of the General Hospital in Vienna, patients were divided into four classes who paid hospital fees according to the rates set by the provincial authorities. The comprehensive financial responsibility for the treatment of impoverished inhabitants lay entirely with the (lack of) provincial budget (for additional insight on this topic also see chapter by Franaszek).

For the successful establishment of a hospital, it was necessary for charitable individuals to take the initiative. The Habsburg Monarchy and the Russian Empire did not have a surplus of capital that would have allowed a group of entrepreneurs to raise and invest funds as a corporate entity or trust. Examples of factory hospitals in industrial cities, established under pressure from the imperial and provincial authorities showed that the business class was able to raise the money to build and operate hospitals for the short-term benefit of their employees (for additional insight on this topic also see chapter by Franaszek).[10] Over time, the interest from the money invested in the new hospital foundations contributed less and less to the running of the hospitals. They ran

10 Nebřenský, *Katedrály industriálního věku*, 140–141. Nebřenský, Herc. Empire in the Cottage, 107. Nebřenský, The Civil Service in the Factory, 132–137.

deficits and had to cut back on services time and again. State health policy threw the hospitals a lifeline and corporate sickness funds had to be forcibly set up for both white and blue-collar workers.[11] Although they were formally private hospitals, some of them also received financial support from the provincial budget and later from public health insurance funds (for additional insight on this topic also see chapter by Franaszek).

In examining health policy, funding, hospital administration, and the epistemic community, factors that contributed to the emergence of medical modernity, this volume shows that healthcare facilities in Central Europe were not fundamentally different from those in Western Europe. Public hospitals evolved from early modern models that could be rebuilt on a large scale. They offered a reference point, a model that successors could imitate and adapt. More immediate practical precedents were provided by the new general hospitals, funded by public subscription that were established in the wake of the voluntary hospital movement in the main provincial towns.[12] The voluntary hospitals that were widespread in England and Scotland did not exist in the Habsburg Monarchy and the Russian Empire. As in France, the Netherlands, Belgium and Germany, hospitals in Central Europe were mostly set up and administered by state, provincial and municipal authorities. The convent hospitals run by the church remained very important, especially for the care of long-term patients. Prague, Pest and Kraków benefited in the design of modern hospitals and their treatment from the fact that they were provincial capitals and centers for the mobilization of national movements. In addition, Vilnius and Brno were also production and transportation hubs, which further strengthened their position nationwide (for additional insight on this topic also see chapters by Kušniráková, Hajdinová, Tinková, Nebřenský, Jakulis, Franaszek).

Western and Central Europe differed in the temporal and geographical embedding of these factors. While the adjustments in health policy and hospital administration took place more or less simultaneously, modern hospital layout and treatment were applied unevenly and became established in different parts of Central Europe with a certain time lag. Moreover, they encountered not only political obstacles but also economic constraints. The provincial authorities complained about the lack of financial resources. The level of the monarch's support depended on the political importance and population of the city and did not necessarily reach all healthcare facilities. This assistance

11 Cf. Vogel, *The Transformation of the American Hospital*, 42–43. See also Snow, The Kokovtsov Commission, 780–796.

12 Smith, The architecture of confinement, 41–61, here 42.

also reflected the connections of the provincial representatives to the court circles. Although the provincial government tried to follow the official health policy, the people in the province asserted their own interests at the expense of imperial projects, such as the construction of a new hospital.

Before there was a public consensus on the importance of building a hospital, the authorities haggled with the provincial estates for every gulden. The general hospital in Zagreb and elsewhere was only opened after respected individuals were convinced and willing to spend more of their money on healthcare. After the economic crisis subsided in the 1890s, the consequences of provincial self-government in the Habsburg Monarchy became clear. The tightening of budgets due to the introduction of public health insurance and the cheapening of building materials had an impact on the design of hospitals. In Kraków and Zagreb, new buildings were constructed for specialized medical departments in which the latest medical knowledge was applied (for additional insight on this topic also see chapters by Horbec, Franaszek).[13]

The volume indicates that medical communities in Central Europe were familiar with Western medical knowledge and practices. However, this did not mean that the doctors accepted them without reservation. In some places, such as Hungary and Croatia, there were not enough professionals. In Bohemia, Moravia and Galicia, doctors had imposed modern treatment based on the clinical experience they had gained working in hospitals. Adjustments in medical treatment could not be introduced immediately, but they were adapted to institutional settings. Despite the proclaimed openness to Western modernity, the staff in the Central European hospitals had to respect established official and professional procedures. Even when some of the doctors became heads of hospital departments, they came up against boundaries established by authorities and colleagues when modifying treatment. Sometimes it was easier to change the treatment and set-up of the provincial hospitals. These institutions served as experimental fields from which enlightened doctors came to the hospitals in the heart of the empire. In fact, the history of these institutions, as detailed in this volume, highlights that Central Europe developed a degree of distinctiveness in terms of the emergence of medical modernity in comparison with Western models. The volume demonstrates that instead of applying diffusionist frameworks for understanding the history of hospitals in Europe, one should rather compare and historicize the different provinces of health care on the continent, from Western to Central, from Eastern to Southern Europe.

13 Nebřenský, *Katedrály industriálního věku*, 154–155.

Bibliography

Archival Sources

Archive of Charles University

Verzeichnis der ordentlichen und außerordentlichen Vorlesungen, welche an der Universität zu Prag gehalten werden, box 89, 90.

Austrian State Archives, Vienna

Finanz- und Hofkammerarchiv, Ungarisches Kamerale

Croatian State Archives, Zagreb

HDA-1 (Croatian-Slavonian Parliament)

HDA-12 (Croatian Royal Council)

HDA-34 (Zagreb County)

HDA-430 (Generalate of Slavonia)

Magyar Nemzeti Levéltár Országos Levéltára [National Archives of Hungary, Central Archives]

C 66 Helytartótanácsi Levéltár [Archives of the Locumtenential Council], Departamentum sanitatis

D 210 Magyar Királyi Helytartótanács [Locumtenential Council] XX. Közegészségügyi Osztály [Department of Public Health]

D 217 Magyar Királyi Helytartótanács [Locumtenential Council] IV. Egészségügyi kútfő [Medical records]

H 1848/1849-i Levéltár [Archives of the 1848/1849 Ministries] 52 Egészségügyi Osztály [Department of Health]

K 150 Belügyminisztériumi levéltár [Archives of the Ministry of the Interior], Általános iratok [General documents]

Masarykův ústav a Archiv Akademie věd České republiky [Masaryk Institute and Archive of the Czech Academy of Sciences]

387 – Josef Pelnář.

Moravský zemský archiv [Moravian Provincial Archive].

A8 – Zemská registratura

A9 – Zemský výbor

A45 – Zemský ústav pro choromyslné

E45 – Milosrdní Bratři Brno

Národní archiv [National Archive] – Prague
Department I, fonds České gubernium – Publicum [Czech Gubernium – Publicum].
Chodovec branch, fonds Zemský ústav pro choromyslné Praha [Provincial Mental Asylum]
Fonds Konvent Milosrdní bratři Praha [Convent of the Brothers of Mercy, Prague-further as KMB Praha], books 104, 115, 529, 533, 534, box 155–156
Fonds Archiv konventu alžbětinek v Praze 1719 –1948(1949) [Archive of the Convent of Sisters of St Elizabeth, Prague – AKA Praha], books 25–26, box 4
Fonds České gubernium, Zemský protomedikát, 1775–1863 [Czech Gubernium, Provincial Protomedicate], boxes 7, 17
Fonds Archiv pražského arcibiskupství II [Archives of the Prague Archbishopric – APA II], sign X: box 59, 1364, 1428

Österreichisches Staatsarchiv, Haus-, Hof- und Staatsarchiv, Kabinettsarchiv, Staatsrat

Haus A – Hofreisen, Sign. 44–1-103

Österreichisches Staatsarchiv, Allgemeines Verwaltungsarchiv, Unterricht und Kultus, Studienhofkommission Akten Teil 2
Semmelweis Orvostörténeti Múzeum, Könyvtár és Levéltár [Semmelweis Medical History Museum, Library, and Archives]
I. Magyar Orvosok és Természetvizsgálók Vándorgyűlései [Society of Hungarian Physicians and Naturalists]
I. Budapesti Királyi Orvosegyesület [Royal Budapest Society of Physicians]

Stadtarchiv Würzburg
Archiv des Bürgerspitals

State Archives of the Hungarian National Archives, Budapest
C-66 (Hungarian Lieutenancy Council, Departamentum sanitatis)

Printed Primary Sources

Bayer, Thaddäus von. *Beschreibung der öffentlichen Armen-Versorgungsanstalten in der könliglichen Hauptstadt Prag,* Prag (printer not listed), 1793.

Bene, Ferenc. A lélekgyógytan (psychiatria) köréből szedett vázlatok. In: Halász, G. (ed.): *A Magyar Orvosok és Természetvizsgálók 1847. augusztus 11–17. Sopronban tartott VIII. nagygyűlésének történeti vázlata és munkálatai,* 79–85. Pest: Nyomtatott Emich Gusztáv M. Akad nyomdásznál, 1863.

Bernt, Joseph. *Systematisches Handbuch des Medicinal-Wesens nach den k. k. Österreichischen Medicinalgesetzen* (Wien 1819), (DFG-Viewer: Systematisches Handbuch des Medicinal-Wesens [Medizinalwesens], Access 11 July 2024).

Bittner, Imre. *Eszmék a közorvostan szabályozására Magyarországban.* Pest: Trattner, 1848.

Boener, Johann Alexander. *Nürnbergische Kleider-Trachten, der Manns- und Weibs-Personen, denen zu mehrerer Ergötzung und Beygefüget sind etliche der vornehmsten Plätze und Gebäude in und an der Stadt, wie auch der Grund-Rieß und doppelter Prospect Derselbigen.* Nuremberg, 1689.

Bolyó, Károly. Elmebetegeinket küldjük kellő időben jól szervezett tébolydába, ha sikert ohajtunk. *Gyógyászat* 2/36 (1862): 741–743.

Bolyó, Károly. Utazási napló-töredékek. (Folytatás). Bolyó Károly tr. a budai tébolyda másodorvosátol. *Gyógyászat* 2/35 (1862): 724–727.

Bolyó, Károly. Utazási napló-töredékek. Bolyó Károly tr. a budai tébolyda másodorvosátol. (Folytatás.) *Gyógyászat* 2/37 (1862): 765–768.

Bolyó, Károly. Utazási napló-töredékek. Bolyó Károly tr. budai őrüldei m. orvostol. *Gyógyászat* 2/2 (1862): 43–46.

Bolyó, Károly. Miként lehetne hazánk szegénysorsu elmebetegeit jutányosan s gyógyápolási szempontból czélszerün elhelyezni? In: Kanka, K. – Rómer, F. (eds.): *A Magyar Orvosok és Természetvizsgálók 1865. Augustus 28-tól September 2-ig Pozsonyban tartott XI. Nagygyülésének történeti vázlata s munkálatai.* Pozsony: [s. n.] (1866).

Bolyó, Károly. Az elmebetegek társas élete és ennek erkölcsi gyógyelőnye jól rendezett tébolydák körében. *Orvosi Hetilap* 12 No. 2 (1868): 25–30.

Bouček, František. *Zápisky praktického lékaře dr. Františka Boučka 1841–1880,* Poděbrady: Bohumil Bouček, 1901.

Brdlík, Jiří. *Padesát let dětským lékařem.* Praha: SZdN, 1961.

Brodowicz, Józef. *Rys Historyczny Zakładów Klinicznych przy Uniwersytecie Jagiellońskim przez Profes. Dra Józefa Brodowicza. Dyrektora Kliniki lekarskiej.* Kraków w drukarni Uniwersyteckiéj 1845.

Bugát, Pál. Őrjintézet Pesten. *Orvosi Tár* 6/25 (1841): 399–400.

Časopis lékařů českých, 1942–1962.

Charvát, Josef. *Můj labyrint světa,* Prague: Galén, 2005.

Chyzer, Kornél. *A Magyar Orvosok és Természetvizsgálók Vándorgyűléseinek története 1840–től 1890–ig.* Sátoraljaújhely: Zemplén Nyomda, 1890.

Csorba, József. *Észrevételek az álladalmi egésség' rendezéséről hazánkban.* Pécs: nyomatott a lyceumi nyomdában, 1848.

Czermak, Josef. Die mährische Landen-Irrenanstalt bei Brünn, ihre bauliche Einrichtung, Administration, ärztliche Gebahrung und Statistik, Wien: K. Czermak, 1866.

Damerow, Heinrich. 'Einleitung: Probleme bei der Gründung der Zeitschrift und Übersicht zum Stand der Psychiatrie (national und international)'. *Allgemeine Zeitschrift für Psychiatrie* 1 (1844): I–XLVIII.

De Deo Sobel, Johannes. *Geschichte und Festschrift der österr.-böhm. Ordens-Provinz der Barmherzigen Brüder*. Vienna: Barmherzigen Brüder, 1892.

Deyl, Zdeněk, *Die Deutsche Karl-Ferdinands-Universität in Prag unter der Regierung Seiner Majestät des Kaisers Franz Josef I.*, Prag: Verlag der J.G. Calve'schen k.u.k. Hof- u. Universitätsbuchhandlung (Josef Koch), 1899.

Einholm, Elias. *Organizacya dla szpitala generalnego wilenskiego*. Wilno: w Drukarni Akademickiey, 1800.

d'Elvert, Christian. *Geschichte der Heil- und Humanitats-Anstalten in Mähren und Oesterr. Schlesien* (Brünn 1858).

Esze, Gábor. Az elmekórházakról. *Orvosi Tár* 3 No. 1 (1844): 11–13.

Fischel, Jakob. 'Aus dem Berichte über die k. k. Irrenanstalt zu Prag für die Jahr 1846, 1847, 1848, 1849 und 1850'. *Allgemeine Zeitschrift für Psychiatrie* 9 (1852): 62–79.

Fischel, Jakob. *Prags k. k. Irrenanstalt und ihr Wirken seit ihrem Entstehen*, Erlangen: Verlag von Ferdinand Enke, 1853.

Frank, Johann P. *Ankündigung des klinischen Instituts zu Göttingen* (…). Göttingen: Johann Christian Dieterich, 1784. Available at https://iiif.wellcomecollection.org/pdf/b21364138, (Accessed 8 Nov. 2023).

Grósz, Lipót. *Emlékirat a hazai betegápolási ügy keletkezése, fejlődése, s jelenlegi állásáról, különös tekintettel a betegápolási költségekre*. Buda: A Magyar Királyi Tudom. Egyetemi Nyomdából, 1869.

Haas, Hermann. *Das Krankenmaterial des Spitals der Barmherzigen Brüder zu Prag vom Jahre 1670 bis auf unsere Zeit mit besonderer Berücksichtigung der Variola*. Prague: H. Dominicus, 1882.

Haffner, Michael. *Versuch eines Vorschlages an dem löblichen Magistrat und das Publicum der königlichen Freystadt Pest zur Errichtung, Einrichtung, und Unterhaltung eines zweckmäßigen Krankenspitales*, Pesth: [s. n.], 1793.

Haffner, Mihály. *Szabad királyi Pest városa neme tanátsának és közönségének szólló projectum egy alkalmatos Beteyek Ispotályának fol állításáro*. Pest: [s. n.], 1793.

Heinroth, Johann Christian. *Lehrbuch der Störungen des Seelenlebens oder der Seelenstörungen und ihrer Behandlung*. Leipzig: Vogel, 1818.

Held, Johann Theobald. *Kurze Geschichte der Heilanstalt der Barmherzigen Brüder in Prag: nebst Rückblicken auf Entstehung, Verbreitung und Schicksale dieses Ordens überhaupt zum besten dieser Anstalt herausgegeben von deren Physikus Johann Theobald Held*. Prague: Gottlieb Haase, 1823.

Held, Jan Theobald. *Jan Theobald Held, Fakta a poznámky k mému budoucímu nekrologu I: vzpomínky pražského lékaře na léta 1770–1799* [Jan Theobald Held. Facts and notes for my future obituary. Part I: Memoirs of a Prague physician, 1770–1799], ed. by Jindřich Květ and Daniela Tinková. Prague: Academia, 2017.

Hőgyes, Endre. *Emlékkönyv a Budapesti Királyi Magyar Tudomány Egyetem Orvosi Karának multjáról és jelenéről*. Budapest: Az Athenaeum részvénytársulat könyvnyomdája, 1896.

Jakubowski, Maciej L. *Szpital św. Ludwika dla dzieci w Krakowie. Jego powstanie, rozwój i działalność dziesięcioletnia 1876–1885* (*St. Louis Children's Hospital in Krakow: Its Establishment, Development, and Ten-Year Activity 1876–1885*). Kraków: Czas Press, 1886.

John, Johann Dionys. *Lexikon der K. K. Medizinalgese[t]ze: T–Z: Nebst der systematischen und chronologischen Uebersicht des ganzen Werkes*. Part 4. Prague: Johann Gottfried Calve, 1791, 271–272.

Kasparek, Jan Rudolf. *Zbiór ustaw administracyjnych w Królestwie Galicji i Lodomerii z Wielkim Księstwem Krakowskim* (*The Compilation of Administrative Statutes in the Kingdom of Galicia and Lodomeria with the Grand Duchy of Krakow*). Kraków: Wydawnictwo Uniwersytetu Jagiellońskiego, 1868.

Kneidl Cyrill. Péče o choromyslné na Moravě. *Časopis lékařů českých*, 42/51 (1903): 1307–1309.

Knörlein, Anton. *Die Irren-Angelegenheiten Ober-Oesterreichs* (Linz 1851).

Knörlein, Anton. *Kurzgefasste Geschichte der Heilanstalten und des Medicinalwesen in Linz*, Linz, 1885.

Kopetz, Wenzel Gust. *Österreichische politische Gesetzkunde, oder systematische Darstellung der politischen Verwaltung in den deutschen, böhmischen und galizischen Provinzen des österreichischen Kaiserthumes*, Wien, 1819.

Kossakowski, Jan Nepomucen. "Kazanie Jana Nepomucena Korwina Kossakowskiego, biskupa wileńskiego przy otwarciu nowego szpitala wileńskiego SS. Filipa i Jakuba dnia 16 czerwca roku 1799 miane." In *Kazania świąteczne i przygodne z rękopismow wydrukowane*, 418–32. Wilno: w Drukarni Dyecezalney, przy kościele świętego Kazimierza zgromadzenia XX. Missionarzów, 1824.

Kossakowski, Jan Nepomucen. "Kazanie Jana Nepomucena Kossakowskiego, biskupa wileńskiego przy poświęceniu cmentarza Swiętego Szczepana wWilnie dnia 6 lipca roku 1795 miane." In *Kazania świąteczne i przygodne z rękopismow wydrukowane*, 433–48. Wilno: w Drukarni Dyecezalney, przy kościele świętego Kazimierza zgromadzenia XX. Missionarzów, 1824.

Kovács, Sebestény Endre. *Javaslat az álladalmi közegészség és az orvosi ügy rendezéséről hazánkban*. Pest: Landerer & Heckenast, 1848.

Kurczewski, Jan. *Biskupstwo wileńskie: od jego założenia aż do dni obecnych, zawierające dzieje i prace biskupów i duchowieństwa diecezji wileńskiej, oraz wykaz kościołów, klasztorów, szkół i zakładów dobroczynnych i społecznych*. Wilno: Nakładem i drukiem Józefa Zawadzkiego, 1912.

Linhartová, Věra. *Jan Bělehrádek a jeho cesta k svobodě ducha*, Prague: Galén, 2003.

Linzbauer, Franciscus Xaver. *Codex sanitario-medicinalis Hungariae*. Tomus II. Budae: Typis Caesareo-regiae scientiarum universitatis, 1852.

Linzbauer, Franciscus Xaver. *Codex Sanitario-Medicinalis Hungariae*, Tomus III, Sectio I. Budae: Typis Caesareo-Regiae Scientiarum Universitatis, 1853.

Linzbauer, Franciscus Xaver. *Codex Sanitario-Medicinalis Hungariae*, Tomus III, Sectio II. Budae: Typis Caesareo-Regiae Scientiarum Universitatis, 1855.

Linzbauer, Franciscus Xaver. *Codex Sanitario-Medicinalis Hungariae,* Tomus III, Sectio III. Budae: Typis Caesareo-Regiae Scientiarum Universitatis, 1860.

Linzbauer, Franciscus Xaver. *A magyar korona országainak nemzetközi egésségügye. Az egyes igazgatási tárgyak fejlődésének történetével – hivatalos adatok nyomán.* Pesten: Kugler Adolf könyvkereskedő bizományában, 1868.

Mařatka, Zdeněk. *Medicína, umění a život v osmi politických režimech,* Prague: Karolinum, 1997.

Mařatka, Zdeněk and Hlaváčková, Ludmila. *Josef Pelnář (1872–1964): osobnost a dílo,* Karolinum: Praha, 2000.

Matoušek, Josef. Vzrůst počtu choromyslných na Moravě a jeho příčiny. *Revue v neuropsychopathologii, therapii, veřejné hygieně a lékařství sociálním* 3/2 (1906): 80–81.

Matoušek, Josef. Vzrůst počtu choromyslných na Moravě a jeho příčiny (dokončení), *Revue v neuropsychopathologii, therapii, veřejné hygiene a lékařství sociálním* 3/3 (1906), 131–134.

Mazzura. Šime. *Javna bolnica na Jelačićevu trgu u Zagrebu. Izvješće na Gradsko poglavarstvo* [1891] [The Public Hospital on Jelačić Square in Zagreb: Report to the City Council] (Zagreb, 1909).

Moravský zemský ústav pro choromyslné u Brna. *Časopis lékařů českých* 5, 1866, č. 38, s. 304.

Moravský zemský ústav pro choromyslné u Brna. *Časopis lékařů českých* 5, 1866, č. 39, s. 311–312.

Moravský zemský ústav pro choromyslné u Brna. *Časopis lékařů českých* 5, 1866, č. 40, s. 319–320.

Neue Courier aus Ungarn, No. 9, 19 January 1799.

N. N. Viszánik külföldön. *Orvosi Tár* 7, No. 3 (1843): 125–126.

Nowak, Aloys. *Notizen über die Prager k. u. k. Irrenanstalt und die Veränderungen in derselben,* Prague 1835.

Otto Hassmann, Otto. 'Die steiermärkische Landes-Irren-Heil- und Pflege-Anstalt "Feldhof"', In *Die Irrenpflege in Österreich in Wort und Bild,* ed. Heinrich Schlöss, 297–301. Halle: Marhold, 1912.

Pándy, Kálmán. *Gondoskodás az elmebetegekről más államokban és nálunk.* Gyula: Corvina, 1905.

Pándy, Kálmán. *Emlékkönyv a nagyszebeni m. k. állami elmegyógyintézet ötven éves fennállásának évfordulójára.* Nagyszeben: Nyomatott Haiser György könyvnyomdájában, 1914.

Preininger, Vladimír. *Sbírka zákonů a nařízení o zdravotnictví se zvláštním zřetelem na země koruny české.* Praha, 1900.

Provinzialnachrichten aus den k. k. Staaten, 58, 21 July 1784, 172.

Purjesz, Ignaz. *Beiträge zur Geschichte der Gründung des Sankt-Rochusspitals im XVIII. Jahrhundert.* Budapest: 1914.

Puschmann Theodor. *Die Medizin in Wien während der letzten 100 Jahre.* Wien 1884.

Riedel, Josef Gottfried. *Erfahrungen über die Wirksamkeit der versendeten karlsbader Mineral-Wässer.* Karlsbad: Gebr. Franieck, 1843.

Riedel, Josef Gottfried. *Prag's Irrenanstalt und Ihre Leistungen*, Prague: Gedruckt in der Sommerschen Buchdruckerei, 1830.

Riedel, Josef Gottfried. *Ärztliche Berichte über die kaiserlich-königliche Irren-Heil- und Pflegeanstalt zu Wien in den Jahren 1852, 1854, 1855 und 1856.* Wien: Aus der K. K. Hof- und Staatsdruckerei, 1858.

Rostafiński, Józef. *Kraków pod względem lekarsko-przyrodniczym* (*Krakow in the Context of Medical and Natural Sciences*). Kraków: Czas Press, 1900.

Rozsay, Joseph. Das Pester städtische Versorgungshaus Elisabethineum. Ein geschichtlicher Rückblick auf das Entstehen dieser Anstalt, sammt einem ausführlichen Ausweise über die Leistungen derselben im Verwaltungsjahre 1855/56. Pest 1857.

Sámuel, Alois. Das Pesther Krankenhaus zu St. Rochus. In *Gemeinnützige Blätter zur Belehrung und Unterhaltung*, 30, n. 7, 21.1.1840, 30.

Schäffner, Joseph A. *Geschichte des Ordens und der Heilanstalt des Elisabethiner – Klosterfrauen in Prag.* Prague: Druck der fürsterzbischöflichen Buchdruckerei, 1845.

Stadler, Antal. A pesti polgári kórház. *Orvosi Tár*, No. 22 (1840): 340–344.

Stráner, Katalin. Város és tudomány. A Magyar Orvosok és Természetvizsgálók Vándorgyűlései Pesten, Budán és Budapesten (1841–1896). *Korall Társadalomtörténeti Folyóirat* (74): 93–113.

Syllaba, Jiří. *Vzpomínky a úvahy lékaře*, Prague: Avicenum, 1992.

Supplementum Codicis Austriaci, oder Chronologische Sammlung aller vom 1-ten Jänner 1759 bis letzten Dezember 1770 erlassenen Generalien, Patenten, Satzordnungen, Rescripten, Resolutionen, dann Landesobrichkeitlichen Edikten, Mandaten und Dekreten, Part VI. Wien, 1777.

Szabad Királyi Pest Város "Szent Rókus" polgári kórháza részére 1842. és 1868. évek között kiadott alapszabályok és szolgálati utasítások. [Pest] : [s.n.], [1842-1868].

Tekieliński, Władysław, ed. *Opis dzienny szkół wileńskich Akademii i Uniwersytetu oraz Diarjusz znaczniejszych wypadków w Wilnie od r. 1781 po rok 1824 nastałych.* Wilno: Drukiem Józefa Blumowicza, 1876.

Thomayer, Josef. *Ze zápisků lékaře*, Praha: Avicenum, 1977.

Töltényi, Szaniszló. Közlemények Töltényi Szaniszló cs. kir. tanácsos s bécsi egyetemi tanár utazási naplójából. (I-ső Értekezés.) A vezelési rendszerről. (Poenitantiarsystem). *Orvosi Tár* 3/22 (1844): 337–345.

Töltényi, Szaniszló. Közlemények Töltényi Szaniszló cs. kir. tanácsos s bécsi egyetemi tanár utazási naplójából. A vezeklési rendszerről. (Vége.) *Orvosi Tár* 3/23 (1844): 354–362.

Töltényi, Szaniszló. Közlemények Töltényi Szaniszló cs. kir. tanácsos s bécsi egyetemi tanár utazási naplójából. (II-dik értekezés). Az elmekórosok ápolási rendszeréről. *Orvosi Tár* 3/1 (1845): 2–8.

Töltényi, Szaniszló. Közlemények Töltényi Szaniszló cs. kir. tanácsos s bécsi egyetemi tanár utazási naplójából. Az elmekórosok ápolási rendszeréről. *Orvosi Tár* 3/2 (1845): 17–26.

Töltényi, Szaniszló. Közlemények Töltényi Szaniszló cs. kir. tanácsos s bécsi egyetemi tanár utazási naplójából. (III-dik értekezés). Az elmekórosok ápolásbani nevelési rendszerről. *Orvosi Tár* 3/15 (1845): 226–223.

Töltényi, Szaniszló. Közlemények Töltényi Szaniszló cs. kir. tanácsos s bécsi egyetemi tanár utazási naplójából. (III-dik értekezés). Az elmekórosok ápolásbani nevelési rendszerről. Vége. *Orvosi Tár* 3/16 (1845): 242–248.

Töltényi, Szaniszló. Közlemények Töltényi Szaniszló cs. kir. tanácsos s bécsi egyetemi tanár utazási naplójából. (IV-dik értekezés.) A buzditó rendszerről. *Orvosi Tár* 3/24 (1845): 370–377.

Topographia Nesocomii et Ptochotrophii Regio-Civilis Pestani ad Sanctum Rochum. [Pest]: [s.n.], 1798.

Ústav dějin Univerzity Karlovy a archiv Univerzity Karlovy, Matriky Univerzity Karlovy, Matriky doktorů, Inv. č. 1 Matrika doktorů české Karlo-Ferdinandovy univerzity I. (1882–1900) s. 1–589.

Ústav dějin Univerzity Karlovy a archiv Univerzity Karlovy, Matriky Německé univerzity v Praze, Matriky doktorů, Inv. č. 2 Matrika doktorů německé Karlo-Ferdinandovy univerzity v Praze (1892–1904) s. 1–370.

Viszánik, Michael. *Die Irrenheil- und Pflegeanstalten Deutschlands, Frankreichs, sammt der Cretinen Anstalt auf dem Abendberge in der Schweiz: mit eigenen Bemerkungen.* Wien: Druck und Verlag von Carl Gerold, 1845.

Viszánik, Michael. *Leistungen und Statistik der k. k. Irrenheilanstalt in Wien seit ihrer Gründung 1784 bis 1844.* Wien: Im Verlage von Mörschner's Witwe und W. Bianchi, 1845.

Volumina Legum, VIII. Petersburg: Nakładem i drukiem Jozafata Ohryzki, 1860.

Vondráček, Vladimír. *Lékař vzpomíná (1920–1938)*, Prague: Avicenum, 1973.

Vondráček. *Lékař dále vzpomíná (1920–1938)*, Praha: Avicenum, 1978.

Vondráček. *Konec vzpomínání (1938–1945)*, Prague: Avicenum, 1988.

Vondráček. *Fantastické a magické vzpomínání*, Praha: Colombus, 2014.

Weiß, Karl. *Geschichte der öffentlichen Anstalten, Fonde und Stiftungen für die Armenversorgung in Wien.* Wien, 1867. (Geschichte der öffentlichen Anstalten, Fonde und Stiftungen für die … – Karl Weiss – Knihy Google, 10 July 2024).

Weitenweber, Rudolf. *Die medicinischen Anstalten Prags.* Prague: Borrosch & André, 1845.

Wiener Zeitung, No. 58 (21. July 1784): 10–11. No. 59. (24 July 1784), 10–12. No. 60 (28 July 1784).

Windisch, Leopold. *Gründliche Darstellung der Einrichtung des bürgerlichen Krankenhauses in der königl. Freystadt Pesth.* Pesth 1829.

Wölfler, Bernhard. *Das alte und neue Wiener Israeliten-Spital nach authentischen Quellen dargestellt.* Wien, 1873.
"Z Wilna V. S. 8 N. S. 19 Czerwca." *Kuryer Litewski*, June 19, 1799.

Secondary Sources

Ackerknecht, Erwin Heinz. *La médecine hospitalière à Paris (1794–1848).* Paris: Payot, 1967.
Ackerknecht, Erwin H. *Medicine at the Paris Hospital, 1794–1848.* Baltimore: The John Hopkins University Press 1967.
Aderbauer, Herbert. *Vom Pfründnerheim zur Arbeits- und Armenanstalt. Das Tübinger Spital und der Wandel seiner sozialen Funktion in der Frühen Neuzeit.* Tübingen: Wbg Theiss in Wissenschaftliche Buchgesellschaft, 1996.
Altın, Burçak Özlüdil. *Psychiatry, Space, and Time: Case of an Ottoman Asylum. In Journal of the Ottoman and Turkish Studies Association* 1 (2018): 67–89.
Andriušis, Aurimas and Tadeusz Srogosz. "Litewska administracja opieki społecznej (szpitalnej) na przełomie w. XVIII i XIX." *Biuletyn Instytutu Filozoficzno-Historycznego WSP w Częstochowie* 15, no. 5 (1998): 29–31.
Ankele, Monika. *Alltag und Aneignung in Psychiatrien um 1900. Selbstzeugnisse von Frauen aus der Sammlung Prinzhorn.* Wien, Köln, Weimar, Böhlau, 2009.
Ansari, Emily Abrams. Shaping the Policies of Cold War Musical Diplomacy: An Epistemic Community of American Composers, *Diplomatic History* 1/36 (2012), 41–52.
Arndt, Agnes. Pahl, Kerstin Maria. *Capitalist Cold. Emotions and the Economy in Europe and the United States.* London, Routledge, 2025.
Bach, Otto. '*Die "Heil- und Pflegeanstalt Sonnenstein"', Ärzteblatt Sachsen* 6 (2010): 288–290. https://www.aerzteblatt-sachsen.de/pdf/sax10_288.pdf (accessed 23 August 2023).
Balázs Peter *Generale Normativum in Re Sanitatis 1770. Orvosok, sebészmesterek, patikusok, bábák, és a járványügy a XVIII. század magyar jogalkotásában* [Doctors, surgeons, pharmacists, midwives, and epidemiology in 18th-century Hungarian legislation]. Piliscsaba-Budapest, 2004.
Bazala Vladimir, *Poviestni razvoj medicine u hrvatskim zemljama* [The historical development of medicine in Croatian lands]. Zagreb, 1943.
Bęczkowska, Urszula. "Gmach kliniczny przy ul. Kopernika 7 (1827, 1840–1843)" ("The-Clinical Edifice at 7 Kopernika Street (1827, 1840–1843)". In *Kliniki i zakłady teoretyczne. Collegium Medicum Uniwersytetu Jagiellońskiego w krakowskiej dzielnicy Wesoła. Gmachy i ludzie* (*Clinics and Theoretical Departments: Collegium Medicum of Jagiellonian University in the Wesoła District of Krakow. Buildings and People*), edited by Piotr Franaszek, 45–60. Kraków: Księgarnia Akademicka, 2016.

Bęczkowska, Urszula. "Rozbudowa szpitala powszechnego św. Łazarza przy ul. Kopernika 17, 19, 21A (1871–1879) oraz wzniesienie szpitala św. Ludwika przy ul. Strzeleckiej 2 (1874–1876)" ("The Expansion of St. Lazarus General Hospital at 17, 19, 21A Kopernika Street (1871–1879) and the Establishment of St. Louis Hospital at 2 Strzelecka Street (1874–1876)") In *Kliniki i zakłady teoretyczne. Collegium Medicum Uniwersytetu Jagiellońskiego w krakowskiej dzielnicy Wesoła. Gmachy i ludzie* (*Clinics and Theoretical Departments: Collegium Medicum of Jagiellonian University in the Wesoła District of Krakow. Buildings and People*), edited by Piotr Franaszek, 75–80. Kraków: Księgarnia Akademicka, 2016.

Bęczkowska, Urszula. "Budowa nowych gmachów dla kliniki chirurgicznej, okulistycznej, chorób wewnętrznych, oraz siedziby zakładów teoretycznych Wydziału Lekarskiego tzw. Collegium Medicum (1887–1901) ("Construction of New Facilities for the Surgical, Ophthalmological, Internal Medicine Clinics, and Headquarters for Theoretical Departments of the Medical Faculty, Referred to as Collegium Medicum (1887–1901)"). In *Kliniki i zakłady teoretyczne. Collegium Medicum Uniwersytetu Jagiellońskiego w krakowskiej dzielnicy Wesoła. Gmachy i ludzie* (*Clinics and Theoretical Departments: Collegium Medicum of Jagiellonian University in the Wesoła District of Krakow. Buildings and People*), edited by Piotr Franaszek, 81–117. Kraków: Księgarnia Akademicka, 2016.

Bęczkowska, Urszula. "Kliniki po II wojnie światowej" ("Clinical Establishments in the Post-World War II Era"). In *Kliniki i zakłady teoretyczne. Collegium Medicum Uniwersytetu Jagiellońskiego w krakowskiej dzielnicy Wesoła. Gmachy i ludzie* (*Clinics and Theoretical Departments: Collegium Medicum of Jagiellonian University in the Wesoła District of Krakow. Buildings and People*), edited by Piotr Franaszek, 153–58. Kraków: Księgarnia Akademicka, 2016.

Becker, Hans-Jürgen. 'Pfründe'. In *Handwörterbuch der Deutschen Rechtsgeschichte*, ed. Erler, Adalbert. Kaufmann, Ekkehard. Vol. III (Berlin, Erich Schmidt Verlag 1984): 1743–1745.

Becker, Hans-Jürgen. 'Laienpfründe'. In *Handwörterbuch der Deutschen Rechtsgeschichte*, ed. Erler, Adalbert. Kaufmann, Ekkehard. Vol. II (Berlin, Erich Schmidt Verlag 1978): 1353–1355.

Begon, Sabine. *De iure hospitalium. Das Recht des deutschen Spitals im 17. Jahrhundert unter besonderer Berücksichtigung der Abhandlungen von Ahasver Fritsch und Wolfgang Adam Lauterbach*. Marburg: Tectum Verlag, 2002.

Bell, Adrian. Sutcliffe, Charles. 'Valuing Medieval Annuities: Were Corrodies Underpriced?'. In *Explorations in Economic History*, 47 (2010): 142–157.

Bergerhausen, Hans-Wolfgang. Wagner, Ulrich. *Quellen zur Geschichte des Bürgerspitals Würzburg 1500–1650*. Würzburg: Schöningh, 2014.

Bernard, Paul P. The Limits of Absolutism: Joseph II and the Allgemeines Krankenhaus. In *Eighteenth-Century Studies* Winter 9/2 (1975/1976): 193–212.

Besold-Backmund, Marlene. *Stiftungen und Stiftungswirklichkeit. Studien zur Sozialgeschichte der beiden oberfränkischen Kleinstädte Forchheim und Weismain.* Neustadt an der Aisch: Degener, 1986.

Białoń, Józef. "Organizacja zespołu klinik Akademii Medycznej w Krakowie" ("The Organization of the Clinical Department at the Medical Academy in Krakow"). *Szpitalnictwo Polskie*, 1/8 (1964): 13–15.

Blackthorne-O'Barr, Erik. Journals of the Plague Year: The Ottoman Press and the Istanbul Cholera Outbreak of 1871, *Journal of the Ottoman and Turkish Studies Association* 1 (2022), 203–230.

Blasius, Dirk. *Der verwaltete Wahnsinn. Eine Sozialgeschichte des Irrenhauses.* Frankfurt: Fischer Taschenbuch Verlag, 1980.

Blasius, Dirk. *Umgang mit Unheilbarem. Studien zur Sozialgeschichte der Psychiatrie.* Bonn: Psychiatrie Verlag, 1986.

Blessing, Bettina. *Katholische Krankenpflege im Sapnnungsfeld säkularer Tendenzen: Die Münchener Barmherzigen Brüder und Elisabethinerinnen von der Mitte des 18. bis zum Beginn des 19. Jahrhunderts.* Stuttgart: Kohlhammer Verlag, 2024.

Bogar, Benedict František. *Milosrdní bratři* [Brothers of Mercy]. Prague: Order of the Brothers of Mercy, 1934.

Bogavčić, Iva Salopek. 'Od kontumca to bolnice: javnozdravstveni uvjeti gradiške Posavine 18. i 19. Stoljeća' *Povijesni prilozi* 62 (2022): 263–294.

Bokesová-Uherová, Mária. *Zdravotníctvo na Slovensku v období feudalizmu.* Bratislava 1973.

Borgolte, Michael. *Stiftung Und Memoria.* Berlin: De Gruyter, 2012.

Bourdieu, Pierre. "The Forms of Capital." In *Cultural Theory: An anthology*, edited by Imre Szeman, and Timothy Kaposy, 241–58. New York: John Wiley & Sons, 1986.

Brooks, Willis E. Reform in the Russian Army, 1856–1861, *Slavic Review* 1 (1984): 63–82.

Broman Thomas H. *The Transformation of German Academic Medicine.* Cambridge: Cambridge University Press, 1996.

Brown, Michael. 'Medicine, Reform and the "End" of Charity in Early Nineteenth-Century England', *The English Historical Review* CXXIV, no. 511 (December 2009): 1353–1388.

Bryant, Chad. *Habsburg History, Eastern European History … Central European History?* Central European History 1/51 (2018), 56–65.

Buben, Milan. *Encyklopedie řádů, kongregací a řeholních společenství katolické církve v českých zemích* [Encyclopaedia of Orders, Congregations, and Monastic Congregations of the Catholic Church in the Czech Lands], Part III, Volume 2. Prague: Libri, 2007, pp. 368–406.

Buczynski Alexander. 'Kuga, kontumaci i karantena: epidemiološke mjere u Vojnoj krajini u 18. i 19. stoljeću' [The plague, kontumaz, and quarantine: epidemiological measures in the Military Frontier in the 18th and 19th centuries], *Narodna umjetnost* 58/1 (2021), 191–208.

Buczynski Alexander. *Pa to su samo Hrvati! Građa za povijest kantonske reorganizacije Vojne krajine 1787. godine* [Those are just Croatians! Materials for the history of the cantonal reorganization of the Military Frontier in 1787]. Zagreb: Hrvatski institut za povijest, 2011.

Butterwick, Richard. *The Polish-Lithuanian Commonwealth, 1733–1795: Light and Flame.* New Haven and London: Yale University Press, 2020.

Bynum, William F. *Science and the Practice of Medicine in the Nineteenth Century*, Cambridge: Cambridge University Press 1999.

Castel, Robert. *Le psychanalysme: l'ordre psychanalytique et le pouvoir*, Paris : Éditions Maspero 1973.

Castel, Robert. *L'Ordre psychiatrique. L'âge d'or l'aliénisme.* Paris: Les Editions de Minuit 1977.

Cavallo, Sandra. *Charity and Power in Early Modern Italy. Benefactors and Their Motives in Turin, 1541–1789*. Cambridge: Cambridge University Press, 1995.

Cavallo, Sandra. "The Motivations of Benefactors: An Overview of Approaches to the Study of Charity." In *Medicine and Charity Before the Welfare State*, edited by Jonathan Barry and Collin Jones, 46–62. London and New York: Routledge, 1991.

Csáky, Moritz. Middle Europe/Central Europe. A Complex Cultural System, in Music in Central Europe. Special *Österreichische Musikzeitschrift* 48/2005, 9–16.

Černoušek Michal. 'Nárys historického vývoje psychiatrických klasifikací' [An Outline of the Historic Development of Psychiatric Classification]. Series Studie k dějinám psychiatrického myšlení II. *Zprávy* 85 (1988): 51–101.

Černoušek, Michal. *Šílenství v zrcadle dějin: pojednání pro inteligentní čtenáře* [Madness in the Mirror of History: An Exposition for Intelligent Readers]. Prague: Grada, 1994.

Černoušek, Michal. *Studie k dějinám psychiatrického myšlení* [Studies on the History of Psychiatric Thought], Vols. I–II. Prague: Novinář, 1987–1988.

Černoušek, Michal. *Studie k dějinám psychiatrického myšlení: určeno pro odborníky psychiatrických a psychologických pracovišť* [Studies on the History of Psychiatric Thought: Intended for Professionals in Psychiatric and Psychological institutions]. Vol. III: *Historie pojmu duševní zdraví a duševní nemoc* [History of the Terms 'Mental Health' and 'Mental Illness']. Prague: Novinář, 1990.

Černý, Karel, ed. *Lékařství: Tématická řada Velké dějiny zemí Koruny České.* Prague: Paseka, 2023.

Cetinoglu, Olivia. A History of the Barbados General Hospital, 1844–1910. In *Caribbean Quarterly* 1 (2014): 96–97.

Chaloupková, Petra. *Správa a fungování Zemského ústavu pro choromyslné v Praze v letech 1791–1886* [Administration and Functioning of the Provincial Institution for the Mentally Ill, 1791–1886]. Unpublished MA Thesis. Prague: Charles University, Faculty of Arts and Philosophy, 2008.

Chwalba, Andrzej. *Historia Polski 1795–1918* (*History of Poland 1795–1918*). Kraków: Wydawnictwo Literackie, 2000.

Clark, Hannah-Louise. Barry Doyle, Barry. Imperial and post-imperial healthcare before welfare states. *European Revue of History* 5–6 (2021): 617–834.

Clavarino, Lodovica. Italian Physicists and the Bomb: Edoardo Amaldi's Network for Arms Control and Peace during the Cold War, *Journal of Contemporary History* 3/56 (2021): 665–692.

Comlos, John. *Nutrition and Economic Development in the Eighteenth-Century Habsburg Monarchy: An Anthropometric History*. Princeton: Princeton University Press, 1989.

Collins, Julie. *The Architecture and Landscape of Health: A Historical Perspective on Therapeutic Places, 1790–1940*. London: Routledge, 2020.

Conrad, Christoph. *Vom Greis zum Rentner. Der Strukturwandel des Alters in Deutschland zwischen 1830 und 1930*. Göttingen: Vandenhoeck & Ruprecht, 1994.

Cotoi, Calin. Cholera, Health for All, Nation-Building, and Racial Degeneration in Nineteenth-Century Romania. *East Central Europe* 43, No 1–2 (2016), 161–187.

Cross, Mai'a K. Davis. Rethinking epistemic communities twenty years later, *Review of International Studies* 1/39 (2013), 137–160.

Curtiss, John Shelton. Russian Sisters of Mercy in the Crimea, 1854–1855. *Slavic Review* No. 1 (1966): 84–100.

Czech, Herwig. Venereal Disease, Prostitution, and the Control of Sexuality in World War II Vienna. *East-Central Europe* 38, No. 1 (2011), 64–78.

Daday, András. Adatok a magyarországi elmebetegek gyógyitásának történetéhez. *Gyógyászat* 76 No. 29–30 (1936): 449–451.

Dawson, Gowan. Lightman, Bernard. Shuttleworth, Sally. Topham, Jonathan R. eds. *Science Periodicals in Nineteenth-Century Britain: Constructing Scientific Communities*. Chicago: The University of Chicago Press, 2020.

Deak, John. *Forging a Multinational State: State Making in Imperial Austria from the Enlightenment to the First World War*, Standford, Stanford University Press, 2015.

Digby, Anne. *Madness, Morality and Medicine: A Study of the York Retreat, 1796–1914*. New York: Cambridge University Press, 1985.

Dirmeier, Artur. *Das St. Katharinenspital zu Regensburg von der Stauferzeit bis zum Westfälischen Frieden. Eine Wohlfahrtseinrichtung im Spannungsfeld zwischen Reichsstadt, Hochstift und Herzogtum*. Regensburg: University of Regensburg, 1988.

Doboș, Corina. Global Challenges, Local *Knowledges*: Politics and Expertise at the World Population Conference in Bucharest, 1974. *East Central Europe* 45 (2018): 215–244.

Dörner, Klaus. *Bürger und Irre. Zur Sozialgeschichte und Wissenschaftssoziologie der Psychiatrie*. Frankfurt am Main: Europäische Verlagsanstalt, 1969.

Dross, Fritz. "Health Care Provision and Poor Relief in Enlightenment and 19th Century Prussia." In *Health Care and Poor Relief in 18th and 19th Century Northern Europe*, edited by Ole Peter Grell, Andrew Cunningham and Robert Jütte, 69–111. Aldershot and Burlington: Ashgate, 2002.

Dross, Fritz. *Krankenhaus und lokale Politik 1770–1850: das Beispiel Düsseldorf*, Essen: Klartext, 2004.

Dugački Vladimir. 'Zagrebačka Zakladna bolnica na Harmici (Jelačićevu trgu), 1804–1931. Ususret 200. obljetnici'[The Zagreb Foundation Hospital on Harmica (Jelačić Square), 1804–1931: Approaching its 200th Anniversary], *Gazophylacium* 8 (2003): 3–4, 74–79.

Ebelová, Ivana. 'Úroveň diagnostiky v 17. až 19. století na základě protokolů nemocných pražských nemocnic milosrdných bratří a alžbětinek' [The quality of diagnostics in the 17th–19th century based on protocols of patients in Prague hospitals of the Brothers of Mercy and Sisters of St Elizabeth]. *Dějiny věd a techniky* 41, No. 3 (2008): 185–198.

Ebelová, Ivana. 'Die Entstehung der ersten Krankenhäuser – Das Krankenhaus der Barmherzigen Brüder und der Elisabethinerinnen.' In Martin Scheutz, Andrea Sommerlechner, Herwig Weigl, and Alfred Stefan Weiss (eds.), *Europäisches Spitalwesen. Institutionelle Fürsorge in Mittelalter und Früher Neuzeit*, 403–408. Munich: Oldenbourg, 2008.

Ehmer, Josef. 'Altersstrukturen Im Historischen Wandel. Demografische Trends Und Gesellschaftliche Bewertung'. In *Alter(n) Anders Denken. Kulturelle und biologische Perspektiven*, ed. Brigitte Röder, Willemijn de Jong, and Kurt W. Alt. Wien/Cologne/Weimar: Böhlau Verlag, 2012.

Ehmer, Josef. 'The Life Stairs: Aging, Generational Relations, and Small Commodity Production in Central Europe'. In *Ageing and Generational Relations over the Life Course. A Historical and Cross-Cultural Perspective*, ed. Tamara K. Hareven. Berlin: De Gruyter, 1996.

Engstrom, Eric J. *Clinical Psychiatry in Imperial Germany: A History of Psychiatric Practice*. Ithaca, NY–London: Cornell University Press 2003.

Fasora, Lukáš. Malíř, Jiří (eds). *Dějiny Brna 4: Modernizace města 1790–1918*. Brno: Archiv města Brna, 2020.

Faure, Olivier. The Social History of Health in France: A Survey of Recent Developments. In *Social History of Medicine* 3/3 (1990): 437–451.

Fekete, J. Intézetünk megalapítása és működése 1900–ig. In Böszörményi, Z. (ed.) *Az Országos Ideg- és Elmegyógyintézet 100 éve*. 67–82. Budapest: Nyomdaipari Szakmunkásképző Intézet, 1968.

Firinger Kamilo and Utvić Vladimir, *Povijest bolničkih ustanova u Osijeku od 1739–1930* [The History of Hospital Institutions in Osijek from 1739 to 1930]. Osijek, 1970.

Foucault, Michel. *Discipline and Punish: The Birth of the Prison*. New York: Pantheon, 1977.

Foucault, Michel. *The Birth of the Clinic: An Archaeology of Medical Perception*. New York: Pantheon, 1973.

Foucault, Michel. *Les Machines à guérir, aux origines de l'hôpital moderne. Bruselas*: E. Mardara, 1979.

Franaszek, Piotr. "Szpitale galicyjskie w drugiej połowie XIX i na początku XX wieku" ("The Galician hospitals during the second half of the 19th and early 20th centuries"), [w:]. *Zeszyty Naukowe Uniwersytetu Jagiellońskiego, Prace Historyczne*, MCCXXX, No. 126 (1999): 125–143.

Franaszek, Piotr. "Krajowy szpital powszechny we Lwowie na przełomie XIX i XX wieku" ("The National General Hospital in Lviv at the turn of the 19th and 20th centuries"), *Zeszyty Naukowe Uniwersytetu Jagiellońskiego*, Prace Historyczne, MCCXXXIII, No. 127 (2000), 121–135.

Franaszek, Piotr. *Zdrowie publiczne w Galicji w dobie autonomii* (*Public Health in Galicia in the Age of Autonomy*) Kraków: Wydawnictwo Uniwersytetu Jagiellońskiego, 2002.

Franaszek, Piotr. "Publiczna ochrona zdrowia w Galicji w dobie autonomii" ("Public Healthcare in Galicia during the Period of Autonomy"). In *Przełom nowożytny w nauce europejskiej i jego kontekst społeczno-kulturowy* (*The Epochal Transition in Early Modern European Science and Its Socio-Cultural Context*), edited by. Bożena Płonka-Syroka, Andrzej Syroka, 133–157. Wrocław: Oficyna Wydawnicza Arboretum, 2004.

Franaszek, Piotr. "Wybrane problemy publicznej ochrony zdrowia w Galicji w dobie autonomii" ("Selected Issues in the Public Health System of Galicia during the Period of Autonomy"). In *Zdrowie i choroba. Wpływ jakości życia na kulturę w Europie Środkowej* (*Health and Illness: The Influence of Quality of Life on Culture in Central Europe*), ed. Antoni Barciak, 157–173. Katowice-Zabrze: Studio Noa, 2013.

Franaszek, Piotr. "O początkach szpitalnictwa krakowskiego i historii krakowskiego zespołu szpitalnego w dzielnicy Wesoła" ("The Origins of Healthcare in Krakow and the Historical Development of the Krakow Hospital Complex in the Wesoła District"). In *Kliniki i zakłady teoretyczne. Collegium Medicum Uniwersytetu Jagiellońskiego w krakowskiej dzielnicy Wesoła. Gmachy i ludzie* (*Clinics and Theoretical Departments: Collegium Medicum of Jagiellonian University in the Wesoła District of Krakow. Buildings and People*), edited by Piotr Franaszek, 15–40. Kraków: Księgarnia Akademicka, 2016.

Frank, Joseph. *Atsiminimai apie Vilnių*. Translated by Genovaitė Dručkutė. Vilnius: Mintis, 2001.

Franz, Albert K. *Aus Vier Jahrhunderten Innerer Geschichte Des Bürgerspitals Zum Hl. Geist in Würzburg*. Würzburg: Freunde mainfränkischer Kunst und Geschichte, 1951.

Frevert, Ute. *Krankheit als politisches Problem, 1770–1880: soziale Unterschichten in Preußen zwischen medizinischer Polizei und staatlicher Sozialversicherung*. Göttingen: Vandenhoeck & Ruprecht, 1984.

Frohman, Larry. *Poor Relief and Welfare in Germany from the Reformation to World War 1*. Cambridge/London: Cambridge University Press, 2008.

From Western Medicine to Global Medicine: The Hospital Beyond the West, ed. Margaret Harrison, Margaret Jones, and Helen Sweet, New Delhi: Orient Blackswan, 2009.

Frieden, Nancy M. *Russian Physicians in an Era of Reform and Revolution, 1856–1905*. Princeton: Princeton University Press, 1981.

Froide, Amy. *Never Married: Single Women in Early Modern England*. Oxford: Oxford University Press, 2005.

Gabriel, Eberhard. Psychiatrische Einrichtungen im Erzherzogtum unter der Enns (Niederösterreich) im 19. Jahrhundert. Vom Irrenturm in Wien zu den Heil- und Pflegeanstalten für Geisteskranke im Licht zeitgenössischer Darstellungen. *Virus. Beiträge zur Sozialgeschichte der Medizin*, No. 16 (2017): 193–207.

Gárdonyi, Albert. A Rókus-kórház s a régi pesti kórházak. *Városi Szemle*, 15, No. 5 (1929): 980–997.

Gavin, Magdalena. Early Twentieth-Century Eugenics in Europe's Peripheries: The Polish Perspective. *East Central Europe* 3 (2011): 1–15.

Geyer-Kordesch, Johanna. German Medical Education in the Eighteenth Century: the Prussian context and its Influence. In Bynum, William F. and Porter, Roy, eds. *William Hunter and the Eighteenth Century Medical World*, 177–205. Cambridge: Cambridge University Press, 2002.

Gelfand, Tobby. A Clinical Ideal: Paris 1789, *Bulletin of the History of Medicine* 3/51 (1977), 397–411.

Grell, Ole Peter, and Andrew Cunningham. "Health Care and Poor Relief in 18th and 19th Century Northern Europe." In *Health Care and Poor Relief in 18th and 19th Century Northern Europe*, edited by Ole Peter Grell, Andrew Cunningham and Robert Jütte. Aldershot and Burlington: Ashgate, 2002, 3–14.

Gillispie, Charles Coulston. *Science and Polity in France: The End of the Old Regime*, Princeton: Princeton University Press, 1981.

Godsey, William D. *The Sinews of Habsburg Power: Lower Austria in a Fiscal-Military State 1650–1820*. Oxford: Oxford University Press, 2018.

Goffman, Erving. *The presentation of self in everyday life*. New York: Garden City – Double Day, 1959.

Golden, Janet Lynne. Long, Diana E. *The American General Hospital: Communities and Social Contexts*, Ithaca, Cornell University Press 1989.

Golden Juliet D. "Show that you are really alive": Sara-Zofia Syrkin-Binsztejnowa's Emergency Medical Relief and Public Health Work in Early Interwar Poland and the Warsaw Ghetto, *Medizinhistorisches Journal* 2/53 (2018), 125–162.

Goldstein, Jan E. *Console and Classify. The French Psychiatric Profession in the Nineteenth Century.* Chicago, IL: The University of Chicago Press 2001.

Gordziejew, Jerzy. *Komisje Porządkowe Cywilno-Wojskowe w Wielkim Księstwie Litewskim w okresie Sejmu Czteroletniego (1789–1792).* Kraków: Wydawnictwo Uniwersytetu Jagiellońskiego, 2010.

Granshaw, Lindsay-Porter, Roy, ed. *The Hospital in History.* London: Routledge, 1989.

Greenbaum, Louis S. "Measure of Civilization": The Hospital Thought of Jacques Tenon on the Eve of the French Revolution, Bulletin of the History of Medicine 1/49 (1975), 43–56.

Greenbaum, Louis S. Thomas Jefferson, the Paris Hospitals, and the University of Virginia, *Eighteenth-Century Studies* 4/26 (1993), 607–626.

Grmek, Mirko D. *Histoire de la pensée médicale en Occident. 2. De la Renaissance aux Lumières*, Paris: Seuil, 1997.

Grois, Bernhard. *Das Allgemeine Krankenhaus in Wien und seine Geschichte.* Wien: W. Maudrich-Verlag, 1965.

Gryglewski, Ryszard W. "Trudne początki – kliniki lekarskiej Akademii Krakowskiej w szpitalu św. Łazarza" ("Formative Challenges – The Genesis of the Medical Clinic at the Krakow Academy within the St. Lazarus Hospital"). In *Kliniki i zakłady teoretyczne. Collegium Medicum Uniwersytetu Jagiellońskiego w krakowskiej dzielnicy Wesoła. Gmachy i ludzie* (*Clinics and Theoretical Departments: Collegium Medicum of Jagiellonian University in the Wesoła District of Krakow. Buildings and People*), edited by Piotr Franaszek, 161–176. Kraków: Księgarnia Akademicka, 2016.

Health Care and Poor Relief in 18th and 19th Century Southern Europe, ed. Ole Peter Grell. Andrew Cunningham. Bernd, Roeck. Aldershot: Ashgate, 2005.

Guthrie, Douglas. *A History of Medicine.* London: Thomas Nelson and Sons, Ltd. 1945.

Haas, Peter M. Introduction: Epistemic Communities and International Policy Coordination. *International Organization: Knowledge, Power and International Policy Coordination* 1/46 (1992): 1–35.

Habek Dubravko. *Iz povijesti zdravstva Bjelovar*a [From the history of healthcare in Bjelovar]. Zagreb-Bjelovar, 2013.

Habek Dubravko. 'O prvoj bjelovarskoj bolnici' [About the first hospital in Bjelovar], *Radovi Zavoda za znanstvenoistraživački i umjetnički rad u Bjelovaru*, No. 9 (2015), 21–30.

Hádlík, Josef. Poznámky k vývoji péče o duševně nemocné na území Moravy a Slezska. In *1863–1963. 100 let psychiatrické léčebny v Brně.* Brno: [nákl. vl.], 1963.

Hajdinová, Eva. 'Léčba nebo náprava? Choromyslní kněží v první polovině 19. století. Pražský špitál milosrdných bratří' [Therapy or correction? Mentally ill priests in the first half of the 19th century. The Prague hospital of the Brothers of Mercy]. *Moderní dějiny* No. 1 (2024): 9–54.

Hajdinová, Eva. 'Obrazy ze sociálního a duševního života moravského kněžstva. Péče o choromyslné duchovní v brněnském špitále milosrdných bratří na přelomu 18. století' [Images from the social and spiritual life of Moravian clergy. Care for mentally ill clergy in the Brno Hospital of the Merciful Brothers at the turn of the 18th century]. *Časopis Matice Moravské* 143/2024: 25–54.

Hartely, Janet M. "Philanthropy in the Reign of Catherine the Great: Aims and Realities." In *Russia in the Age of Enlightenment: Essays for Isabel de Madariaga*, edited by Roger Bartlett and Janet M. Hartley, 167–202. London: Palgrave Macmillan, 1990.

Held, Thomas. 'Ausgedinge und ländliche Gesellschaft. Generationenverhältnisse im Österreich des 17. bis 19. Jahrhunderts.' In *Gerontologie und Sozialgeschichte. Wege zu einer historischen Betrachtung des Alters. Beiträge Einer internationalen Arbeitstagung am Deutschen Zentrum für Altersfragen, Berlin 5–7. Juli 1982*, ed. Christoph Conrad and Hans-Joachim von Kondratowitz, 151–186, Berlin: DZA, 1983.

Henderson, John. Horden Peregrine. Pastore, Alessandro (ed.). *The Impact of Hospitals 300–2000*. Berlin, Bern, Bruxelles: Peter Lang, 2007.

Heveroch, Antonín et al. *Zemské ústavy pro choromyslné v Čechách* [Provincial Institutes for the Mentally Ill in Bohemia]. Prague: Zemský správní výbor v Čechách, 1926.

Hickman, Clare. *Therapeutic Landscapes: A History of English Hospital Gardens since 1800*. Manchester: Manchester University Press, 2013.

Hilber, Marina. Obstetric expertise in the Austrian periphery: Ludwig Kleinwächter's practice in Czernowitz, Bukovina (1884–1906). *European Review of History* No. 5–6 (2021): 663–688.

Hirc Dragutin. 'Bolnica milosrdne braće' [The hospital of the Hospitaller Brothers]. *Stari Zagreb*, vol. II (2008): 541–550.

Hlade, Josef. *Theodor Meynerts (1833–1892) Physikalisierung des Ich: die Zweite Wiener Medizinische Schule und die österreichische Philosophie*. Würzburg: Königshausen & Neumann, 2022.

Hlaváčková, Ludmila. Česká a německá psychiatrická klinika pražské lékařské fakulty do roku 1918 [The Czech and German psychiatric clinic of the Prague Medical Faculty until 1918]. In *Historia – Medicina – Cultura. Sborník k dějinám medicíny*, eds. Karel Černý – Petr Svobodný, 133–159. Prague: Karolinum, 2006.

Hlaváčková, Ludmila. *Dějiny všeobecné fakultní nemocnice v Praze 1790–2010*. Praha: Maxdorf, 2011.

Hlaváčková, Ludmila. Druhá česká a německá interní klinika v Praze v dobách přednostenství E. Maixnera, J. Thomayera a R. Jaksche, In *Acta universitatis carolinae*, (2011): 11–43.

Hlaváčková, Ludmila. *History of the General Univeristy Hospital in Prague*. Týn nad Vltavou: Nová forma, 2014.

Hlaváčková, Ludmila. 'Nemocnice milosrdných bratří a Celestýn Opitz' [The hospital of the Brothers of Mercy and Celestýn Opitz]. *Sborník lékařský* 97, No. 1 (1996): 161–166.

Hlaváčková, Ludmila and Petr Svobodný. *Pražské špitály a nemocnice* [Prague hospitals and infirmaries]. Prague: NLN, 1999.

Hlaváčková, Ludmila. 'Das Spitalwesen in Böhmen und Mähren vom Beginn des Dreißigjährigen Kriegs bis zu den Josephinischen Reformen (1620–1780)'. In Martin Scheutz, Andrea Sommerlechner, Herwig Weigl, and Alfred Stefan Weiss (eds.), *Europäisches Spitalwesen. Institutionelle Fürsorge in Mittelalter und Früher Neuzeit*, 381–402. Munich: Oldenbourg, 2008.

Hlaváčková, Ludmila and Petr Svobodný. *Všeobecná nemocnice v Praze 1790–1952* [The general hospital in Prague, 1790–1952]. Prague: Karolinum,1990.

Hlaváčková, Ludmila and Petr Svobodný. 'Vznik a vývoj novoměstského nemocničního centra od konce 18. století do současnosti' [The Origins and Development of the Hospital Compound in the New Town of Prague Since 18th Century Until the Present]. In Václav Ledvinka and Jiří Pešek (eds.), Nové Město pražské ve 14.–20. století: sborník referátů a diskusních příspěvků ze 16. vědeckého zasedání Archivu hlavního města Prahy. Prague: Scriptorium, 1998.

Hlaváčková, Ludmila and Petr Svobodný. *Pražské špitály a nemocnice*. Prague: NLN, 1999.

Hlaváčková, Ludmila. Veřejné zdravotnictví od osvícenských reforem do roku 1848. In *Velké dějiny zemí koruny české: lékařství*. Praha: Paseka, 2023.

Hochedlinger, Michael. Die Sanitätshofdeputation. In *Verwaltungsgeschichte der Habsburgermonarchie in der Frühen Neuzeit. Band 1/1. Hof und Dynastie, Kaiser und Reich, Zentralverwaltungen, Kriegswesen und landesfürstliches Finanzwesen*. ed. Michael Hochedlinger, Petr Maťa und Thomas Winkelbauer. Wien: Vandenhoeck & Ruprecht, 2019.

Holzwart-Schäfer, Iris. 'Pfründner und Bedürftige im Esslinger Katharinenspital. Soziale Schichtung, Versorgung Und Alltag im 15. und 16. Jahrhundert.' *Esslinger Studien* 44 (2005): 7–35.

Hollán, Henrik. *Adatok és szemelvények a Szent Rókus Közkórház és fiókjai alapításának és fejlődésének történetéből*. Budapest : Medicina; [Pécs] : Pécsi Szikra Ny, 1967.

Horáčková, Ladislava. Menšíková, Miroslava. Vargová, Lenka. *Zdravotní péče o brněnské obyvatele v 18. a 19. století*. Brno: Oddělení lékařské antropologie Anatomického ústavu Lékařské fakulty Masarykovy univerzity, 2011.

Horánszky, Nándor. Schwartzer Ferenc javaslata 1848–ból az országos tébolyda ügyében. *Orvostörténeti Közlemények* 29 (1963): 257–269.

Horánszky, Nándor. A magyar elmegyógyászat a XIX. században. In *Az Országos Ideg- és Elmegyógyintézet 100 éve.* ed. Zoltán Böszörményi, 37–53. Budapest: Nyomdaipari Szakmunkásképző Intézet, 1968.

Horbec Ivana. Skenderović Robert, 'The Quarantines of the Croatian and Slavonian Military Frontier and their Role in the 18th Century Epidemic Control.' In *Plague between Prague and Vienna. Medicine and Infectious Diseases in Early Modern Central Europe* eds. Karel Černý and Sonia Horn, 190–230. Prague: Karolinum, 2018.

Horbec Ivana. *Zdravlje naroda – bogatstvo države. Prosvijećeni apsolutizam i počeci sustava javnog zdravstva u Hrvatskoj* [The Health of the People – the Wealth of the State: Enlightened Absolutism and the Beginnings of Public Health Care System in Croatia]. Zagreb, 2015.

Horváth, Alice. A Pesti Rókus-Kórház. *Építés-Építészet Tudomány*, 14. kötet, 1–2 szám (1982): 321–371.

Hroch, Miroslav. *Na prahu národní existence.* Praha: Mladá fronta, 1999.

Hudson, Geoffrey L. 'Disabled Veterans and the State in Early Modern England'. In *Disabled Veterans and the State*, ed. David A. Gerber, 117–144. Ann Arbor: Michigan University Press, 2012.

Hüntelmann, Axel C. The shifting politics in public health in Germany between the 1890s and 1920s. *European Review of History* 5–6 (2021): 636–662.

Iacob, Bogdan C. Doboș, Corina. Grosescu, Raluca. Iacob, Viviana. Pașca, Vlad. State Socialist Experts in Transnational Perspective. East European Circulation of Knowledge during the Cold War (1950s-1980s). *East Central Europe* 45 (2018): 145–159.

Iacob, Bogdan C. Together but Apart: Balkan Historians, the Global South, and UNESCO's History of Humanity, 1978–1989. *East Central Europe* 45 (2018): 245–278.

Iacob, Bogdan C. Malariology and Decolonization: Eastern European Experts from the League of Nations to the World Health Organization. *Journal of Global History* 17/2 (2022), 233–253.

Iacob, Viviana. Scenes of Cold War Diplomacy: Romania and the International Theatre Institute, 1956–1969. *East Central Europe* 45 (2018): 184–214.

Imbert, Jean. *Histoire des hôpitaux en France.* Toulouse: Privat, 1982.

Imhof, Arthur E. The Hospital in the 18th Century: For Whom? The Charite Hospital in Berlin, the Navy Hospital in Copenhagen, the Kongsberg Hospital in Norway, *Journal of Social History* 4/10 (1977), 448–470.

Jahn, Hubertus. "Health Care and Poor Relief in Russia, 1700–1856." In *Health Care and Poor Relief in 18th and 19th Century Northern Europe*, eds. Ole Peter Grell, Andrew Cunningham and Robert Jütte, 157–71. Aldershot and Burlington: Ashgate, 2002.

Jakulis, Martynas. *Špitolės Vilniuje: labdara, gydymas ir skurdas XVI–XVIII a.* Vilnius: Vilniaus universiteto leidykla, 2019.

Janáčková, Jaroslava, ed. *Nedosněné sny: korespondence bratří Mrštíků*, Praha: Odeon, 1978.

Janicka, Iwona. *Kultura higieniczna Wilna w latach 1795–1915.* Gdańsk: Wydawnictwo Uniwersytetu Gdańskiego, 2009.

Jelínek, Petr. Klášterní nemocnice řádu Milosrdných bratří ve Valticích a její knihy nemocných – The Monastery Hospital of the Brothers of Mercy in Valtice (Feldsberg) and Its Books of the Sick (1661–1780). *Časopis matice Moravské* 128, No. 1 (2009): 47–80.

Jelínek, Petr. 'Klášterní nemocnice řádu Milosrdných bratří v Brně a její knihy nemocných (1748–1780)' [Convent hospital of the Order of the Brothers of Mercy in Brno and its patient registers, 1748–1780]. *Časopis Matice Moravské* 130, No. 1 (2011): 41–77.

Jelínek, Petr. Milosrdní bratři v Prostějově a jejich klientela – Brothers of Mercy in Prostějov and their clientèle (1740–1780). *Časopis matice Moravské* 131 No. 1 (2012): 3–38.

Jeziorowski, Tadeusz. "Order Świętego Stanisława Biskupa i Męczennika 1765–1795." In *Praemiando incitat. Order Świętego Stanisława 1765–1831: w 250. rocznicę powołania orderu*, edited by Michał Zawadzki and Dariusz Nowacki, 52–110. Warszawa: Zamek Królewski w Warszawie – Muzeum, 2015.

Johanson, Christine. Autocratic Politics, Public Opinion, and Women's Medical Education during the Reign of Alexander II, 1855–1881. *Slavic Review* 38, No. 3 (1979): 426–443.

Jones, Colin. The Construction of the Hospital Patient in Early Modern France. In *Institutions of Confinement: Hospitals: Hospitals, Asylums, and Prison in Western Europe and North America, 1500–1950*, ed. Norbert Finzsch, Robert Jütte, 55–74. Cambridge, New York, and Melbourne: Cambridge University Press, 1996.

Jones, Colin. Sonenscher, Michael. The Social Functions of the Hospital in Eighteenth-Century France: The Case of the Hôtel-Dieu of Nîmes, *French Historical Studies* 2/13 (1983), 172–214.

Judson, Pieter M. *The Habsburg Empire: A New History*. Cambridge, Massachusetts, Harvard University Press, 2016.

Jütte, Robert. *Poverty and Deviance in Early Modern Europe*. Cambridge: Cambridge University Press, 1994.

Jütte, Robert. Vom Hospital zum Krankenhaus: 16. bis 19. Jahrhundert. In *"Einem jeden Kranken in einem Hospitale sein eigenes Bett": zur Sozialgeschichte des Allgemeinen Krankenhauses in Deutschland im 19. Jahrhundert*, ed. Alfons Labisch, Reinhard Spree, 31–50. Frankfurt am Main: Campus Verlag, 1996.

Kalkan, Hasibe. Metin And: Creating A Theatrical Epistemic Community in Turkey. In: *Developing Theatre in the Global South: Institutions, networks, experts*. Eds. Nic, Leonhardt and Balme Christopher B. London, UCL Press, 2024, 171–189.

Karenberg, Axel. Lippert, Marcella. 'Irrenhäuser in Prag (1600–1900).' *Würzburger medizinhistorische Mitteilungen* 13 (1995): 331–340.

Karenberg, Axel. 'Retrospective Diagnosis: Use and Abuse in Medical Historiography'. *Prague Medical Report* 110/2 (2009): 140–145.

Kaufmann, Doris. *Aufklärung, bürgerliche Selbsterfahrung und die "Erfindung" der Psychiatrie in Deutschland, 1770–1850*. Göttingen: Vandenhoeck & Ruprecht, 1995.

Keel, Othmar. *L'avènement de la médecine clinique et moderne en Europe 1750–1815*. Montréal: Presses de l'Université de Montréal, 2002.

Kemenah-Stanislaw, Alexandra Kathrin. "An die nechsterledigte Stelle darauff hiebeuor keiner Vorströstung erlangt aus Gnaden einnehmen zu lassen bewilliget" – Die Aufnahme in das Dresdner Jakobsspital Anhand von Supplikationen des 16. und 17. Jahrhunderts, In *Leben im Spital. Pfründner und ihr Alltag 1500–1800*, ed. Artur Dirmeier, 85–104. Regensburg: Verlag Friedrich Pustet, 2018.

Kemper, Claudia. "The Nuclear Arms Race is Psychological at Its Roots": Physicians and Their Therapies for the Cold War. In *Understanding the Imaginary War: Culture, Thought and Nuclear Conflict, 1945–1990*. Eds. Matthew Grant, Benjamin Ziemann, Manchester: Manchester University Press, 213–237.

Kirk, Stuart A., Gomory, Tomi, Cohen, David. The History and Historians of Madness. In: Kirk, Stuart A., Gomory, Tomi, Cohen, David. *Mad Science. Psychiatric Coercion, Diagnosis, and Drugs*. New Brunswick, NJ–London, 2013.

Kisacky, Jeanne. *Rise of the Modern Hospital: An Architectural History of Health and Healing, 1870–1940*. Pittsburgh: University of Pittsburgh Press, 2017.

Kinzelbach, Annemarie. Leprosaria: The Simultaneity of Segregation and Integration in Early Modern Southern German Towns, *Tracing Hospitals Boundaries: Integration and Segregation in Southeastern Europe and Beyond, 1050–1970*, eds. Jane L. Stevens Crawshaw, Irena Benyovsky Latin, and Kathleen Vongsathorn, 46–66. Leiden: Brill, 2020.

Kolda, Jindřich. 'Zárodky zdravotnických knihoven českých milosrdných bratří v 18. století'. [The beginnings of Czech medical libraries of the Brothers of Mercy in the 18th century]. *Česká a slovenská farmacie* 67, No. 5–6 (2018): 216–220.

Kopytko, Adam. *Służba zdrowia w Galicji doby autonomicznej* (*The Healthcare System in Galicia during the Period of Autonomy*), MA thesis. Kraków : Jagiellonian University, 2000.

Korybut-Marciniak, Maria. *Dobroczynne Wilno. Pomoc ubogim i potrzebującym w Wilnie w pierwszej połowie XIX wieku.* Olsztyn: Centrum Badań Europy Wschodniej Uniwersytetu Warmińsko-Mazurskiego w Olsztynie, 2012.

Kovács, Janka. Elmebetegügy a 18–19. század fordulóján: elméleti keretek, koncepciók, megoldási javaslatok. *Korall Társadalomtörténeti Folyóirat* 71 (2018): 7–26.

Kovács, Janka. "Érzelmi nyavalyák" és "ész-tébolyodások": A lélek betegségei az orvosi disszertációkban a 18–19. század fordulóján. In Aetas Történettudományi Folyóirat 34, No. 2 (2019): 67–84.

Kovács, Janka. *A lélek tudománya. Diszciplinarizálódás, medikalizáció és tudásterjesztés Magyarországon (1770–1830)*. Budapest, HUN-REN Bölcsészettudományi Kutatóközpont, 2024.

Kovács, Janka. 1798: Megnyílik a Rókus kórház. Az intézményi elmebeteg-ellátás kezdetei Magyarországon. In *Magyarország globális története a kezdetektől 1868–ig.* Ed. Laczó, F. – Vadas, A. – Varga, B., 416–420. Budapest: Corvina, 2023.

Kovács, Janka. "Finding a Place for the Most Unfortunate?" Madness, Institutionalization, and the Obstacles of Care I the Late Eighteenth- and Early Nineteenth-Century Habsburg Monarchy." In: Ureczky, E. (ed.) *Crises of Care: Pandemic Cultures, Biopolitics and the Medical Humanities.* Debrecen: University of Debrecen, 2024. (Forthcoming.).

Kovács, Janka. The darkest field of medicine? The integration of psychological knowledge into medical education in the Habsburg Monarchy (1780s–1840s). *European Review of History: Revue européenne d'histoire* 31 No. 1 (2024): 17–46.

Krász, Lilla. The Circulation of Medical Knowledge in Eighteenth-Century Hungary. *East Central Europe* 3 (2013): 268–295.

Křečková, Jitka. Kuchařová, Hedvika. *Dějiny konventu alžbětinek v Praze. 300 let od jejich příchodu* [The history of the convent of Sisters of St Elizabeth in Prague. 300 years since their arrival]. Prague: Konvent sester alžbětinek v Praze, 2020.

Kretschmayr, Heinrich (ed.). *Die österreichische Zentralverwaltung. II. Abt. Von der Vereinigung der österreichischen und böhmischen Hofkanzlei bis zur Errichtung der Ministerialverfassung. 2. Band: Die Zeit des Directoriums in Publicis et Cameralibus.* Wien: Adolf Holzhausen, 1925.

Kurucz, György. Standards of Observation and Representation: Travel Instructions for a Technological Journey in 1820. In *Wissenschaften zwischen Tradition und Innovation – Historische Perspektiven/Sciences between Tradition and Innovation – Historical Perspectives.* ed. Lilla Krász, 123–139. Wien: Praesens Verlag, 2022.

Kurucz, György. "In the Interest of the Homeland and His Lordship's Domains": The Study Tours of the Professors of Hungary's First College of Farming. In *The Culture of the Aristocracy in the Habsburg Monarchy, 1750–1820*, ed. Gábor Vaderna, 205–212, Wien: Praesens Verlag, 2022.

Kušniráková, Ingrid. 'Pacienti a zdravotnícky personál bratislavskej nemocnice milosrdných bratov v ranom novoveku' [Patients and the nursing staff of the Brothers' of Mercy hospital in Bratislava in the Early Modern Period]. *Theatrum historiae* 11 (2012): 69–80.

Labisch, Alfons. Spree Reinhard. Die Kommunalisierung des Krankenhauswesens in Deutschland während des 19. und frühen 20. Jahrhundert. In *Kommunalisierung im Spannungsfeld von Regulierung und Deregulierung im 19. und 20. Jahrhundert*, ed. Josef Wysocki, 7–48. Berlin: Duncker & Humblot, 1995.

Lafferton, Emese. *Hungarian Psychiatry, Society and Politics in the Long Nineteenth Century.* Cham: Palgrave Macmillan, 2022.

Lakomá, Lena. *Ústavní péče o choromyslné na Moravě v letech 1863–1892 na příkladu Černovic* (bakalářská diplomová práce). Brno: Masarykova univerzita, Filozofická fakulta Brno, 2020.

Lambacher, Hannes. *Das Spital der Reichsstadt Memmingen. Geschichte einer Fürsorgeanstalt, eines Herrschaftsträgers und wirtschaftlichen Großbetriebs und dessen Beitrag zur Entwicklung von Stadt und Umland.* Kempten: Verlag für Heimatpflege, 1991.

Lamber, William de Jong. Eugenics and Lysenkoism in Interwar and Postwar Polish Biology. *East Central Europe* 1/38 (2011): 115–132.

Lane, Hugo. Austrian Officials and the Making of the Polish-Ruthenian Divide, 1815–1848. In *Habsburg Civil Servants: Between Civil Society and the State.* Eds. Alexander Maxwell and Daša Ličen, New York – Oxford: Berghahn Books, 2025, 25–44.

Lane, Joan. *A Social History of Medicine: Health, Healing and Disease in England, 1750–1950,* Abingdon: Routledge 2001.

Laurenson, Pip. Saaze, Vivian van. Van de Vall, Renée. Bridging the Gaps between Theory and Practice through Cross-Institutional Collaboration in the Conservation of Contemporary Art. In *Engaged Humanities: Rethinking Art, Culture, and Public Life.* Eds. Van de Vall, Renée, Amsterdam: Amsterdam University Press, 2022, 271–304.

Ledebur, S. *Das Wissen der Anstaltspsychiatrie in der Moderne: zur Geschichte der Heil- und Pflegeanstalten Am Steinhof in Wien.* Wien: Böhlau, 2015.

van Leeuwen, Marco H. D. 'Guilds and Middle-Class Welfare, 1550–1800: Provisions for Burial, Sickness, Old Age, and Widowhood', *The Economic History Review* 65, no. 1 (February 2012). 61–90.

Lesky, Erna. Das Wiener Allgemeine Krankenhaus. seine Gründung und Wirkung auf deutsche Spitäler, *Clio Medica* 2 (1967): 23–37.

Lesky, Erna. *Die Wiener medizinische Schule im 19. Jahrhundert,* Graz: H. Böhlaus, 1965.

Lesky, Erna. *Österreichisches Gesundheitswesen im Zeitalter des aufgeklärten Absolutismus.* Wien: Archiv für österreichische Geschichte, 1959.

Lindemann, Mary. *Medicine and Society in Early Modern Europe,* Cambridge: Cambridge University Press 2013.

Lindenmeyr, Adele. *Poverty is Not a Vice: Charity, Society and the State in Imperial Russia.* Princeton: Princeton University Press, 1996.

Lobenwein, Elisabeth. Weiß, Alfred Stefan. 'Frühneuzeitliche Hospitalordnungen und deren Regelung des Alltäglichen Lebens. Eine Annäherung anhand österreichischer

Quellen'. In *Historia Hospitalium. Jahrbuch der Deutschen Gesellschaft für Krankenhausgeschichte*, ed. Gunnar Stollberg, Christina Vanja, Ernst Kraas, 47–86. Münster/Berlin: Lit, 2020.

Lovejoy, David B. The Hospital and Society: The Growth of Hospitals in Rochester, New York, in the Nineteenth Century, *Bulletin of the History of Medicine* 49 (1975): 536–555.

Maingot, Anthony P. *Race, Ideology, and the Decline of Caribbean Marxism*, Gainesville, University Press of Florida, 2015.

Magocsi, Paul Robert. *The Roots of Ukrainian Nationalism: Galicia As Ukraine's Piedmont*, Toronto, University of Toronto Press, 2022.

Małudzińska, Monika. *"Próżnowanie stało się powszechnym nałogiem". Żebracy i włóczędzy w stanisławowskiej Warszawie.* Warszawa: Neriton, 2014.

Manulak, Michael V. Developing World Environmental Cooperation: The Founex Seminar and the Stockholm Conference. In *International Organizations and Environmental Protection: Conservation and Globalization in the Twentieth Century.* Eds. Wolfram Kaiser, Jan-Henrik Meyer. New York – Oxford, Berghahn Books, 2019, 138–162.

Matoušek, Otakar. "The Medical School of Vienna and of Prague." In *Medizinhistorisches Journal* 2, no. 2 (1967): 99–106.

McCants, Anne. 'The Role of the Charitable Institution in the Early Modern Dutch Economy: The Case of the Amsterdam Burgerweeshuis.' Ann Arbor, University of California at Berkeley, 1991.

McMahon, Norbert. *The story of the Hospitallers of St. John of God*, Dublin, M. H. Gill and Son, 1958.

Merkulova, Polina. *Pedagogy and the Building of British Psychiatry at the Age of Asylum, 1792–1914.* Unpublished doctoral thesis, University of Leeds, Leeds, 2022.

Meumann, Markus. *Findelkinder, Waisenhäuser, Kindsmord: Unversorgte Kinder in der Frühneuzeitlichen Gesellschaft*. Munich: R. Oldenbourg Verlag, 1995.

Michalewicz, Jerzy. ed. *Inwentarz akt wydziałów i studiów Uniwersytetu Jagiellońskiego 1850–1939* (*1954*) (*Inventory of Documents of Departments and Studies of Jagiellonian University 1850–1939* (1954). Kraków: Archiwum Uniwersytetu Jagiellońskiego, 1997.

Mieszkowski, Łukasz. A Foreign Lady: the Polish Episode in the Influenza Pandemic of 1918, *Acta Poloniae Historica* 113 (2016), 195–231.

Miller, Ian. Food, Medicine and Institutional Life in the British Isles, 1790–1900. In *The Routledge History of Food*, ed. Carol Helstosky. Abingdon: Routledge, 2014.

Miramon, Charles de. *Les 'Donnés' Au Moyen Âge. Une Forme de Vie Religieuse Laïque v. 1180–v. 1500*. Paris: Les èditions du CERF, 1999.

Mircheva, Gergana. Fighting Social Pathology: Criminology and Eugenics in Bulgaria, 1896–1939. *East Central Europe* 1 (2011): 16–43.

Mitchell, Harvey. Politics in the Service of Knowledge: The Debate over the Administration of Medicine and Welfare in Late Eighteenth-Century France, *Social History* 2/6 (1981), 185–207.

Mitchell, Piers D. 'Retrospective diagnosis and the use of historical texts for investigating disease in the past.' *International Journal of Paleopathology* 1/1(2011): 81–88.

Mitterauer, Michael. 'Familienwirtschaft und Altersversorgung.' In *Vom Patriarchat zur Partnerschaft. Zum Strukturwandel der Familie*, ed. Michael Mitterauer, Reinhard Sieder. Munich: Verlag C. H. Beck, 1980.

Mogilner, Marina. Racial Psychiatry and the Russian Imperial Dilemma of the "Savage Within." *East Central Europe* 1–2 (2016): 99–133.

Moran, James E. Topp, Leslie. Introduction: Interpreting psychiatric spaces. In *Madness, Architecture and the Built Environment: Psychiatric Spaces in Historical Context*, eds. Leslie Topp, James E. Moran, and Jonathan Andrews, New York, Abingdon: Routledge, 2007, 1–16.

Mueller, Lucas M. Risk on the Negotiating Table: Malnutrition, Mold Toxicity, and Postcolonial Development. In *Risk on the Table: Food Production, Health, and the Environment.* Eds. Angela N. H. Creager. Jean-Paul, Gaudilliére. New York, Oxford. Berghahn Books, 2021. 138–162.

Müller, Thomas. Vergleich und Transferanalyse in der Medizingeschichte? Eine Diskussion anhand von Reiseberichten als Quelle. *Medizinhistorisches Journal* 39, No. 1 (2004): 57–77.

Nebřenský, Zdeněk. Civil Service in the Factory: Trade Inspectors and Working-Class Politics in the Habsburg Monarchy, 1884–1914. In Maxwell, Alexander. Ličen, Daša. *Habsburg Civil Servants Between Civil Society and the State*, New York, Oxford: Berghahn Books 2025, 131–151.

Nebřenský, Zdeněk. Herc, Svatopluk. Empire in the Cottage: Welfare Capitalism and Workers' Housing Policy in the Habsburg Monarchy, 1880–1914, *International Labor and Working-Class History* 104 (2023): 103–122.

Nebřenský. *Katedrály industriálního věku: textilní továrny a sociální otázka v českých zemích*. Praha: Nakladatelství Lidové noviny, 2017.

Neumaier, Rudolf. Pfründner. In *Die Klientel des Regensburger St. Katharinenspitals und ihr Alltag (1649–1809)*. Regensburg: Verlag Friedrich Pustet, 2011.

Núñez-García, Víctor M. Los hospitales docentes en la España contemporánea, In *Dynamis,* (2021), 1, 53–77.

Ohngemach, Ludwig. 'Spitäler in Oberdeutschland, Vorderösterreich und der Schweiz in der Frühen Neuzeit'. In *Europäisches Spitalwesen. Institutionelle Fürsorge in Mittelalter Und Früher Neuzeit*. ed. Martin Scheutz et al., 255–291. Munich/Vienna: De Gruyter, 2008.

Ohngemach, Ludwig. *Stadt und Spital. Das Rottweiler Hl.-Geist-Spital bis 1802*. Rottweil: Stadtarchiv Rottweil, 1994.

'O prvoj bjelovarskoj bolnici'. *Radovi Zavoda za znanstvenoistraživački i umjetnički rad u Bjelovaru*, 9 (2015): 21–30.

Osterkamp, Jana. Hyland, Jaime. Cooperative Empires: Provincial Initiatives in Imperial Austria, *Austrian History Yearbook* 47 (2016): 128–146.

Osterkamp, Jana. Imperial Diversity in the Village: Petitions For and Against the Division of Galicia in 1848, *Nationalities Papers* 5/44 (2016): 731–750.

Osterkamp, Jana. Imperial Loyalties: Pluralism of Belonging, Territories, and Spaces in the 19th Century, *Nationalities Papers* 5/50 (2022): 857–870.

Outhwaite, R. B. Objects of Charity: Petitions to the London Foundling Hospital, 1768–72, *Eighteenth-Century Studies* 4/32 (1999), 497–510.

Pan-Montojo, Juan. *Apostolado, profesión y tecnología: Una historia de los ingenieros agrónomos en España*. Madrid: 2005.

Parry-Jones, W. Ll. *The Trade in Lunacy. A Study of Private Madhouses in the Eighteenth and Nineteenth Centuries*. London: Routledge, 1972.

Paşca, Vlad. A Détente Equation: The United Nations Economic Commission for Europe and Socialist Experts before Helsinki (1947–1975). *East Central Europe* 45 (2018): 160–183.

Pauly, Michel. Peregrinorum, Pauperum et Aliorum Transeuntium Receptaculum. Hospitäler zwischen Maas und Rhein im Mittelalter, *Vierteljahrschrift für Sozial- und Wirtschaftsgeschichte* 1/94 (2007): 255–57.

Pauly, Michel. "Von der Fremdenherberge zum Seniorenheim: Funktionswandel in mittelalterlichen Hospitälern an ausgewählten Beispielen aus dem Maas-Mosel-Rhein-Raum," In *Funktions- und Strukturwandel spätmittelalterlicher Hospitäler im europäischen Vergleich*, ed. Michael Matheus. Stuttgart: Franz Steiner Verlag, 2005.

Pawlowsky, Verena. *Mutter ledig – Vater Staat: das Gebär- und Findelhaus in Wien 1784–1910*. Wien: Studien Verlag 2001.

Pelzl, Ludwig J. "Altersvorsorge zwischen Politik, Caritas und Ökonomie – Verkauf und Preisgestaltung von Spitalpfründen im Regensburger Katharinenspital in der Frühen Neuzeit." In *Spital und Wirtschaft in der Vormoderne. Sozial-Karitative Institutionen und ihre Rechnungslegung als Quelle für die Sozial- Und Wirtschaftsgeschichte*. ed. Mark Spoerer, Artur Dirmeier, 207–234. Regensburg: Verlag Friedrich Pustet, 2020.

Pelzl, Ludwig J. Zuijderduijn, Jaco. "Or Do You Prefer Cash? Pensions in Kind in Pre-Modern Germany and the Low Countries." In *Mezzi Di Scambio Non Monetari. Merci e Servizi Come Monete Alternative Nelle Economie Dei Secoli XIII–XVIII/Alternative Currencies. Commodities and Services as Exchange Currencies in the Monetarized*

Economies of the 13th to 18th Centuries. 237–255. Florence: Florence University Press, 2024.

Pelzl, Ludwig J. Zuijderduijn, Jaco. "Saving the Best for Last? Old Age Retirement among the Urban Middle Classes in Leiden and Regensburg," *The History of the Family* 2/27 (2022): 326–349.

Petersson, Erik. "Wounded Veterans and the State: The Precursor of the Veteran's Home in Sweden (1560–1650)," *Scandinavian Journal of History* 2/39 (March 2014): 185–197.

Piasek Gustav and Piasek Martina. "Tradicija hospitala (ksenodohija) u Varaždinu" [The tradition of hospice (xenodochium) in Varaždin], *Arhiv za higijenu rada i toksikologiju* 57 (2006): 459–468.

Piasek Gustav and Piasek Martina. "Varaždinsko zdravstvo u 17. stoljeću" [Healthcare in Varaždin in the 17th century], *Arhiv za higijenu rada i toksikologiju* 55 (2004): 25–34.

Piltz, Jan. *Klinika neurologiczno-psychiatryczna Uniwersytetu Jagiellońskiego* (*The Neurological-Psychiatric Clinic of Jagiellonian University*) Kraków: Jagiellonian University Press, 1929.

Pisarski, Tadeusz. *Sprawozdanie z działalności Oddziału Urologicznego Państwowego Szpitala św. Łazarza w Krakowie od dnia 14-go sierpnia 1929 do 31go grudnia 1931 r.* (*Report on the Activities of the Urological Department of the State St. Lazarus Hospital in Krakow from August 14, 1929, to December 31, 1931*). Kraków: Unknown Publisher, 1932.

Poitras, Geoffrey. The Early History of Financial Economics, 1468 to 1776. From Commercial Arithmetic to Life Annuities and Joint Stocks. Cheltenham: Edward Elgar Publishing, 2000.

Polonsky, Anton. The Revolutionary Crisis of 1846–1849 and Its Place in the Development of Nineteenth-Century Galicia, *Harvard Ukrainian Studies* 22 (1998), 443–469.

Porter, Dorothy. *Health, Civilization, and the State: A History of Public Health from Ancient to Modern Times*, London: Routledge, 1999.

Porter, Roy. *Mind Forg'd Manacles: A History of Madness in England from the Restoration to the Regency*. Ann Arbor, MI: University of Michigan Press 1987.

Porter, Roy. The gift relation: philanthropy and provincial hospitals in eighteenth-century England. In *The Hospital in History*, ed. Lindsay Granshaw, Roy Porter, 149–178. London, New York: Routledge, 1989.

Postřihač, Antonín. Lenz, Jaroslav. *Dějiny kláštera a nemocnice alžbětinek v Praze na oslavu dvěstěletého trvání* [The history of the convent and hospital of the Sisters of St Elizabeth in Prague commemorating 200 years of their existence]. Prague: Self-published, 1922.

Praspaliauskienė, Rima. *Nereikalingi ir pavojingi: XVIII a. pabaigos – XIX a. pirmosios pusės elgetos, valkatos ir plėšikai Lietuvoje*. Vilnius: Žara, 2000.

Quellen zur europäischen Spitalgeschichte in Mittelalter und Früher Neuzeit – Sources for the History of Hospitals in Medieval and Early Modern Europe, ed. Martin Scheutz,

Andrea Sommerlechner, Herwig Weigl, Alfred Stefan Weiß. Wien: München, 2010.

Rambousková, Barbora and Martykánová, Darina. Social Class in the Czech Physicians' Quest for Professional Authority and Social Acknowledgement, 1830s–1930s, In *Hungarian Historical Review*, no. 3 (2023): 363–394.

Reddig, Wolfgang F. *Bürgerspital und Bischofsstadt. Das St. Katharinen- und das St. Elisabethenspital in Bamberg vom 13.–18. Jahrhundert. Eine Vergleichende Studie zu Struktur, Besitz und Wirtschaft*. Bamberg; Frankfurt an der Oder: Scripvaz Verlag, 1998.

Redon, Odile. "Autour de l'hôpital Santa Maria Della Scala à Sienne au XIIIe Siècle," *Ricerche Storiche* XV (1985): 17–34.

Reinarz, Jonathan. *Health Care in Birmingham: The Birmingham Teaching Hospitals, 1779–1939*, Woodbridge: Boydell Press, 2009.

Reinarz, Jonathan. The transformation of medical education in eighteenth-century England: international developments and the West Midlands, *History of Education* 4/37 (2008), 549–566.

Reicke, Siegfried. *Das Deutsche Spital und sein Recht im Mittelalter*. Stuttgart: Verlag von Ferdinand Enke, 1932.

Ress, Imre. Niessen, James P. Hungary, *Austrian History Yearbook* 29, No. 1 (1998): 43–81.

Rigó, János. *A Budapesti Orvostudományi Egyetem jubileumi évkönyve az Orvosi Kar alapításának 200. évfordulója alkalmából.* Budapest: Kossuth Nyomda, 1969.

Riley, James C. *The Eighteenth-Century Campaign to Avoid Disease.* Houndmills, Basingstoke, Hampshire and London: The Macmillan Press, 1987.

Risse, Guenter B. Before the Clinic Was "Born". Methodological Perspectives in Hospital History. In *Institutions of Confinement: Hospitals: Hospitals, Asylums, and Prison in Western Europe and North America, 1500–1950*, ed. Norbert Finzsch, Robert Jütte, 75–96. Cambridge, New York, and Melbourne: Cambridge University Press, 1996.

Risse, Guenter B. *Mending Bodies, Saving Souls: A History of Hospitals*, New York, Oxford: Oxford University Press 1999.

Rose, Christopher S. Implications of the Spanish Influenza Pandemic (1918–1920) for the History of Early Twentieth-Century Egypt, *Journal of World History* 4/32 (2021), 655–684.

Rosen, George. Hospitals, Medical Care and Social Policy in the French Revolution, *Bulletin of the History of Medicine* 2/30 (1956), 124–149.

Rosenberg, Charles E. And Heal the Sick: The Hospital and the Patient in the 19th Century America, *Journal of Social History* 4/10 (1977), 428–447.

Rosiak, Stefan. *Bonifratrzy w Wilnie (1635–1843–1924). Szkic z dziejów opieki społecznej w Wilnie.* Wilno: Wydane staraniem konwentu wileńskiego OO. Bonifratrów, 1928.

Rosiak, Stefan. *Prowincja Litewska Sióstr Miłosierdzia. Szkic z dziejów martyrologji Kościoła katolickiego pod zaborem rosyjskim.* Wilno: Księgarnia św. Wojciecha, 1933.

Sannwald, Wolfgang. *Spitäler in Pest Und Krieg. Untersuchungen Zur Wirtschafts- und Sozialgeschichte Südwestdeutscher Spitäler Im 17. Jahrhundert*. Gomaringen: Gomaringer Verlag und Druck, 1993.

Safley, Thomas Max. *Children of the Labouring Poor*. Leiden/Boston: Brill, 2005.

Safley, Thomas Max. *Kinder, Karitas und Kapital. Studien zur Wirtschafts- und Sozialgeschichte des frühmodernen Augsburg*. Augsburg: Wißner-Verlag, 2009.

Salacz, P. ed. *A Budapesti Királyi Orvosegyesület jubiláris évkönyve, 1837–1937*. Budapest, [s. n.], 1937.

Šámal, Jindřich. *Klášter a nemocnice Alžbětinek na Slupi* [The convent and hospital of Sisters of St Elizabeth na Slupi]. Prague: Vyšehrad, 1941.

Seidman, Naomi. Legitimizing the Revolution: Sarah Schenirer and the Rhetoric of Torah Study for Girls, in *New Directions in the History of the Jews in the Polish Lands*, eds. by Antony Polonsky, Hanna Węgrzynek, Andrzej żbikowski, Boston, Academic Studies Press, 2018, 356–365.

Schelleová, Ilona. Schelle, Karel. *Civilní kodexy 1811–1950–1964*. Brno: Doplněk, 1993.

Scheutz, Martin. 'Supplikationen an den "ersamen" Rat um Aufnahme ins Bürgerspital. Inklusions- und Exklusionsprozesse am Beispiel der Spitäler von Zwettl und Scheibbs'. In *Armen und ihre Lebensperspektiven in der Frühen Neuzeit*, ed. Sebastian Schmidt, 157–206. Frankfurt am Main: Peter Lang, 2008.

Scheutz Martin. Weiß Alfred Stefan. *Spital als Lebensform: Österreichische Spitalordnungen und Spitalinstruktionen der Neuzeit*. Wien: Böhlau, 2015.

Scheutz Martin. Weiß Alfred Stefan. 'Spitalordnungen als essentielle Grundlage der Organisation der Spitäler der Frühen Neuzeit – Eine Leerstelle der komparatistischen Spitalforschung'. In *Historia Hospitalium. Jahrbuch der Deutschen Gesellschaft für Krankenhausgeschichte*, ed. Gunnar Stollberg, Christina Vanja, and Ernst Kraas, 151–190. Münster/Berlin: Lit, 2012.

Schlumbohm, Jürgen. "The Pregnant Women are here for the Sake of the Teaching Institution": The Lying-In Hospital of Göttingen University, 1751 to c. 1830, *Social History of Medicine*, 1 (2001): 59–78.

Schott, Herbert. *Das Verhältnis der Stadt Würzburg zur Landesherrschaft im 18. Jahrhundert*. Würzburg: Freunde Mainfränkischer Kunst und Geschichte, 1995.

Schott, Herbert. 'Fürstlicher Absolutismus und Barocke Stadt'. In *Geschichte der Stadt Würzburg*, ed. Ulrich Wagner, 130–202. Stuttgart: Theiss, 2001.

Scull, A. *The Most Solitary of Afflictions. Madness and Society in Britain 1700–1900*. New Haven – London: Yale University Press, 1993.

Sechel, Teodora Daniela. Networks of Medical Knowledge in Eastern and Central Europe: Introduction to the Thematic Bloc. *East Central Europe* 3 (2013): 207–214.

Shorter, Edward. *A History of Psychiatry. From the Era of the Asylum to the Age of Proza*. New York, NY: Wiley 1997.

Signori, Gabriela. 'Kontingenzbewältigung durch Zukunftshandeln: Der spätmittelalterliche Leibrentenvertrag.' In *Ermöglichen und Verhindern. Vom Umgang mit Kontingenz*, ed. Stephan Brakensiek, Markus Bernhardt, Benjamin Scheller, 117–142. Frankfurt am Main: Campus Verlag, 2016.

Simon, K. A Budapesti Királyi Orvosegyesület a kezdetektől a forradalomig. *Tanulmányok Budapest Múltjából* 38 (2013): 131–174.

Sinkulová, Ludmila. *Lékaři, stát a zdraví lidu: z historie zdravotní služby v českých zemích.* Praha: Státní zdravotnické nakladatelství, 1959.

Skulimowski, Mieczysław. "Zarys rozwoju szpitalnictwa akademickiego w Krakowie" ("An Overview of the Evolution of Academic Hospital System in Krakow"), *Szpitalnictwo Polskie* vol. 8, no. 1 (1964): 7–11.

Sloane, David. "Not Designed Merely to Heal": Women Reformers and the Emergence of Children's Hospitals, The Journal of the Gilded Age and Progressive Era 4/4 (2005), 331–354.

Šmigelskytė-Stukienė, Ramunė, Eduardas Brusokas, Liudas Glemža, Robertas Jurgaitis, and Valdas Rakutis. *Modernios administracijos tapsmas Lietuvoje: valstybės institucijų raida 1764–1794 metais.* Vilnius: Lietuvos istorijos institutas, 2014.

Smith, Leonard. The architecture of confinement: Urban public asylums in England, 1750–1820. In *Madness, Architecture and the Built Environment: Psychiatric Spaces in Historical Context*, eds. Leslie Topp, James E. Moran, and Jonathan Andrews, 41–61. New York, Abingdon: Routledge, 2007.

Smith, Leonard. *Private Madhouses in England, 1640–1815. Commercialised Care for the Insane.* Cham: Palgrave Macmillan, 2020.

Snow, George Edward. The Kokovtsov Commission: An Abortive Attempt at Labor Reform in Russia in 1905, *Slavic Review* No. 3 (1972): 780–796.

Sonderegger, Stefan. 'Wirtschaften Mit Sozialem Auftrag. Zur Wirtschaftsführung Des St. Gallener Heiliggeistspitals Im 15. Jahrhundert.' In *Orte der Verwahrung. Die innere Organisation von Gefängnissen, Hospitälern und Klöstern seit dem Spätmittelalter*, ed. Gerhart Ammerer et al., 191–216. Leipzig: Leipziger Universitätsverlag, 2010.

Spang, Rebecca L. *Stuff and Money in the Time of the French Revolution*, Cambridge (Mass.)/London: Harvard University Press, 2015.

Spree, Reinhard. Krankenhausentwicklung und Sozialpolitik in Deutschland während des 19. Jahrhunderts, *Historische Zeitschrift*, No. 1, vol. 206 (1995): 75–105.

Spree, Reinhard. Sozialer Wandel im Krankenhaus während des 19. Jahrhunderts. Das Beispiel des Münchner Allgemeinen Krankenhauses, *Medizinhistorisches Journal*, 3/4 (1998): 245–291. Available at JSTOR, http://www.jstor.org/stable/25805219 (Accessed December 8, 2023).

Srogosz, Tadeusz. "Próby reform szpitalnictwa w Wilnie u schyłku I Rzeczypospolitej." In *Studia z dziejów Wielkiego Księstwa Litewskiego (XVI–XVIII wieku)*, edited by Sławomir Górzyński and Mirosław Nagielski, 403–13. Warszawa: Wydawnictwo DiG, 2014.

Stauter-Halsted, Keely. Bio-Politics between Nation and Empire. *East Central Europe* 1–2 (2016): 134–160.

Stauter-Halsted, Keely. Moral Panic and the Prostitute in Partitioned Poland: Middle-Class Respectability in Defense of the Modern Nation. *Slavic Review* 3/68 (2009): 557–581.

Steinberg, Holger. 'Die Errichtung des ersten psychiatrischen Lehrstuhls: Johann Christian August Heinroth in Leipzig.' *Nervenarzt* 75(3) (March 2004): 303–307. https://link.springer.com/article/10.1007/s00115-003-1605-3.

Steinberg, Holger. 'Johann Christian August Heinroth (1773–1843). Der erste Lehrstuhlinhaber für Psychiatrie und sein Krankheitskonzept'. In: M. C. Angermeyer and Holger Steinberg (eds.), *200 Jahre Psychiatrie an der Universität Leipzig. Personen und Konzepte*, 1–80. Heidelberg: Springer Medizin Verlag 2005.

Stolberg, Michael. "Health Care Provision and Poor Relief in the Electorate and Kingdom of Bavaria." In *Health Care and Poor Relief in 18th and 19th Century Northern Europe*, edited by Ole Peter Grell, Andrew Cunningham and Robert Jütte, 112–35. Aldershot and Burlington: Ashgate, 2002.

Strohmayer, Hermenegild. *Der Hospitalorden des Hl. Johannes von Gott. Barmherzige Brüder*. Regensburg: Johann von Gott Verlag 1978.

Strohmayer, Hermenegild. *Krankenpflegeschulen im Hospitalorden des hl. Johannes von Gott.* Munich: Johann von Gott Verlag, 1986.

Stuckert, Howard Morris. *Corrodies in the English Monasteries. A Study in English Social History of the Middle Ages*. Philadelphia: University of Pennsylvania Press 1923.

Stunz, Holger R. 'Hospitäler im deutschsprachigen Raum im Spätmittelalter als Unternehmen für die caritas – Typen und Phasen der Finanzierung'. In *Funktions- und Strukturwandel spätmittelalterlicher Hospitäler im europäischen Vergleich*, ed. Michael Matheus, 129–159. Stuttgart: Franz Steiner Verlag, 2005.

Surman, Jan. *Universities in Imperial Austria 1848–1918: A Social History of a Multilingual Space*. Purdue University Press, 2019.

Szasz, Thomas. *Coercion as Cure: A Critical History of Psychiatry.* New Brunswick, NJ–London: Transaction Publishers 2007.

Szasz, Thomas. *Psychiatry: The Science of Lies*, Syracuse: New York Press, 2008.

Szpak, Ewelina. Industrialization: The Environmental End of Old Krakow?, in *Krakow: An Ecobiography*, eds. Adam Izdebski, Rafał Szmytka, Pittsburgh: Pittsburgh University Press, 2021.

Terpstra, Nicholas. *Abandoned Children of the Italian Renaissance: Orphan Care in Florence and Bologna*. Baltimore: The Johns Hopkins University Press, 2005.

Ther, Philipp. Beyond the Nation: The Relational Basis of a Comparative History of Germany and Europe, *Central European History* 1/36 (2003), 45–73.

Tinková, Daniela. 'Selbstmordstrieb auf den Leib eingeschrieben. Selbsttötungsdebatte in der französischen und deutschen medizinischen Literatur an der Wende des 18 und 19 Jahrhundert,' *Brünner Beiträge zur Germanistik und Nordistik* 32, supplement Literatur und Suizid (2018): 11–33.

Tinková, Daniela. '"Šílenství" a "psychiatrie" jako předmět kritické historické reflexe posledního půlstoletí' ['Madness' and 'psychiatry' as subjects of critical historial investigation of the last half-a-century], *Dějiny – teorie – kritika* 2 (2023): 11–39.

Tinková, Daniela. *Tělo, věda, stát: zrození porodnice v osvícenské Evropě*, Praha: Argo, 2010.

Thompson, John D. Goldin, Grace. *Hospital: A Social and Architectural History,* New Haven: Yale University Press, 1975.

Topp, Leslie. *Freedom and the cage: modern architecture and psychiatry in Central Europe, 1890–1914*. Pennsylvania: Pennsylvania State University Press, 2017.

Tošovský, Václav. *Neboj se, nic nebude bolet! (O první éterové narkóze v Čechách.)* [Do not worry, nothing will hurt! (On the first aether anaesthesia in Bohemia]. Prague: Aleko, 1992.

Ueno, Masayuki. *Managing Religious Diversity in the Ottoman Empire: Experiences of Istanbul Armenians in the Nineteenth Century*, Edinburg, Edinburgh University Press, 2025.

Ulbricht, Otto. 'The Debate about Foundling Hospitals in Enlightenment Germany: Infanticide, Illegitimacy, and Infant Mortality Rates.' *Central European History* 3–4/18 (1985): 211–256.

Unowsky, Daniel. *The Plunder: The 1898 Anti-Jewish Riots in Habsburg Galicia*, Stanford: Stanford University Press 2018.

Vacek, Jaroslav. *O nemocech duše. Kapitoly z psychiatrie* [On the illnesses of the soul. Chapters from psychiatry]. Prague: Mladá fronta, 1996.

Vacek, Jaroslav. *Velké psychiatrické případy* [The great psychiatric cases]. Prague: Paseka, 2001.

Vencovský, Eugen. *Čtení o psychiatrii* [Readings from Psychiatry]. Prague: Avicenum, 1983.

Venclovský, Eugen. *Počátky české psychiatrie XVIII. a XIX. století* [The beginnings of Czech psychiatry, 18th and 19th century]. Prague: Státní zdravotnické nakladatelství, 1957.

Vencovský, Eugen. *Psychiatrie dávných věků* [Psychiatry in ancient times]. Prague: Karolinum, 1996.

Vikár, Gy. Az elmeápolás kezdetei Magyarországon. In *Az Országos Ideg- és Elmegyógyintézet 100 éve*, ed. Zoltán Böszörményi, 37–53. Budapest: Nyomdaipari Szakmunkásképző Intézet, 1968.

Vitecek, Daniel. *Der Wiener Narrenturm: Die Geschichte der niederösterreichischen Psychiatrie von 1784–1870*, Wiesbaden: Springer, 2023.

Vlček, Jaroslav. 'Nemocnice alžbětinek' [The Hospital of Sisters of St Elizabeth]. *Praktický lékař* 67, No. 7 (1987): 274–277 and *Praktický lékař* 67, No. 18 (1987): 693–695.

Vogel, M. *The invention of the modern hospital: Boston 1870–1930*. Chicago: Chicago University Press, 1980.

Voth, Hans Joachim. Height, Nutrition, and Labor: Recasting the "Austrian Model." *The Journal of Interdisciplinary History* 25, No. 4 (1995): 627–636.

Vushko, Iryna. *The Politics of Cultural Retreat: Imperial Bureaucracy in Austrian Galicia, 1772–1867*, Yale: Yale University Press, 2015.

Wachholz, Leon. *Szpitale krakowskie 1220–1920* (*Krakow Hospitals 1220–1920*). Kraków: Wydawnictwo W.L. Anczyca, 1921–1924.

Waszczyszyn, Elżbieta. The 19th century Medical Clinic of Collegium Medicum of the Jagiellonian University in Krakow. An outline of conservation problems in the light of requirements of a modern university hospital. *Wiadomości Konserwatorskie/Conservation News* 27/210, 51–66.

Watzka, Carlos. *Arme, Kranke, Verrückte. Hospitäler und Krankenhäuser in der Steiermark vom 16. bis zum 18. Jahrhundert und ihre Bedeutung für den Umgang mit psychisch Kranken* (Veröffentlichungen des Steiermärkischen Landesarchivs 36). Graz: Böhlau, 2007.

Watzka, Carlos and Petr Jelínek. 'Krankenhäuser in Mitteleuropa vor der Aufklärung: Das Beispiel des Ordenshospitals der Barmherzigen Brüder in Feldsberg/Valtice und seiner Patienten 1630–1660.' *Medizinhistorisches Journal* 44, No. 3–4 (2009): 235–273.

Watzka, Carlos. 'Die Krankenprotokolle der Barmherzigen Brüder in Graz 1730–1759. Ein Beitrag zur steirischen Sozial- und Medizingeschichte des 18. Jahrhunderts.' In: Meinhard Brunner, *Rutengänge, Studien zur geschichtichen Landeskunde, Festgabe für Walter Brunner zum 70. Geburtstag*, 316–337. Graz: Historische Landeskommission für Steiermark, 2010.

Watzka, Carlos. 'Die "Landes-Irrenanstalt Feldhof bei Graz" und ihre Insassen 1874–1913. Eine Skizze zur Entstehung der "modernen" Anstaltspsychiatrie in der Steiermark.' In *Psychiatrische Institutionen in Österreich um 1900*. ed. Eberhard Gabriel, Gamper Martina, 14–40. Vienna: Verlaghaus der Ärtze, 2009.

Watzka, Carlos. 'Die Landesirrenanstalt Feldhof bei Graz und ihre Patienten vor 1914. Übersicht und neue historisch-soziologische Forschungsergebnisse'. In *Psychiatrische Institutionen in Österreich um 1900*, ed. Eberhard Gabriel, Gamper Martina, 143–160. Vienna: Verlaghaus der Ärtze, 2009.

Watzka, Carlos. Psychiatrische Anstalten in Österreich, 1780–1850: Eine Übersicht aus wissenschaftsgeschichtlicher und soziologischer Perspektive, in *Österreich in Geschichte und Literatur* 53, No. 4 (2009): 356–372.

Watzka, Carlos. *Seelenheil und Seelenleid: Die Diatetik der Emotionen im Fruhneuzeitlichen Katholizismus in Bayern und Osterreich* (Medizin, Gesellschaft Und Geschichte – Beihefte 78), Stuttgart: Franz Steiner Verlag, 2021.

Watzka, Carlos. *Vom Hospital zum Krankenhaus. Zum Umgang mit psychisch und somatisch Kranken im frühneuzeitlichen Europa*. Cologne: Böhlau, 2005.

Weindling, Paul J. *Health, Race and German Politics between National Unification and Nazism, 1870–1945*. Cambridge: Cambridge University Press, 1989.

Wilson, Adrina. Conflict, Consensus and Charity: Politics and the Provincial Voluntary Hospitals in the Eighteenth Century. *English Historical Review* 442 No. 3 (1996): 599–619.

Witecki, Stanisław. "Healthcare and Catholic Enlightenment in the Polish-Lithuanian Commonwealth." *Studies in Church History* 58 (2022): 150–172.

Wollf, Larry. *The Idea of Galicia: History and Fantasy in Habsburg Political Culture*. Stanford: Stanford University Press, 2010.

Zsakó, István. Az egykori országos tébolyda keletkezésének története. *Orvostörténeti Közlemények* No. 4 (1956): 84–107.

Zuijderduijn, Jaco. "Good Fresh Air and Expert Medical Service": Old Age Pensioners in Leiden's St. Hiëronymusdal Retirement Home, Sixteenth Century.' *The History of the Family* 21 (2015): 195–213.

Zuijderduijn, Jaco. De Moor, Tine. 'Spending, Saving, or Investing? Risk Management in Sixteenth-Century Dutch Households.' *The Economic History Review* 1/66 (2013): 38–56.

Żytkowicz, Leonid. *Zburzenie murów obronnych Wilna (1799–1805)*. Wilno: Wydawnictwo magistratu m. Wilna, 1933.

Index of Names

Index of Places

Index of Subjects

www.ingramcontent.com/pod-product-compliance
Ingram Content Group UK Ltd.
Pitfield, Milton Keynes, MK11 3LW, UK
UKHW022219051026
15624UKWH00001B/232

9 789004 755055